The Physiological Effects
of Wheat Germ Oil
on Humans in Exercise

The Physiological Effects
of Wheat Germ Oil
on Humans in Exercise

Forty-two Physical Training Programs
Utilizing 894 Humans

By

THOMAS KIRK CURETON, Ph.D.(D.Sc. hon.), F.A.C.S.M.

Professor Emeritus and Director
Physical Fitness Institute
University of Illinois
Urbana, Illinois

With a Foreword by

Ezra Levin

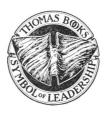

CHARLES C THOMAS · PUBLISHER
Springfield · Illinois · U.S.A.

Published and Distributed Throughout the World by

CHARLES C THOMAS • PUBLISHER

Bannerstone House

301-327 East Lawrence Avenue, Springfield, Illinois, U.S.A.

Natchez Plantation House

735 North Atlantic Boulevard, Fort Lauderdale, Florida, U.S.A.

© *1972, by* CHARLES C THOMAS • PUBLISHER

ISBN 0-398-02270-4

Library of Congress Catalog Card Number: 70-180810

With THOMAS BOOKS *careful attention is given to all details of manufacturing and design. It is the Publisher's desire to present books that are satisfactory as to their physical qualities and artistic possibilities and appropriate for their particular use.* THOMAS BOOKS *will be true to those laws of quality that assure a good name and good will.*

Printed in the United States of America

C-1

*... Those whose curiosity is satisfied with observing what happens have occasionally done service by directing the attention of others to the phenomena they have seen; but it is to those who endeavor to find out how much there is of anything that we owe all the great advances in our knowledge.**

---

* J. C. Maxwell: *Theory of Heat*. London, Lagerman, Green and Company, 1888, p. 74.

Foreword

DISCOVERY of a scientific fact involves two elements: (1) the discovery of the fact; and (2) determination of the rationale for the fact.

Doctor Cureton's work of twenty years has established the fact that wheat germ oil extracted with ethylene dichloride will improve endurance and relieve heart stress, as evaluated by controlled experiments using precise measurements. This fulfills the requirement of the discovery of a scientific truth.

The second requirement, "Why does it work?" has not yet been fully elucidated. There are scientists who will not accept a new truth because the rationale is not clear. Such a position has unfortunately too often obstructed progress. The history of medical science is replete with acceptance of discoveries of treatment of disease, reached empirically. Long-term study followed to determine the rationale. It is redundant to point to forms of treatment, proved to be effective, for which the rationale is even yet unknown.

Now that Doctor Cureton has established the facts, the reasons "why" must be pursued. In this connection, we may find direction by outlining the work done with wheat germ oil, revealing its biological characteristics. Such knowledge may lead to building the structure for understanding the results obtained by Doctor Cureton.

Following is a brief outline of literature and unpublished studies that emphasize biologically significant entities in wheat germ oil in addition to vitamin E.

Levin[22] reviewed literature to emphasize the dichotomy of vitamin E and wheat germ oil.

Vogt-Moeller[41] demonstrated the effects of wheat germ oil on neuromuscular disorders of dogs.

Goettsch and Ritzman[18] reported tocopherol as not identical with neurotrophic factors in wheat germ oil.

Milhorat[29, 30] reported curing of dermatomyositis with wheat germ oil extracted with ethylene dichloride and showed that hexane extracted wheat germ oil is not effective. He also showed that treatment with tocopherols is ineffective.

Blumberg[6] and Martin[28] identified growth factors in wheat germ oil.

Pergallo and Fiori[33] claimed a hematopoietic factor in wheat germ oil.

Ershoff and Levin[16] showed wheat germ oil contains an unidentified factor improving the swimming performance of guinea pigs.

Alfin-Slater[2] reported an unidentified factor in wheat germ oil that reduced the liver cholesterol in animals and showed later[3] that treatment with alpha tocopherol was negative.

Levin et al.[23] reported octacosanol isolated from wheat germ oil as a substance of biological significance.

Levin[24] assayed synthesized octacosanol for androgenic stimulation, using the Dorfman chick comb technique, indicated a highly significant response in minute doses. This work was confirmed by Dorfman.

Dukelow, in unpublished studies, found that feeding octacosanol to sows increased the percentage of sows that farrowed, compared to the controls.

Farrell[17] showed that experimental rats receiving octacosanol required less time for reproduction and reflected higher conception rates than the controls.

Risse[34] reported ten out of sixty infertile cows conceived after treatment with wheat germ oil.

Vogt-Moeller and associates[42, 43] published studies showing the positive effects of wheat germ oil with cattle and human reproduction.

Tutt,[39, 40] Moussu,[31] Jones,[19] Strassl[38] and McIntosh[26] reported positive results in aiding the conception of cows that were functionally sterile.

In this connection, the carefully controlled study by Marion[27] is especially significant. This three-year work confirmed the findings of the previous workers to prove that administration of wheat germ oil will statistically decrease the number of services required for conception.

Bonadonna and Kaan[7] showed that wheat germ oil treatment to bulls resulted in a larger amount of semen of better quality and of greater viability.

Dukelow and Erickson[12] reported that wheat germ oil produced greater numbers of spermatozoa in the second ejaculates in two of three experimental periods.

Dukelow and Matalamaki[14] reported an increase in number of lambs per one hundred ewes bred and per one hundred ewes lambing, respectively.

Using the same methods, Abdulgani *et al.*[1] reported almost identical results.

Aubel *et al.*,[4] Bay and Vogt-Moeller,[5] Lentz,[21] Crampton[8, 9] and Dukelow[13] showed beneficial effects of wheat germ oil in the breeding performance of swine.

In human experimentation, McEachern[25] working in the Montreal Neurological Institute, published studies to indicate that wheat germ oil contains factors that affected the neurological mechanism. He confirmed Milhorat's findings that VioBin wheat germ oil is a specific in the treatment of dermatomyositis. The study shows significant values in several cases of atypical muscular dystrophy, progressive muscular dystrophy and menopausal muscular dystrophy. His plans for continuing this work were terminated by his untimely death.

Currie's work[10] clearly established that a concentrate of wheat germ oil aided women who had a history of habitual abortion to give birth to living children. This work has been confirmed by Silbernagel,[35] Silbernagel and Patterson,[36] Silbernagel and Patterson[37] and Patterson and Silbernagel.[32]

Dukelow and Chernoff[11] in a study published in the Proceedings of the VI International Congress of Animal Reproduction and Artificial Insemination, 1968, show that octacosanol overcomes the embryonic death in rabbits artificially induced by an intra-uterine device.

A review, *Wheat Germ Oil and Reproduction*, by Dukelow[15] is an excellent bibliography.

Keane[20] showed that laboratory animals given wheat germ oil produced larger litters, and more of the young survived than the controls.

In unpublished work, Ershoff and Levin showed that liver glycogen levels were approximately four times greater in rats on a highly purified diet injected with wheat germ oil compared to controls injected with saline solution.

In unpublished studies, Ershoff and Levin, feeding (a) trilaurate, (b) corn oil and (c) wheat germ oil respectively, showed an increase in glycogen in testes (a) 141, (b) 156, (c) 209. Increased weight of seminal vesicles (a) 137, (b) 140, (c) 236.

In a subsequent work, Ershoff and Levin repeated the experiment using immature rats. Two series were evaluated changing the carbohydrate in the diet. Series 1. Feeding refined cottonseed oil and wheat germ oil respectively, total glycogen 66, 140; glycogen per gram of tissue 36, 63. Series 2: Total glycogen 116, 165; glycogen per gram of tissue 54, 79; all values expressed as micrograms per gram.

In an unpublished work, Ershoff and Levin showed that 5 per cent wheat germ oil added to the diet resulted in a highly significant increment in uterine weight compared to controls given cottonseed oil, 106.7 mgs compared to 39.4 mg.

In an unpublished study, Ershoff and Levin, feeding refined cottonseed oil and VioBin wheat germ oil, respectively, showed ovarian and uterine weights increased in animals given wheat germ oil; ovarian weights 33.3, 44.3; uterine weights 138.1, 188.7 mg.

Significant unfinished work by George Wright, George Wolf and B. Connor Johnson are reviewed in Addendum II. The significance of these studies is reflected in the quotation from the original report: "General Conclusions: It can now be stated with certainty that octacosanol exerts a profound effect on the metabolic machinery of the rat when present at low levels in the diet."

Work has been done with VioBin wheat germ oil in its effect on liver cholesterol. I refer to a report by Alfin-Slater *et al.* (1960) of an unidentified factor in wheat germ oil that lessened the increase in liver cholesterol caused by cholesterol feeding; and a subsequent report by this worker that alpha tocopherol acetate was negative in similar trials.

This work by Alfin-Slater has renewed significance in view of a remarkable study in press by Gier and Marion, Kansas State University. Addendum I is a review of this paper. It indicates clearly what the authors state, that wheat germ oil "contains an active principle, probably a combination of polyunsaturated fatty acids and octacosanol, that aid in the degradation and elimination of excess cholesterol."

The reason "why" for Doctor Cureton's work is beginning to be understood. We see in wheat germ oil, and probably in other unrefined vegetable oils, substances that profoundly affect metabolism. The fact that the unrefined vegetable oils have been removed from the American diet through degermination of seeds, and refining the oil derived from such seeds, points to the possibility that there may be a deficiency in the American diet of substances essential to maintenance of efficient metabolism.

Many of these experiments stimulated Doctor Cureton to undertake the pioneering research which has been reported in numerous scientific publications and which is so well summarized in this book.

With his associates, Doctor Cureton has studied the effect of wheat germ oil and octacosanol on a variety of subjects ranging from young boys to businessmen to athletes. His work has utilized standard measures of endurance (treadmill run, etc.) as well as complex physiological measurements, including the brachial pulse wave and oxygen debt studies.

He was honored upon his retirement from academic life on April 25-26, 1969, when a special Symposium on Physical Fitness was conducted at the University of Illinois. Every scientific paper at the symposium was authored and presented by one of Doctor Cureton's former students (Ph.D.s).

This volume will also serve to honor Doctor Cureton for his efforts in the field of research on unrefined vegetable oils and, particularly, wheat germ oil. This volume represents the most complete collection of scientific research data ever assembled on the physiological effects of wheat germ oil on human endurance.

In these twenty years, this scientist has kept his mind's "eye" on his controlled experiments. His *facts* will be a basic reference when future students follow the path he has paved for them.

EZRA LEVIN, M.S.

REFERENCES

1. Abdulgani, I., Ross, C. V. and Riley, J. C.: 9th Annual Sheep Day Program, University of Missouri, Columbia, Missouri, 1965, p. 37.
2. Alfin-Slater, R. B.: Factors affecting EFA utilization. Proc. of the Symposium on Drugs Affecting Lipid Metabolism. Amsterdam, Elsevier Publishing Co., 1960, p. 111.
3. Alfin-Slater, R. B., Auerbach, S. and Shull, R. L.: *Fed. Proc.*, 19:18, 1960.
4. Aubel, C. E., Hughes, J. S. and Lienhardt, H. F.: *Proc. Amer. Soc. Anim. Prod.*, 1929, p. 133.
5. Bay, F. and Vogt-Moeller, P.: *Vet. J.*, 90:288, 1934.
6. Blumberg, H.: *J. Biol. Chem.*, 108:127, 1935.
7. Bonadonna, T. and Kaan, I.: *Zootec. Vet.*, 9:148, 172 and 206, 1954.
8. Crampton, E. W.: *Sci. Agri.*, 21:750, 1941.
9. Crampton, E. W.: *Sci. Agri.*, 23:161, 1942.
10. Currie, D.: *Brit. Med. J.*, 2:1218, 1937.
11. Dukelow, W. R. and Chernoff, H. N.: *Proc. VI International Congress of Animal Reproduction and Artificial Insemination,* 1968.
12. Dukelow, W. R. and Erickson, W. E.: *Proc. V International Congress Animal Reproduction and Artificial Insemination* (Toronto), 4:601, 1964.
13. Dukelow, W. R.: *J. Reprod. Fertil.*, 10:441, 1965.
14. Dukelow, W. R. and Matalamaki, W.: *J. Anim. Sci.*, 22:1137, 1963.
15. Dukelow, W. R.: Wheat germ oil and reproduction. A review. Supplementum 121, *Acta Endocrinol. Periodica,* Copenhagen, 1967.
16. Ershoff, B. M. and Levin, E.: *Fed. Proc.*, 14:431, 1955.
17. Farrell, P. R.: The effects of octacosanol on conception and reproduction, on maintenance and growth of young, and on oxygen uptake in the white rat. M. S. Thesis, Kansas State University, Manhattan, Kansas, 1965.
18. Goettsch, M. and Ritzman, J.: *J. Nutr.* 17:371, 1959.
19. Jones, I. R.: *Proc. West Div. Amer. Dairy Sci. Ass.,* October, 1939.
20. Keane, K. W., Cohn, Eva M. and Johnson, B. Connor: Reproductive failure of rats on glyceryl trilaurate containing diets and its prevention by certain natural fats. *J. Nutr.* 45:275-288, 1951.
21. Lentz, R. W.: *Berl. Tierartz. Wschr.*, 201, April 8, 1938.
22. Levin, E.: *Amer. J. Dig. Dis.*, 12:20, 1945.
23. Levin, E.: Collins, V. K., Varner, D. S. and Mosser, J. S.: Compositions

comprising octacosanol, triacontanol, tetracosanol, or hexacosanol, and methods employing same. U. S. Patent Office 3,031,376, 1962.

24. Levin, E.: *Proc. Soc. Exp. Biol. Med.* (New York), 112:331, 1963.
25. McEachern, D., Rabinovitch, Reuben and Gibson, William C.: Neuromuscular disorders amenable to wheat germ oil therapy. *J. Neurol. Neurosurg. Psychiat.*, 14:95, 1951.
26. McIntosh, R. A.: *Canad. J. Comp. Med. Vet. Sci.*, 4:342, 1940.
27. Marion, G. B: *J. Dairy Sci.*, 45:904, 1962.
28. Martin, G. J.: *J. Nutr.*, 13:679, 1937.
29. Milhorat, A. T.: *Science*, 101:93, 1945.
30. Milhorat, A. T., Toscani, V. and Bartels, W. E.: *Proc. Soc. Exp. Biol. Med.* (New York), 59:40, 1945.
31. Moussu, R.: *Rec. Med. Vet.*, 111:905, 1935.
32. Patterson, J. B. and Silbernagel, W. M.: *J. Int. Coll. Surg.*, 35:335, 1961.
33. Pergallo, I. and Fiori, E.: *Z. Vitamin-, Horman- u. Fermentforsch.*, 8:136, 1938.
34. Risse, W.: Behandlung der Unfruchtbarkeit mit standardisierten Weizenkeimol (Vitamin E) and Hormovilan bei kindern. Diss. Hannover, 1926 (An. Breed. Abstr. 7), 1939, p. 220.
35. Silbernagel, W. M.: *Ohio State Med. J.*, 43, 1947, p. 739.
36. Silbernagel, W. M. and Patterson, J. B.: *Ohio J. Sci.*, 49:195, 1949.
37. Silbernagel, W. M. and Patterson, J. B.: *J. Int. Coll. Surg.*, 23:719, 1955.
38. Strassl: *Berl. u. Munch. Tierartzl. Wschr.*, 1938, p. 397.
39. Tutt, J. F. D.: *Vet. J.*, 89:416, 1933.
40. Tutt, J. F. D.: *Vet. Rec.*, 49:568, 1937.
41. Vogt-Moeller, P.: *Tierartzl. Rundschau*, 48:274, 1942.
42. Vogt-Moeller, P.: Vitamin E, a Symposium, Society of the Chemical Industry, London, 57, 1939.
43. Vogt-Moeller, P. and Bay, F.: *Vet. J.*, 87:165, 1931.

Preface

THE practical coach and director of physical fitness exercise programs is not greatly concerned with the chemistry of muscle enzymes or of vitamin supplements but with its practical effects upon performance, feelings of added physiological reserves and speeds in various reactions. While there are physiological effects, the coach is not overly concerned whether the effects are psychological or physiological. He is concerned mainly that performances improve coincidental with taking wheat germ, wheat germ oil or octacosanol. Many have demonstrated such favorable changes occurring. We have conducted forty-two experiments to check the effects of these dietary supplements provided by the VioBin Corporation of Monticello, Illinois.

It is very clear that there will be no unanimity in the way these experiments will be viewed. It is unreasonable to expect that the nutritionist will settle for anything less than biological evaluation of the ingredients of wheat germ oil, octacosanol or wheat germ; or will medical and public health scientists settle for less than knowledge of the long-range health and survival effects. Such studies would be valuable, but in the meantime, we feel that students of physical fitness should see the data we have accumulated over the past twenty years.

We are dealing here with the difficulties of assessing mathematical significance in comparatively small groups of persons who eat anything they want and who are subject to psychological pressures affecting their performance. Calculations for reliability are varied according to whether the data were skewed or not (Cf. Appendix A), since few of the samples were strictly random.

It is clear that an experiment can be made invalid by subjects dropping out of matched group experiments; sometimes soreness or fatigue may interfere; or psychological difficulties may arise, such as in one of our experiments with a team losing most of the meets and some team members refusing to keep up the regular amount of practice, with unequal effects in two matched groups. This one experiment was disqualified. In the university there are problems of vacations, examinations and various types of anxieties which may affect results. Consequently, when a difference shows up *significantly* over and above *ad libitum* feeding and all other variations that would increase the standard errors of measurement, *the difference between the supplement and the placebo is real.* Not all experiments can be kept under perfect control. Our experiments have shown results distinctly favoring the experimental treatments, and we believe that psychological influences have not affected one group any more than another. So, we are impelled to lay out the data of the various experiments to stand for what they are really worth, no more, no less.

The results, as described in this monograph, certainly would never have been brought out to the extent that they have except that a basic type of nutritional deficiency must exist in the foodstuffs available to the subjects used in these experiments—and most probably in the whole United States. While there is no feasible way to determine such subclinical dietary deficiencies, because of the cost per person and the lack of available scientific techniques, a review of recent nutritional materials indicates a great and growing problem in this area because of the following situations and most probable causes of nutritional deficiencies:

1. Unequal distribution of foods, due to economics (poor groups).
2. Old foods, spoilage of food on shelves.
3. Processing and adulteration for preservation, biological antipathy.
4. Cooking and reheating, storing and thawing, reheating.
5. Poor choices, preference to taste and style, social patterns, dieting leading to chemical imbalance.
6. Restriction of food to curb overweight, lack of balance and bulk.
7. Poor food (empty calories), low in vitamins, minerals and trace elements.
8. Induced deficiencies due to sickness, overstress, alcoholism, confinement, drugs and hospitalization.

9. Indoor confinement (lack of vitamin D) and absence of irradiation.
10. Lack of enough exercise to use the food day by day, proper stimulation of the lymph flow, and oxygen intake associated with poor fitness.
11. Biological individuality—people being different in body type, digestive and assimilatory apparatus, enzymes and cellular needs.
12. Bias and wrong beliefs, folk lore of the erroneous type.

We have found that in twenty years of working with people who have taken WGO or the related substances, there are measurable benefits and, unquestionably, benefits which cannot be measured, and no harmful effects which have ever been observed from the capsulated materials used (toxic effects).

It is well known too that there is a general shortage of fresh, uncooked polyunsaturated acids in the diet of modern, urban man—and the effects are probably as disastrous as that observed when cattle are long without fresh, green food—they usually die prematurely of heart disease. While this research has not been on heart disease per se, the lowered cardiovascular fitness and poorer relative motor performances which result from a) inactivity, b) withdrawal of the WGO and other dietary supports, and c) grossly poor diet—all of which carry strong inference. We have shown that WGO and octacosanol, taken in moderate amounts, will enable most human subjects to bear stress better (according to the stress indicators used). This is undoubtedly true of some other good nutrients also.

These types of experiments to improve human subjects in the various physical fitness tests used would have been conducted anyway as part of my charged responsibilities of the Physical Fitness Research Laboratory at the University for twenty-five years, whether we had used the dietary substances or not. It is part, however, of trying to find the ways to make human beings fitter. Forty of these experiments show that we improved the humans, by both the exercise and improved nutrition.

The thirty-one abstracts in Part Two describe in detail the *group experiments* carried out under my direction, as part of the work of the Physical Fitness Research Laboratory, University of Illinois, from 1950 through 1970. In Part One the results were collated around each major test used, showing the agreement of the evidence. The two parts mutually support each other. While each experiment should be seen for itself, the meaning of the work is not clear for most until all of the experiments are seen under one cover. Part One is essentially the author's interpretation of all of the experiments, summarized in that part. The original theses are in the library at the University of Illinois, in Urbana.

THOMAS KIRK CURETON, JR.

Acknowledgments

FIRST of all, I acknowledge the contribution made by my doctoral students and some students at the master's degree level, who have contributed to this work. Their names are found in Part Two with the work which they contributed. Their theses have been used in this collation; all were completed under my supervision and sponsorship in the Graduate College, University of Illinois.

Some of the explanatory materials relative to the tests used have been taken from my own publications to which cross references have been made, to clarify the methods used in testing the human subjects.

Several medical doctors have been involved with this work, and their names are mentioned in the particular experiments in which they participated. For the first ten years Dr. Norris Brookens was the part-time medical doctor of our laboratory in Urbana. He was mostly involved with the design of the experiments in that he controlled the feeding (usually double-blind method). Col. James Tuma, United States Marines, and Dr. E. H. Lanphier, Little Creek Underwater Demolition Unit, United States Marine Base, Virginia, deserve special mention for their assistance, as does the Bureau of Medicine and Surgery, United States Navy, for approving the experiments and providing some financial assistance.

I would like to acknowledge my colleagues in the Physical Fitness Research Laboratory who participated in the work: Dr. R. H. Pohndorf, Dr. Alan Barry, Dr. Bruce Noble, Dr. Bradley Rothermel, Dr. Ben Williams and Mrs. Betty Frey.

The articles, authored by Dr. Roger Williams and Professor H. F. Kaiser, are acknowledged with appreciation. Their principles seem to be illustrated by this series of studies, and I wish to point to the truth of those basic principles in biological individuality and in the setting of statistical standards, respectively.

I was guided by the reaction of Dr. Philip Rasch on the appropriateness of the statistical level of 0.10.

The experimental work could not have been accomplished without the encouragement of Mr. Ezra Levin and the financial assistance of the VioBin Corporation. Mr. Levin has carefully prepared the Foreword which documents the animal studies of a correlative nature. V. K. Collins, biochemist, read the entire manuscript.

My appreciation is also expressed for the great assistance of Mrs. Betty Woodward, Associate Editor, the staff of Charles C Thomas, Publisher, and Mary Lee Jewett, who drew the graphs.

Thomas Kirk Cureton, Jr.

Contents

PART ONE

The Physiological Effects
of Wheat Germ Oil
on Humans in Exercise

Part One

Introduction to the Problem, and Research Methods Used for Separating the Effects of Physical Training from the Unique Effects of Wheat Germ Oil and Related Substances (Octacosanol and Wheat Germ) with Humans

THE research methods used in this series of investigations, especially the work on humans, is a bit unorthodox, or at least undeveloped. This is because the investigations have not been directed toward internal chemical analysis of the dietary supplements used, although a certain amount has been known about this aspect, but have been directed toward the effect upon the body in various types of physical performances and physical fitness tests. This area is certainly new, and few other investigations are to be found. Nevertheless, the practical effects are discovered, which should only enhance and stimulate the more profound biochemical studies to be carried further. The facts are plain, wheat germ oil is a valuable ergogenic aid to health and to physical performance.

It has long been controversial that any dietary supplement (vitamin, oil or nutrient, *not drug*) would improve the athletic endurance, strength or speed. This is perhaps due to the known and anticipated difficulty of *controlling* the human subjects, with their very great variability in living habits, psychological inhibitions and adherences, right and wrong beliefs, religious dictates and built-in preferences associated with diverse family background and diverse anthropological types (ectomorphs, mesomorphs, medials and endomorphs, etc.). The devotion to any led or prescribed physical exercise program varies in itself, as does the environment (temperature, barometric pressure, relative humidity) winter to spring and summer, which variations do complicate the problem. Some of the physical tests also may be judged to be very crude, and these have appreciable variation too. Some of the tests used are very reliable (consistent in reproducible results), and some are not very reliable in this sense. Willpower affects some of the results and must be accounted for and partialed out or controlled in some manner. Such obstacles have been considered virtually insurmountable by some but better to see the results as can be obtained than to assume that animal results will forecast accurately the most probable effects on humans. This is not certain at all.

Several comprehensive reviews have been written of the related literature, so it will not be labored in this volume, except for a few very pertinent and overlapping experiments which bear exactly on what we have been doing. It is fortunate that these experiments do support the main thesis of our experiments, and reinforce the concept that we have long had, that something important is here, but hard to isolate and pin down. It is easy for people who have not done any of this type of work to say that these are poor experiments but let them try for twenty years, as we have, and then see what they say! It may be sufficient to refer to the background work published by Keys,[1] Henschel,[2] Karpovich[3] and Cureton.[4] This outlines the rather negative results which have come from some similar investigations, but *not* on WGO, octacosanol or wheat germ supplements which we used, but outlines the work and results of various experiments with dietary supplements of a great variety of other kinds. Most investigations of this type have become controversial (vitamin B_1, vitamin C, vitamin E, etc.).

The author began experimenting with diet and performance as a research problem in 1934.[5] His interest has continued unabated until the present time. After being an athlete, then a coach and for the last thirty years a research laboratory director, this problem has always been pressing and demanding more investigation than should be found available. The direct research with humans under stress of athletics or physical fitness programs and tests has been seldom encountered, with such exceptions as the work of Prokop,[6] Tuttle, *et al.*,[7] Keys,[8] Johnson, *et al.*,[9] and Yakolev.[10] More recently, the work of Bergstrom, *et al.*,[11] has attracted attention, in which alternate depletion, then filling the "muscle reservoirs" with glycogen from a carbohydrate-rich diet for several days, demonstrated the validity of the concept that it is

possible to affect the physical performances by deliberate variations in the training alimentation with significant results.

Our own work has stirred some controversy and has stimulated
additional research as typified by the investigations of Yakolev
(summarized by Brozek),[12] Poiletman,[13] Farrell[14] (and Gier) and
Consolazio, *et al.*[15]

THE RESEARCH METHODS

Our research methods have been limited to the use of certain
physiological tests which have long been used in the Physical
Fitness Research Laboratory at the University of Illinois (Urbana), on *normal* human subjects. Some types of tests have been
used which are not too well known in medical or nutritional cir-
cles, so these are especially explained in small summary chapters
concentrated upon each test and the literature related to the reliability and validity of each test. The tests have long been used
to evaluate the status and improvement of human subjects quite
apart from this dietary supplement research. The longitudinal
evaluations of *changes* in various physiological parameters has
been the principal type of research carried out for the past
twenty-five years in our laboratory, so it was natural that we
should add the studies of dietary supplements (WGO), octacosanol (OCTCNL), and wheat germ cereal (WGC) to what we
were doing. This involved us in collaboration with several other
disciplines (anthropology, physiology, psychology, medicine, bio-
chemical-nutritional work, along with our own).* Many of the
theses drawn upon are graduate student theses, done by invita-
tion to get the work done under our direction, and at the same
time to help a needy student financially and supervise his work
as faculty sponsors, in the usual University of Illinois degree
process. In the Ph.D. work, the kindly help of specialists from
other departments, especially educational statistics and also the
University of Illinois computer facilities has always been present.
The work throughout has been directed by the author, but with

---

* These associates are named in the prefaces of the original studies and those
most involved are named in the author's "special acknowledgment" (author's
reviews) and in this chapter.

the help of other faculty members and the laboratory medical consultant, associated physiologists and medical doctors.

The experiments with wheat germ oil utilizing human subjects began at the University of Illinois, in our laboratory, in 1949-50, when Mr. Ezra Levin came to Professor T. K. Cureton and asked him if we could involve wheat germ oil (VioBin® brand) in our work, and compare our human subjects with and without it, to see if it affected human performance and physiological efficiency in any way. We began, and have continued the work for twenty years. The abstracts of all of the studies done in our department are given in Part Two, arranged as nearly as possible on a progressive chronological basis, to show the evolution of the work, and the progressive improvement of the research methods. The interpretations of these researchers are given in the abstracts (Part Two) as made by the original investigators, but tempered by the available consultants: Dr. Norris L. Brookens (M.D., Ph.D.), Professor Fred Kummerow (Ph.D.), Mr. Ezra Levin, Professor Connor Johnson, and others, named on the thesis committees, especially Professor R. E. Pingry (educational statistics), Professors O'Kelly (physiological psychology), F. R. Steggerda (physiology), R. H. Pohndorf (physical education), B. D. Franks (physical education) and B. L. Rothermel (physical education). As twenty years have passed one study has reinforced another, so that additional confidence has been gained as to the overall meaning of the many works. The collation of these forty-two separate studies is the job at hand.

SEVERAL RESEARCH DESIGNS

The *matched, parallel groups design* is perhaps the best, in which subjects have been tested and matched at T_1, usually with double testing, or retesting, for consistency checks, and determination of the standard errors of measurement (S.E._meas.).[16] The same program was then given to the subjects, usually under a competent instructor to see that they did it, and who also accounted for attendance and completion of all aspects of the program; and then retests (T_2) and sometimes after a rest-break of a few days, again retests for consistency purposes. In this pattern, two and sometimes three or four groups have been used. More than two groups has usually been unsatisfactory because of reducing the numbers in each group, thus hurting the reliability calculations. Six to twelve weeks have usually been used for the controlled program of activity, but a few longer studies have been conducted. The capsules of WGO, OCTCNL and placeboes (cottonseed oil, vitamin E in refined corn oil or cottonseed oil, devitaminized lard with E added to equal that in the WGO) were administered usually "double-blind" fashion for the same length of time as the activity program. It was found that twelve weeks were sufficient to eliminate the training effect (learning and familiarity with the work and tests) before a plateau would be reached, after which it was very hard to make any additional change. The second main *pattern* was the *single group pattern*, pretested at T_1, the subjects worked out regularly on the program for twelve weeks, then tested again (T_3), the tests sometimes being given both at ground level and at 10,000 feet of simulated altitude in the available decompression chamber (United States Air Force Chamber, located in the Atmospheric Environment Laboratory, in the School of Mechanical Engineering), which permitted precise control of the environmental conditions when testing was done. Once a group was trained very well, progressively over twelve weeks, and a plateau reached on both performance and naive "stress indicator tests," such training curves usually turned downward after a week or two on "plateau," and it would be most unusual if in the same experiment involving day-to-day continuous training for such a curve to *rise upward again,* associated with the addition of WGO or OCTCNL, which did occur in certain experiments. Yet, this experimental pattern is not quite as fully "fool-proof" as the *parallel group pattern,* although care was taken to see that the intensity or duration of the day-to-day work was not increased. Experiments were run on the basis of tests at 0, 10 and 20 weeks, this being toward the end of the series, as a double check on a control group "in training" gaining after ten weeks. Usually, this was not so, at least not within the same six month period.

The work hinges on using certain types of tests, classified and known as "fatigue indicators," or suitably reliable tests for endurance, response tests to given stimuli (reaction time tests);

challenge type (all-out) strength, endurance or speed tests (mile run time, 600-yard run time, all-out treadmill run (8.6% grade, 7 mile/hour); reactions of the cardiovascular system to standardized amounts of stress or load; the "peak" oxygen intake and net oxygen debt tests; the quiet, standardized basal metabolism tests (BMR) lying and sitting; pulse rate response and recovery tests (as the Cureton progressive pulse ratio, or Harvard five-minute step test, 17-inch bench). These types of physiological responses have long been studied in our laboratory, although the treadmill test, the brachial pulse wave (sphygmogram) or (BPW), the Garrett- Cureton total body reaction time test (TBRT) Krasno-Ivy flicker fusion frequency (FFF) and the Cureton progressive pulse ratio tests (PPRT) were originated and standardized at the University of Illinois. These tests are in print in other materials, and are briefly described herein, with references given to additional published research studies of these tests and their interpretation. The use of these tests may be confusing to a chemist, a nutritionist, or even a medical doctor but more familiar to a researcher in physical education or stress psychology.*

Individual longitudinal case studies have also been added to the study, which have a definite value, not evaluated by group statistics methods at all, but with graphs show the concomitant variations nicely, as the dietary supplements were varied from WGO, to placeboes, to nothing, and to wheat germ cereal in some predetermined order of alternation to observe the effects.

Matching Groups

The methods used for matching groups were a) to test everybody on the critical tests, b) to alternately rank the subjects in the most important test, this usually declared as the main object of study, c) arrange the two groups by alternate selection and systematic rotation, d) compute the means and sigmas of each group, if not matched to make slight adjustments and e) compute the significance of the difference between the means, by the $D/S.E._{diff.}$ or t test, and refer to appropriate small sample statistical tables for the probability (.10, or .05 or .01) of there

---

* See references: 17, 18, 19, 20, 21, 22, 23, 24, 25.

being a real difference between the means not due to chance. If all of this were done, the matching procedure is called "proved."[26]

Equalizing the Work of Matched Groups

It has always been a principal problem to equalize the work done by the two groups being compared in the matched group type of experiment. Usually all subjects were led by an instructor and the work as standardized by the instructor was required of all, attendance was checked, and the work of the men noted. Only two experiments, those by Mayhew and Wiley, Experiments 29 and 30 did the testing on a calibrated ergometer bicycle (Hellebrandt-Kelso type), so that the load could be exactly measured. For the program itself, the men were not interested in machines but wanted to walk and jog, run, swim, row, play games and do calisthenics in a natural way under an experienced leader. The day-to-day work was done on the track or in the gymnasium, not on machines, to make the results meaningful as a physical education experience. It was usual to have the work moderately "paced" so that all men could keep up, at least do all of the work, but they could "let out" on a test if they wanted to go all-out, and were encouraged to do so. It has always been the concept that hard work was needed but built up to on a gradual progressive basis. The effects have seemed small on sedentary subjects, and in one experiment in which the work was "voluntary" (laissez-faire) the results are not very good (Exp. 11). The kilocalorie level in this was much less.

Time and Nature of the Feeding

The subjects were fed at the end of their work, in general, but the boys in the Sports Fitness School were fed in the middle of the afternoon, at 3:15 PM, after two periods and with three more periods to go. This "break period" being for the purpose of giving the capsules (A, B or C) and the milk to wash them down (½ pint of 2% milk). The number of capsules was 20×3 minims, or 10×6 minims, for all adults and young men, but usually was somewhat less than this for the boys, as described in each experiment. The number of weeks was very important, six weeks at least is required in our opinion, up to as long as twenty weeks in one; ten weeks of pretraining in three with capsules then fed for ten more weeks. In almost all experiments the feeding of the capsules was closely supervised by instructors, the laboratory doctor and nurse being responsible for making up the dosages in bottles containing capsules marked "A," or "B" or "C." The wheat germ cereal could not be so camouflaged.

The Placeboes

The placeboes used in Experiment 1 (Forr-Cureton) were obtained from Hoffmann-La Roche Co., New Jersey (Dr. E. L. Sevringhaus). They contained synthetic vitamin E in amounts equal to 100 mg per capsule. These were matched by using a number of WGO capsules (0.043 mg per 3-minim capsule) sufficient to balance the synthetic vitamin E (checked by Professor E. Connor Johnson) in 1949-50. The details of the Forr experiment are given in the abstract in Part Two.

A letter from the VioBin Corporation (V. K. Collins to Mr. Levin) states, "Our placeboes for wheat germ oil were being prepared by Strong-Cobb. With these we were using natural vitamin E in cottonseed oil, for comparison with wheat germ oil. The natural vitamin E content of cottonseed oil was ignored. The criticism of the other vegetable oils on the basis of their tocopherol content is hardly valid; it is the alpha tocopherol which should be considered; and the wheat germ oil runs higher than the other oils by a factor of 10 or more. In any case, the naturally occurring tocopherol would tend to load the experiment against wheat germ oil."

THE CHARACTERISTICS OF WHEAT GERM OIL (VioBin)

Since VioBin wheat germ oil has been used time and again in the experiments described in this report, it is necessary to make clear as possible the exact nature of what was fed to the subjects. Therefore, the following description of wheat germ oil is given:

VioBin oil is extracted from the embryo of the wheat, extracted with ethylene dichloride, and kept at 0 C until capsulated. Each 3-minim capsule contains 175 mg of oil, high in linoleic acid and containing 0.44 mg of vitamin E. Rancid oil is contraindicated, so it must be refrigerated unless capsulated. The daily dosage of fresh oil was equivalent to one teaspoonful (4 cc), or 20×3 minims, or 10×6 minims.[*]

---

[*] Statement from the VioBin Corp., Monticello, Illinois (by Mr. Ezra Levin).

The following is taken from the *Journal of the American Medical Association*, Vol. 165, No. 1. "Depending upon the variety from which it is obtained, wheat germ oil contains anywhere from 30 to 57 per cent (weight) linoleic acid; in addition wheat germ probably contains small amounts of plant sterols in the form of sitosterol. Some of the other known compounds include naturally occurring vitamins, cholin, inositol, p-aminobenzoic acid and traces of many minerals."

Subjects

The subjects used in the experiments have been students in the University of Illinois, boys in the Sports Fitness School of the University of Illinois, and volunteer adults from the University community, both white and blue collar types. It has not been possible to get "random samples" in the true sense but only approximations (stratified with poor, average and good subjects in groups being compared). This may be a limitation in certain instances where the statistics used demand a "true random sample," and the use of t tests,[22] analysis of variance and covariance always gives results a bit nebulous. Realizing this shortcoming, it is best to look at the actual results of a given group, this in terms of the raw score or standard score data, and not put so much weight on the t tests. It is better too, with these type data to look at the actual errors of the S.E._meas. type,[16] computed from the actual deviations in retests for consistency, and realize that such errors are distributed normally and can be evaluated by the normal probability tables, within the sample itself. The several hundred subjects used in these experiments (721) have not been interested in the capsules used by them, as they were given blind or double-blind but have been interested in *improving themselves* in the various tests of performance and associated physiological type tests. They have viewed the taking of the capsules as an "adjunct" necessary to the experiments, and they were not told, at the time of the experiment, what was in the capsules. Usually

---

Note: VioBin Wheat Germ Oil contains less than 5 part per million of residual ethylene dichloride. Ten 6 min. capsules contain less than 20 micrograms of ethylene dichloride, a completely insignificant quantity.

Ethylene dichloride is broken down in the body to common harmless substances, chloride ions and aldehydes. The reaction involved has been worked out by Heppel and Porterfield in the *Journal of Biological Chemistry*, 176:764-769, 1948.

they were talked of as "vitamins" without any name as to the type being used. The control subjects also thought they were taking "vitamins." The subjects were always willing to cooperate in this respect. The motivation to do well, to improve, was always good too, except in one experiment (Marx, 1952) which was dropped from the list presented because of known irregularities (low morale, irregular attendance at practice, imbalance of groups) which introduced so much interference and irregularity that the results are meaningless. Fortunately, this situation was understood, so that it could be dealt with, without needlessly penalizing all of the other good experiments—an example, however, of what can happen with human subjects when they are completely disinterested or prejudicial to the work. The subjects

---

NOTE: Octacosanol is not included in the list above but the octacosanol in the VioBin WGO is equal to 0.011 per cent, and is the principal ingredient showing positive relationships to the improvements of endurance, T-wave reaction time and various cardiovascular tests used in the University of Illinois experiments. While vitamin E is a constituent of WGO, its effect is discounted on the particular tests used in the Illinois experiments because in the experiments in which WGO was matched with WGO in parallel groups, the desirable effects are attributed to WGO and octacosanol rather than to vitamin E as interpreted by us. Usually in the corn oil, the lard (with added vitamin E) had as much or slightly more vitamin E than the wheat germ oil.

TABLE I

BIOCHEMICAL CONTENTS OF WHEAT GERM OIL[*]
(average values)

Acid (Common Name)	Wheat Germ Oil	Corn Oil	Cottonseed Oil	Lard
Myristic			0.5	1
Palmitic—$C_{12}H_{28}O_2$	11.8	8	21	28
	3.0			
Stearic—Saturated		1.5	2	13
	1.2			
Arochidic		0.5	0.2	
Lignoceric		0.2	0.3	
Palmitoleic				3
Oleic	28.1	46	29	46
Linoleic	52.3	42	45	6
Linolenic	3.5		2	0.7
Arachidonic				2

[*] Data from Sullivan and Bailey, *J. Amer. Chem. Soc.*, 58:383-90, 1936.
[†] Data for corn oil, lard and cottonseed oil are from Armour Chemical Division.

TABLE II

TOCOPHEROL CONTENT OF INDIVIDUAL FATS AND OILS

Taufell K. and Serzisko R. (Germany)—Ernshrungsforschung 6:323, 1961

The authors have studied the tocopherol content and the distribution of the tocopherols in several oils and fats.

Tocopherol Content of Individual Oils

Kind	Total Tocopherol in Micrograms per Gram of Oil	Types of Tocopherol		
		Alpha	Gamma	Delta
Peanut oil	422.0	—	—	—
Peanut oil	348.0	—	—	—
Rape seed oil	600.2	—	—	—
Rape seed oil	561.6	—	—	—
Linseed oil	611.0	—	—	x
Olive oil	143.5	80.5	x	x
Olive oil	128.7	—	—	—
Soya bean oil	780.0	9.7	47.8	29.4
Soya bean oil	749.0	8.7	47.6	26.7
Sunflower oil	596.7	75.5	20.0	x
Sunflower oil	580.7	74.6	19.5	x

There is a wide difference in the tocopherol content of margarines, apparently. The authors have analyzed the total tocopherol content of six commercial types and found that the total tocopherol content varied from 13.7 to 31.5 mg per 100 gm of margarine.

Tocopherol Content of Various Cereal Germ Oils

Kind	Total Tocopherol for 1 gm of Germ in Micrograms	Total Tocopherol per 1 gm of Oil	Percentages of Total Tocopherol			
			Alpha	Beta	Gamma	Delta
Wheat germ oil	268.9	—	9.9	49.3	43.2	—	—
	256.7	—	11.6	50.6	38.0	—	—
Rye germ oil	176.3	—	13.4	55.5	—	30.3	—
	168.4	—	14.0	69.1	—	21.7	—
Rice germ oil	—	1827.5	11.7	56.8	—	24.4	6.6
	—	1687.1	11.4	54.3	—	24.8	9.7

The authors have also studied the tocopherol content of lard, bacon and butter.

Tocopherol in Lard and Butter

Kind	Total Tocopherol per 100 mg per 100 gm of Fat
Lard	2.40
Bacon	1.92
Butter	2.20
Butter	1.20
Butter	1.60
Butter	5.80
Butter	5.70

Characteristically, vegetable fats contain more tocopherol than animal fats. The gamma form is usually richest in plants, whereas animal fats principally contain the alpha form.

---

* From: *The Summary.* Schute Institute for Clinical and Laboratory Medicine, p. 30, Vol. 14:No. 1, June, 1962, London, Canada.

have only been examined as students entering the University, and generally not just before the experiment with the exception that all young boys have been examined before the summer school began by medical doctors, and the adult men have been examined at least once at the time of joining the adult work. Some may have been in the work one or more years, and after some irregular attendance joined a regular experiment.

The Placeboes Used

Since the placeboes used were changed from time to time from 1950 to 1969, it is necessary to deal with this in every experiment separately. The placeboes obtained from the VioBin Corporation are listed in the following letter from Mr. V. K. Collins, biochemist at the VioBin plant, in Monticello, Illinois.

We have looked up the records on placebo capsules delivered to you since 1953.

Date	No Charge Number	Item
5-11-53	9649	14,200 lard placeboes, 6 min.
6-18-53	9718	1 box lard placeboes.
1-15-54	10225	Approximately 60,000 lard placeboes.
12-21-54	10894	30,000 cottonseed oil plus tocopherol placeboes.
5- 2-55	11202	30,000 same as above.
2- 6-56	11655	1 carton placeboes (lecithin).
5- 2-56	11866	1,200 cottonseed oil placeboes, 3 min.
7-17-56	12047	2,000 same as above.
9-17-57	12899	100,000 cottonseed oil placeboes, 6 min.
6-27-58	13451	30,000 cottonseed oil placeboes.
7-13-59	14258	15,000 lard placeboes.
7- 3-63	17459	15,000 cottonseed oil placeboes.
7-19-63	17478	15,000 same as above.
6-26-64	18105	8,000 lard placeboes.

I trust that this is the information you need to complete your records.

The following letter is from Elmer L. Sevringhaus, M.D., Director of Clinical Research at Hoffmann-La Roche Inc.

In response to your note of December 16, I have determined that our alpha tocopherol is mixed with corn oil in the capsules which we shall be sending to you. Under separate cover, therefore, I am shipping 3,600 capsules containing 100 mg each of alpha tocopherol acetate in corn oil. I am glad that this material can be made available to you in the form which you desire and we shall be very much interested to hear of the results that you achieve with it.

Octacosanol, a Crystalline Derivative of Wheat Germ Oil

Octacosanol is an octacosyl alcohol with the formula ($CH_3 \cdot (CH_2)_{26} \cdot CH_2 OH$) with a molecular weight of 410.75 and a melting point of 83.2 to 83.4 C. It can be isolated from a number of plant substances such as wheat wax, candilla wax, wool wax, alfalfa wax, sugar cane cuticular wax, the leaves of *Ginkgo biloba* and *Ephedra gerardina* (Neufeld, 1963), the leaves of *Sancococca pruniformis* (Gopinath, Kohli and Kidwai, 1962) and the cotton plant (Sadykov, Isaw and Isailov, 1963).

Wheat germ and wheat germ oil are known to contain factors which have varied effects. *Octacosanol* appears to be one of the principal factors in wheat germ and in wheat germ oil responsible for some of the effects named in experiments described in this book. The *octacosanol* herein referred to is a component of wheat wax.

Wheat Germ

The wheat germ was obtained from the Kretchmer Corporation, direct from the factory at Carrollton, Michigan. It was not absolutely fresh and, as all wheat germ is, it was baked in rotary ovens before bottling. But it came in bottles, just as bought in any grocery store. The fact that WGO, or octacosanol synthetic, could have an effect greater than wheat germ is hard to believe, but that is just what occurred in eight out of ten experiments. One year, 1958, insistence placed upon getting the wheat germ fresh (just bottled) rather than "stored or shelved" material, resulted in the best results, when it rivaled the effect of WGO/ octacosanol in Hupe's Exp. No. 15. The principal ingredients of wheat germ as announced by the Kretchmer Corp. are included in Table III.

Only in one year did the wheat germ outdo the WGO and the OCTCNL in affecting endurance (Fig. 9) in Hupe's Experiment, 1962. In this year, it was insisted that the WGC be absolutely

---

Note: Reference may be made to the published report, Accepted Foods, Council on Foods and Nutrition, of the American Medical Assn., *Journal of the American Medical Assn.*, 143:1486, Aug. 26, 1950.

TABLE III

WHEAT GERM ASSAY

(Furnished by the manufacturer, 1968)

Calories	125	per ounce, or 4.4 per gram
Riboflavin	0.44	mg/100 gm
Niacin	4.94	mg/100 gm
Pantothenic acid	1.5	mg/100 gm
Folic acid	0.5	mg/100 gm
Biotin	0.0125	mg/gm
Pyradoxine	1.3	mg/100 gm
Choline	425	mg/100 gm
Inositol	750	mg/100 gm
Phosphorus	970	mg/100 gm
Iron	8.8	mg/100 gm
Moisture	3.6%	
Ash	5.0%	
Fat	12.4%	
Protein	34.0%	
Crude fiber	2.0%	
Carbohydrate	43.0%	

fresh, it was sent to us just the week before we began the experiments. It was in the usual bottles. There were definite results from wheat germ in 1960 and 1963 over the placeboes. Fluctuation of the results may be due to many possible factors such as: a) different age of the materials, b) different placeboes, c) different subjects and d) different programs. From an assay report on "Toasted Wheat Germ," made available by the Kretchmer Corporation, dated May 24, 1950, from the Biochemical Laboratory of the University of Wisconsin, Wisconsin Alumni Research, the amount of tocopherols per gram is given as 0.42 mg.

It is important to realize that the average person in the United States gets very little, if any, unrefined polyunsaturated fatty acids in the diet. There are practically no *unrefined* vegetable oils available in the processed, hydrogenated oils used for cooking. All of the fats used are heated to over the boiling point in cooking, and WGO has not been heated to over 100° F. In this series of studies,* the *unrefined* oils have been shown to create an effect on physical fitness tests which is a new type of finding.

---

* The WGO fed per day, 4 to 7 times per week, was 10 × 6 minims capsules (or 20 × 3 minims for children); the 6-minim capsules contained 7.5 mg of vitamin E per capsule of the oil. The principal placebo was devitaminized lard but with 8.5 mg of vitamin E and certain experiments on placebo of cottonseed

TABLE IV

THE PROBABLE ACTION AND THE NATURE OF
THE SUPPLEMENTS FED (WGO, OCTACOSANOL, WGC)

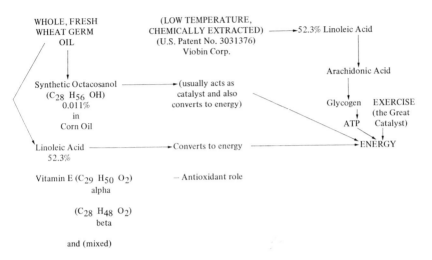

The amazing implications of this work are that the VioBin type of WGO and octacosanol (OCTCNL) as a proved constituent to the extent of 0.011 per cent octacosanol, which outdid wheat germ and corn oil, as far as these experiments go. Since corn oil is refined, we do not consider it a source of octacosanol. Very few people get the unsaponifiable fraction with the phosphatides, phytosterols, now recognized for lowering the cholesterol. The long list of nutrients in wheat germ is impressive but it is baked and also spoils easily. There is more to WGO than meets the eye. The logical explanation of its superiority is not completely formulated and no final attempt at this is presented. Only the grosser aspects are considered. In part, this is due to the nature of our experimental situation, and the dominant interest among all of our subjects "to get fit." If WGO will help, that is good.

---

oil containing 8.5 mg of vitamin E per capsule. The capsules containing the WGO and the placeboes were identical, as were the capsules containing 0.011 per cent octacosanol in refined corn oil, the same amount in wheat germ oil. Each 6-minim capsule contained 175 mg of whole, fresh WGO. The WGO contained 11.8 per cent palmitic acid, 28.1 per cent oleic, 52.3 per cent linoleic, 3.5 per cent linolenic, and other substances in slight amounts including the unsaponifiable fraction with phosphatides, phytosterols and octacosonal (0.011%) Each type of placebo is indicated specifically with each experiment.

REFERENCES

1. Keys, Ancel: Physical performance in relation to diet, *Fed. Proc.*, 2:164-187, Sept., 1943. Contains 410 references.
2. Henschel, Austin F.: Vitamins and muscular fatigue, *Lancet*, 63:355, Nov. 1943; and *Res. Quart.*, 13:280-285, Oct., 1942.
3. Karpovich, P. V.: Ergogenic aids in work and sport, *Res. Quart., Suppl.*, 12:432-450, May, 1941.
4. Cureton, T. K.: Diet related to athletics and physical fitness, *J. Phys. Ed.*, 57:Nos. 2, 3, 4, 5, 1959-60.
5. Cureton, T. K.: Diet as related to success in competitive swimming, *Beach and Pool*, 7:10-14, Jan., 1934.
6. Prokop, L.: Vitamine und Sportleistung, *Med. u. Ernährung*, 1961, No. 2, 174-176, 199-201 (University of Vienna); "Vitamins and Wheat Germ Oil in Sport Performances," *Sport-arztliche*, Heft ¾, 1960, pp. 100-109.
7. Tuttle, W. W., *et al.*: Breakfast and vitamin B-complex related to performance, *J. Amer. Diet. Ass.*, 24:945, 1049, 1948; 25:21, 123, 322, 398, 1949. Reviewed in *Nutr. Rev.*, 8:45, 1950.
8. Keys, A.: Cardiovascular effects of undernutrition and starvation. In *Mod. Conc. Cardiovasc. Dis.*, 17:21-22, Sept., 1948; and also, Nutrition in relation to etiology and course of degenerative disease, *J. Amer. Diet. Ass.*, 24:281-285, April, 1948.
9. Johnson, R. E., *et al.*: The effect of a diet deficiency in part of the vitamin B-complex upon men doing manual labor, *J. Nutr.*, 23:259-269, Mar., 1942.
10. Yakolev, N. M.: The importance of vitamins for sportsmen, *Theory and Practice of Physical Education*. Leningrad, Govt. Ptg., Nov., 1958, pp. 18-19.
11. Bergstrom, J., *et al.*: Diet, muscle glycogen and physical performance, *Acta Physiol. Scand.*, 71:140-150, 1967.
12. Brozek, Josef: Soviet studies on nutrition and higher nervous activity. In *Ann. N. Y. Acad. Sci.*, 93:665-714, 1962.
13. Poiletman, R. N. and H. A. Miller: The influence of wheat germ oil on the electrocardiographic t-wave of the highly trained athlete, *J. Sp. Med. Phys. Fitness*, 8:No. 1, Mar., 1968.
14. Farrell, P. R.: The Effects of Octacosanol on Conception and Reproduction, on the Maintenance and Growth of the Young, and on Oxygen Uptake in the White Rat. Manhattan, Kansas, M. S. thesis, Kansas State University, Dept. of Zoology, 1965, Sponsor: Prof. H. I. Gier.
15. Consolazio, C. F., *et al.*: The effect of octacosanol on the swimming time of rats, *J. Ap. Physiol.*, 19:265, 1964.

16. Goodwin, H. M.: *Elements of Precision Measurements and Graphical Methods.* New York, McGraw-Hill Co., 1920.
17. Cureton, T. K.: *Physical Fitness Appraisal and Guidance.* St. Louis. C. V. Mosby Co., 1947, p. 566.
18. Cureton, T. K.: *Physical Fitness of Champion Athletes.* Urbana, University of Illinois Press, 1951, p. 458.
19. American Assn. for Health, Physical Education and Recreation: *Measurement and Evaluation Materials in Health and Physical Education and Recreation.* Washington, D. C.: 1201 16th St., N.W. (NEA Building), 1950.
20. Cureton, T. K.: *Physical Fitness Workbook.* Champaign, Illinois, Stipes Pub. Co., 1944, p. 150.
21. Cureton, T. K., Huffman, W. J., Welser, L., Kireilis, R. W., and Latham, D. E.: *Endurance of Young Men.* Washington, D. C., National Research Council, Society for Research in Child Development, X:No. 40, No. 1, 1945, p. 284.
22. Cureton, T. K. and Barry, A. J.: *Improving the Physical Fitness of Youth.* Chicago, University of Chicago Press, Publications of the National Society for Research in Child Development.
23. Cureton, T. K.: *The Physiological Effects of Exercise Programs on Adults.* Springfield, Illinois, Charles C Thomas, 1969, p. 217.
24. Cureton, T. K.: *Physical Fitness Workbook for Adults.* Champaign, Illinois, Stipes Pub. Co., 1970, p. 220.
25. Falls, H. B. (Ed.): *Exercise Physiology.* New York, Academic Press, 1968, p. 471.

Chapter II

Summary of the Results of Forty-Two Experiments

RESULTS OF GROUP EXPERIMENTS

THE thirty-one group experiments have produced twenty-one statistically significant returns, with WGO predominant, just because it was used more times. Whenever octacosanol was used, it did as well as the WGO as an average, and they appear to act almost as identical substances. Twenty additional times out of the thirty-one experiments, the raw score results show favorable trends for one or another of the dietary substances used. The seven times no results developed of any consequence probably show no relationship, and one of these was due to the failure of wheat germ to give any result. Once (Hupé, 1958) the wheat germ cereal (WGC) did affect the cardiovascular measures more than either WGO or octacosanol (cf. Tables V-A, V-C).

In these experiments a great deal of variability is to be expected, as they were done under "field" conditions, with no real control over the diet except that it be "constantly the same, week to week." Perhaps the greatest variation is in the fact that the work could not be absolutely controlled, and some day-to-day variation expected in the practical work, and this due to the great preference of the men for such activities as jogging, swimming, calisthenics, handball and other games. Exact quantification of the work was not possible. The meaningful changes occur time and again in the same direction.

While more "reliable" results could be obtained just by using more cases, the more men involved, the harder it is to know just exactly what extraneous things a man may be doing and to know about other interfering causes such as sickness and temporary temperamental indispositions. Humans are very variable, and with more subjects, more extreme subjects are sure to be included, involving many who abhor exercise, drink too much, smoke too much and abuse themselves in overwork at night. Taking tests during an examination week, or even just before it greatly upsets students. Colds interfere also with the regularity of attendance, and the quality of the workouts even if men continue. In the author's opinion, the statistical inference generalizations are of less importance than studying the long time record of each and every individual, over several years, with alternation of the dietary supplements with placeboes. This has been done for a limited number of subjects and will be reported at the end of this section. When the trends are favorable, again and again, the effect is there but somewhat variable. As the controls improved over the experiments, the results are more definite.

The results as a whole show (Tables V-C and VI) that out of thirty-one group experiments conducted, eleven of these used *endurance* as the criterion, with the groups matched to pinpoint whether the WGO, OCTCNL or WGC affected the results. The results show that statistical significance better than the 0.10 level was obtained in five experiments (38.5%) and an absolute advantage of practical value obtained ten out of thirteen times (77%). The only dietary supplement to fail was wheat germ cereal (WGC) in Brown's experiment in 1960, and in this two overweight boys had a lot to do with nullifying the experiment. In any case the advantage for WGC was small, so it has been listed in the NER (no evidence result) column. Eliminating the WGC experiment by Brown, some favorable evidence appeared in ten experiments otherwise for WGO or OCTCNL. The problem of statistical significance has been argued in other places, this being viewed with "tongue in cheek" because of the skewed and relatively small samples. The main point is whether the groups *in hand* benefitted from the WGO or OCTCNL, and to this the answer is, "Yes, they did!" Could these results be duplicated with similar samples ninety out of one hundred times? Significance was obtained <.10 five times out of thirteen experiments (38.5%), so the answer is probably *not*. The samples would have to be larger and the distributions random to replicate ninety times out of one hundred. *This does not mean that the dietary supplements were not advantageous, but only that more cases and normal distributions would be needed for absolute confidence.* All in all, the results are quite impressive to the reviewer.

In the area of "peak" O_2 intake and net O_2 debt, there are only

TABLE V-A

SUMMARY OF STUDIES INVOLVING WHEAT GERM OIL, OCTACOSANOL AND
(Directed by Professor Thomas K. Cureton, Ph.D.)

Exp. No. Date	No. of Exp. Subjects	No. of Controls	Names of the Experimenters	Title of Study
1. (1949)	3×9 / 3×8	3×9 / 3×8	Forr (M.S.) / Cureton (sponsor)	WGO, corn oil and synthetic vitamin E effects on reaction times and CV tests
2. (1951)	6	3	*Harvison (M.S.) / Cureton (sponsor)	WGO effect on breath holding at ground level and at 10,000 feet simulated altitude
3. (1951)	6	3	*Smiley (M.S.) / Cureton (sponsor)	WGO effect on bicycle ergometer all-out ride time, at ground level and 10,000 ft.
4. (1951)	6	3	*Toohey (M.S.) / Cureton (sponsor)	WGO effects on progressive pulse ratio and pulse rates at ground level and altitude
5. (1951)	6	3	*White (M.S.) / Cureton (sponsor)	WGO effect on Schneider index and pulse rates, ground level and 10,000 feet simulated altitude
6. (1951)	6	3	*Ganslen (Ph.D.) / Cureton (sponsor)	WGO effect upon "peak" O_2 intake and sitting metabolic rate at ground level
7. (1952)	8	8+3	Storm (M.S.) / Cureton (sponsor)	WGO effects on adipose tissue, agility and weight residual (Cureton equation)
8. (1952)	9	9+5	Armer (M.S.) / Cureton (sponsor)	WGO effect on reaction times, agility and dynamometer strengths
9. (1952)	6	3	*Constantino (M.S.) / Cureton (sponsor)	WGO effect on the heartometer BPW at ground level and at 10,000 feet altitude
10. (1953)	6	3	*Susic (M.S.) / Cureton (sponsor)	WGO effect on the ECG precordial T-wave at ground level and 10,000 feet altitude
11. (1952)	9	9	Maley (M.S.) / Cureton (sponsor)	WGO effect with adult non-led program and cardiovascular tests
12. (1954)	11	11	Vohaska (M.S.) / Cureton (sponsor)	WGO effects on competitive wrestlers in all-out TM run and CV index
13. (1953-55)	8	8+5	Cureton (Ph.D.) and Pohndorf (M.P.E.)	WGO effects in pool physical conditioning programs upon TM run and BPW

No.	Year	N	N	Investigators	Description
14.	(1958)	5, 5, 5, 5	5, 5, 5, 5	Conner (M.S.) / Cureton (sponsor)	WGO effect in four physical conditioning programs upon dynamometer strength
15.	(1958)	5, 5, 5, 5	5, 5, 5, 5	Hupé (M.S.) / Cureton (sponsor)	Wheat germ, WGO, octacosanol effects in four different programs on CV tests
16.	(1958)	5, 5, 5, 5	5, 5, 5, 5	Tillman (M.S.) / Cureton (sponsor)	Wheat germ, WGO, octacosanol effects in four programs on agility and TBRT
17.	(1959)	16	16	Col. J. Tuma (Ph.D.) / Cureton (sponsor)	WGO and octacosanol effects upon endurance, CV tests and course survival
18.	(1958-59)	6	6	Bernauer (M.S.) and Cureton (staff)	WGO effect upon running times, brachial pulse wave and metabolism
19.	(1960)	10	10	Brown (Ph.D.) / Cureton (sponsor)	WGO effects upon "peak" oxygen intake and all-out treadmill run time
20.	(1963)	16, 16	16, 16	Banister and Cureton (staff)	WGO, octacosanol, wheat germ effects upon 600-yard run time
21.	(1957-63)	12, 12	10	Cureton, Orban, Barry, Phillips, Herden, Carhart	WGO effects on endurance of United States Navy Underwater Swimmers, Key West
22.	(1963)	10, 10	20	Dempsey (Ph.D.) / Cureton (sponsor)	WGO effects on BCG and pulse rate (IJ/t in velocity tracing)
23.	(1964)	1	1	Wiggett (M.S.) / Cureton (staff)	Octacosanol effect on reaction times (TBRT-visual, auditory, combined)
24.	(1964)	37	37	Chen (M.S.) / Cureton (sponsor)	WGO effect upon all-out treadmill run time (8.6% grade, 7 mi/hr)
25.	(1955-56)	16, 19	18	Linda Cundill (M.S.) / Cureton (sponsor)	WGO effects on pre-ejection intervals (ICP and EML, pulse rate of heart cycle)
26.	(1966)	4	5	Johnson (M.S.) / Cureton (sponsor)	WGO effects on total body reaction times (visual, auditory, combined)
27.	(1967)	6, 6	6	Franks (Ph.D.) and Cureton (Ph.D.) staff	WGO and wheat germ cereal effects on flicker fusion frequency and 600-yard run times
28.	(1968)	6, 6, 6	6	Samson (M.S.) / Cureton (sponsor)	WGO effect on basal metabolism
29.	(1968)	6, 6	7	Mayhew (M.S.) / Cureton (sponsor)	WGO effects on the precordial T-wave at rest and in stages of recovery
30.	(1968)	10, 10	12	Wiley (Ph.D.) / Cureton (sponsor)	WGO effects on the pre-ejection intervals of the ECG (ICP and EML)
31.	(1968)	20, 20	20	Milesis (M.S.) / Cureton (Ph.D.) staff	WGO effects upon total body reaction time (visual, auditory, combined)

INDIVIDUAL CASES—LONGITUDINAL

Exp. No. Date	No. of Exp. Subjects	No. of Controls	Names of the Experimenters	Title of Study
32. (1945-59)	1	0 (own control)	Cureton and staff on Cureton	WGO effects contrasted with wheat germ and nothing with variations, alternating
33. (1953-56)	1	0 (own control)	Cureton and staff on Tuckey	WGO effects alternating with nothing, four years, continuous training
34. (1949-58)	1	0 (own control)	Cureton and staff on D. Hubbard	WGO effects alternated with placebo effects and nothing, eight years
35. (1954-56)	1	0 (own control)	Cureton and staff on Skornia	WGO effects alternated with wheat germ and nothing, eight years
36. (1953-56)	1	0 (own control)	Cureton and staff on Birkland	WGO effects alternated with nothing and placeboes, four years
37. (1953-57)	1	0 (own control)	Cureton and staff on Dickey	WGO effects alternated with nothing and placeboes, four years
38. (1953-57)	1	0 (own control)	Cureton and staff on Kummerow	WGO effects alternated with wheat germ, placeboes and nothing, four years
39. (1953-57)	1	0 (own control)	Cureton and staff on Smythe	WGO effects alternated with placeboes, four years
40. (1953-57)	1	0 (own control)	Cureton and staff on Rae	WGO effects alternated with placeboes and wheat germ, four years
41. (1953-57)	1	0 (own control)	Cureton and staff on Steidner	WGO effects alternated with wheat germ and placeboes, four years
42. (1954-63)	1	0 (own control)	Cureton and staff on Joie Ray	WGO effects alternated with nothing, ten years continuously
N =	498	396		

* The same subjects were used in these experiments, with different experimenters responsible for particular measurements named in each study.

three experiments and none of these gave irrefutably favorable results, but only in some cases, so the rating is only moderately favorable. The effect upon net oxygen debt appears to be better than the effect upon aerobic oxygen intake but the former is not statistically significant because of the large variability in the determination of the net O_2 debt. Yet, both Dr. Prokop and Professor Gier have reported experiments which support our less definite results.

As to the supplements affecting *total body reaction time* (Garrett-Cureton test), eight experiments were completed and four times (50%) there was a result better than 0.10 level of significance, and three times the effect of WGO lacked a bit of obtaining this standard of reliability but all eight experiments gave some evidence favorable to the use of WGO (87.5%). All three reaction times (visual, auditory and combined stimuli) were usually affected. This suggests that the nervous system is affected by WGO, which coincides with Brozek's summary of the Russian work. Muscle cells and nervous cells appear to be affected but it is very doubtful if oxygen transport was affected. The efficiency of recovery appears to have been affected. Subjects on WGO or OCTCNL generally stood measured amounts of stress better.

Eleven experiments of the longitudinal type with *individuals*, alternating in different years the use of WGO with placeboes, or nothing, or with WGC, indicate the superiority of WGO, as again and again the improvements were relatively greater than for the placebo substances or nothing, and an effect over and above the exercise effect (cf. Exp. 32 through 42, Part Two).

Biological individuality is to be expected, in accordance with the principles of Roger Williams, who has reported that the enzymatic reactions are very different in different people. It is also true that some people do not use WGO readily but use it much better if they take it right after exercise, when the body is hot and the stomach is empty. In several experiments, to be described in detail, sedentary people have improved less than the active (exercised) subjects, considering only the effects over and above the exercise effect itself. In our experiments the WGO has always been taken in capsules, to prevent spoilage and for camouflage "blind or double-blind" purposes.

TABLE V-B

WHEAT GERM CEREAL (KRETCHMER) AT THE PHYSICAL FITNESS RESEARCH CENTER

Exp. No. (Year)	Type of Placebo	Nature of the Research Methods	Type of Subjects (Age Group)
1. (1949)	Synthetic vitamin E in corn oil and corn oil	Three parallel groups in each of two groups (1) swimming (2) Physical Education	Undergraduate students
2. (1951)	None—pretraining to plateau, then tests at T_2	T_1 to T_2, four weeks of pretesting to T_2 then supplements and T_3, six weeks	Physical Education graduate students
3. (1951)	None—Four weeks pretesting (T_1)	T_1 to T_2, four weeks of pretesting to T_2 then supplements and T_3, six weeks (twelve weeks to plateau, then WGO six weeks)	Physical Education graduate students
4. (1951)	None—Four weeks pretesting (T_1)	T_1 to T_2, four weeks of pretesting to T_2 then supplements and T_3, six weeks (twelve weeks to plateau, then WGO six weeks)	Physical Education graduate students
5. (1951)	None—Four weeks pretesting (T_1)	T_1 to T_2, four weeks of pretesting to T_2 then supplements and T_3, six weeks (twelve weeks to plateau, then WGO six weeks)	Physical Education graduate students
6. (1951)	None—Four weeks pretesting (T_1)	T_1 to T_2, four weeks of pretesting to T_2 then supplements and T_3, six weeks (twelve weeks to plateau, then WGO six weeks)	Physical Education graduate students
7. (1952)	Cottonseed oil (CSO) capsules (20×3 minims)	Two matched groups in parallel program, testing T_1 and T_2, six weeks between	Middle-aged men
8. (1952)	Cottonseed oil capsules (20×3 minims)	Two matched groups in parallel program, in mixed voluntary exercise, six weeks	Middle-aged men
9. (1952)	None—Four weeks pretesting (T_1)	Single group, T_1 to T_2 training (twelve weeks) then six weeks continued program on WGO to T_3	Graduate students
10. (1953)	None—Four weeks pretesting (T_1)	Single group, T_1 to T_2 training (twelve weeks) then six weeks continued program on WGO to T_3	Graduate students
11. (1952)	Cottonseed oil capsules (20×3 minims)	Matched halves of swimming team, exp. group six weeks on WGO versus placebo controls	Undergraduates, varsity men
12. (1955)	Cottonseed oil capsules (20×3 minims)	Matched halves of wrestling team, exp. group four weeks on WGO versus placebo controls	Undergraduates, varsity men

No. (Year)	Substance	Description	Subjects
13. (1953-55)	Cottonseed oil capsules (20 × 3 minims)	Two groups matched on all-out treadmill run, exp. group six weeks on WGO, calisthenics and swim	Middle-aged men
14. (1958)	Lecithin oil capsules (92% CSO) (20 × 3 minims)	Four matched groups by 600-yard run, six weeks on four different activities, WGO on strength	Boys
15. (1958)	Lecithin oil capsules (92% CSO) (20 × 3 minims)	Four matched groups by 600-yard run, six weeks WGO versus OCTACL versus wheat germ on endurance	Boys
16. (1958)	Lecithin oil capsules (92% CSO) (20 × 3 minims)	Four matched groups by 600-yard run, six weeks WGO, OCTACL, WG on agility and TB reaction times	Boys
17. (1959)	Cottonseed oil capsules (20 × 3 minims)	Three matched groups by composite muscular endurance, WGO versus OCTACL versus placebo controls	Navy underwater demolition men
18. (1959)	Devitaminized lard capsules (15 × 3 minims)	Two halves of a track cross-country team, matched by 440-yard run, eight weeks WGO versus control	Undergraduate track men
19. (1960)	None—Each boy retested versus own record	Single group of twenty boys tested four times: T_1 to T_2, repeat in 1 week T_3, after rest T_4	Boys
20. (1963)	Devitaminized lard capsules (15 × 3 minims)	Four matched groups by 600-yard run time, six weeks WGO versus placebo controls, all in S-F	Boys
21. (1957)	Cottonseed oil capsules (20 × 3 minims)	Three groups matched by muscular endurance tests, six weeks on WGO, OCTACL on muscular endurance	Navy underwater men
22. (1963)	Devitaminized lard capsules (15 × 3 minims)	Three groups matched by 600-yard run time, WGO versus placeboes on 600-yard run time	Boys
23. (1964)	Devitaminized lard capsules (15 × 3 minims)	Two groups matched by 600-yard run time, six weeks on WGO versus placebo controls on TM-run time	Boys
24. (1964)	None—one on octacosanol and one on nothing	Two matched track sprinters compared on TB reaction times (visual, auditory, both, twenty-four weeks)	Undergraduate men
25. (1965-66)	Devitaminized lard capsules (15 × 3 minims)	Two matched groups by 600-yard run times, T_1, six weeks in S-F school then T_2, rest and T_3	Boys
26. (1966)	Devitaminized lard capsules (10 × 6 minims)	Two groups of adult men matched by average of TB reaction times, 3/wk. for sixteen weeks OCTACL versus placeboes	Adult men
27. (1967)	Devitaminized lard capsules (15 × 3 minims)	Three groups matched by pretests of flicker FF (Krasno Ivy) six weeks in S-F, WGO versus WG cereal	Boys
28. (1968)	Devitaminized lard capsules (10 × 6 minims)	Tests on basal metabolic rate and R-wave of ECG, eighteen men in pretraining for ten weeks (T_1 to T_2), then split into three matched groups; ten weeks on WGO versus controls	Adult men

Exp. No. (Year)	Type of Placebo	Nature of the Research Methods	Type of Supjects (Age Group)
29. (1968)	Devitaminized lard capsules (10 × 6 minims)	Tests T_1, T_2, T_3 at 0, 10 and 20 weeks experimentals versus two control groups on T-wave of ECG	Adult men
30. (1968)	Devitaminized lard capsules (10 × 6 minims)	Same pattern—tests at 0, 10 and 20 weeks on pre-ejection intervals, exps. versus two control groups	Adult men
31. (1968)	Devitaminized lard capsules (10 × 6 minims)	Three groups matched on total body reaction time, six weeks on WG and WGO versus controls	Boys
32. (1945-49)	None—each man served as own control then alternated	Alternated WGO, nothing, WG used for eighteen years to observe effects on precordial T-wave	Man
33. (1953-56)	Cottonseed oil capsules at times (20 × 3 minims)	Alternated for four years, WGO versus placeboes to observe effects on cardiovascular tests	Man
34. (1949-58)	Cottonseed oil capsules at times (20 × 3 minims)	Alternated for nine years, WGO versus nothing versus placeboes to observe changes in cardiovascular tests	Man
35. (1954-56)	None—each man served as own control then alternated	Alternated for three years, WGO, nothing, wheat germ to observe changes in cardiovascular tests	Man
36. (1953-56)	Cottonseed oil capsules (20 × 3 minims)	Alternated for four years, wheat germ, WGO and placeboes to observe changes in cardiovascular tests	Man
37. (1953-57)	Cottonseed oil capsules (20 × 3 minims)	Alternated for five years, wheat germ, nothing, WGO, placeboes to observe changes in cardiovascular tests	Man
38. (1953-57)	Cottonseed oil capsules (20 × 3 minims)	Wheat germ, nothing, placeboes alternated for five years to observe changes in cardiovascular tests	Man
39. (1953-57)	Cottonseed oil capsules (20 × 3 minims)	Wheat germ, nothing, WGO alternated for five years to observe effects on cardiovascular tests	Man
40. (1953-57)	Cottonseed oil capsules (20 × 3 minims)	Wheat germ, nothing, WGO alternated for five years to observe changes in cardiovascular tests	Man
41. (1953-57)	Cottonseed oil capsules (20 × 3 minims)	WGO, nothing, wheat germ alternated for five years to observe effects on cardiovascular tests	Man
42. (1954-63)	Nothing, own control	Alternated WGO with nothing, ten years to observe effects on mile run time and cardiovascular tests	Man

TABLE V–C
THE UNIVERSITY OF ILLINOIS PHYSICAL FITNESS
RESEARCH LABORATORY, 1949–69

1. (1949) . . . . . ° Significant changes in total body reaction time and T-wave of the ECG attributable to use of WGO; and statistically insignificant changes due to corn oil and vitamin E (synthetic)

2. (1951) . . . . . ° Insignificant effects of WGO on breath holding time at ground level and at 10,000 feet simulated altitude in decompression chamber; but the PT program improved breath holding

3. (1951) . . . . . Some gains possibly attributable to the use of WGO in 6 weeks period after the exp. subjects had trained for 12 weeks and reached a plateau on CV tests and all-out ride time

4. (1951) . . . . . After pretraining for 12 weeks and reaching plateau on CV tests and all-out ride time progressive pulse ratio improved at ground level and at 10,000 feet simulated altitude

5. (1951) . . . . . After pretraining for 12 weeks and reaching plateau on CV tests and all-out ride time Schneider index further improved, significantly

6. (1951) . . . . . After pretraining for 12 weeks and reaching plateau on CV tests and all-out ride time subjects improved further on WGO for 6 weeks of continued training at ground level

7. (1952) . . . . The weight reduced slightly on WGO compared to a gain by control subjects on placeboes; weight residual dropped less in WGO group than placebo group, permitting better norm

8. (1952) . . . . . Exercise did cause significant improvement in visual, auditory and combined total body reaction times: WGO caused further improvement in visual reaction time

9. (1952) . . . . . Significant improvements were made in the brachial pulse wave (Sphygmogram) by training; addition of WGO for 6 weeks of further training failed to improve at ground level or altitude

10. (1952-53) . . . Twelve weeks of physical training made slight improvements (insignificant) in the precordial T-wave of the ECG but the addition of WGO for 6 weeks with continued training did change it (significant)

11. (1952) . . . . . Insignificant changes were made by WGO experimental group on WGO and also control group on synthetic vitamin E in 6 weeks after pretraining (informal nonled) 4 months had made slight changes

12. (1955) . . . . . WGO experimental group made significant changes in composite CV tests while matched control group did not change significantly on placeboes; TM all-out run was insignificantly different

13. (1953-55) . . . WGO experimental group made significant (D/S.E.$_{meas.}$) changes while control group on placeboes did not, on all-out treadmill run, brachial pulse wave (Sphygmogram), and other CV tests

14. (1958) . . . . . WGO experimental group made significant changes in left-

hand grip and back strength dynamometer tests while control group did not; octacosanol experimental group improved leg strength more

15. (1958) ..... Wheat germ, octacosanol and WGO experimental groups improved more than lecithin control group in all-out treadmill run and brachial pulse wave (Sphygmogram), lecithin not placebo

16. (1958) ..... Octacosanol, wheat germ and WGO affected total body reaction tests (visual, auditory, and combined responses)—effect was in order of mention, all significant agility run (insignificant)

17. (1959) ..... Octacosanol and WGO experimental groups made greater relative improvements than controls on muscular endurance, strength and weight residuals, and CV tests than controls

18. (1958-59) ... WGO group improved significantly over control group on placeboes in area of brachial pulse wave (Sphygmogram) and basal metabolic rate; improvement in run time favored WGO group

19. (1960) ..... Training differences between wheat germ cereal and control groups for "peak" O_2 intake were insignificant and only average of 0.9 cc/min/kg difference developed; 7 on WGC, 5 no improvement

20. (1963) ..... WGO exp. group improved more than control group on placeboes and difference was significant by $D/S.E._{meas.}$ ratio on 600-yard run as criterion. WGO did better than OCTACL or lard

21. (1957-63) ... WGO and octacosanol experimental groups bettered the placebo group on four of five muscular endurance tests and on Harvard 5-minute step test—all Navy men on same daily program

22. (1963) ..... WGO group was significantly better in pulse rate reduction and in IJ/t ratio of the ballistocardiogram test than control group on placeboes

23. (1964) ..... WGO experimental group was significantly better on the all-out treadmill run than the matched placebo group by analysis of variance (combining four groups of boys)

24. (1964) ..... One subject on octacosanol improved after 4 weeks preliminary testing period to achieve plateau compared to control subject on visual, auditory and combined TB reaction times

25. (1965-66) ... WGO experimental group improved the amplitude of the brachial pulse wave (Sphygmogram) at 5-minutes post-exercise recovery more than control group and WGO group stood stress better in run

26. (1967) ..... WGO experimental group improved more than control group on total body reaction time (average) and more WGO subjects improved than placebo subjects; one placebo subject bettered WGO

27. (1967) ..... WGO experimental group changed the least (showed stress less) than the wheat germ cereal or placebo groups on Krasno-Ivy flicker fusion frequency test—WGO group stood stress better

28. (1968) ..... After 10 weeks of pretraining as entire group, the split 6 men on WGO improved more than the placebo group

and group on nothing in BMR, R-wave, I_a wave of BCG (significant)

29. (1968) .... After 10 weeks of pretraining as entire group, the split experimental WGO group improved more in T-wave of ECG at fifth, sixth and ninth minute of recovery than control group

30. (1968) .... After 10 weeks of pretraining as entire group, split 7-man group improved the pre-ejection intervals more (significant) than the control group; WGO subjects stood stress better

31. (1968) .... Experimental group on WGO after fourth week of feeding on WGO made significantly better reduction in total body reaction times than control groups on wheat germ and placeboes

INDIVIDUAL CASES—LONGITUDINAL

32. (1945-49) ... One older man, tested at various times over 18 years on the precordial T-wave of the ECG showed the greatest increase on WGO feeding, alternated with nothing and wheat germ

33. (1953-56) ... One middle-aged man, tested for 4 years, made his highest Schneider index and improved the systolic amplitude and area of the brachial pulse wave more on WGO

34. (1949-58) ... One middle-aged man, tested for 9 years, made his highest scores on the all-out treadmill run and improved his T-wave of the ECG more while on WGO than while on PLAC

35. (1954-56) ... One middle-aged man, tested for 3 years, improved his precordial T-wave of the ECG relatively more on WGO and on wheat germ than on nothing

36. (1953-56) ... One middle-aged man, tested for 4 years, improved his Schneider index relatively more while on WGO than while on wheat germ, placeboes or nothing

37. (1953-57) ... One middle-aged man, tested for 4 years, improved his precordial T-wave of the ECG relatively more while on WGO and wheat germ than while on nothing or placeboes

38. (1953) .... One middle-aged man, tested for 5 years, improved his T-wave of the ECG relatively more while on WGO, and also the amplitude and area of the BPW than while on placeboes

39. (1953-57) ... One middle-aged man, tested for 5 years, improved the area of the brachial pulse wave (Sphygmogram) relatively more while on WGO than while on placeboes or nothing

40. (1953-57) ... One middle-aged man, tested for 5 years, improved his all-out treadmill run relatively more while on wheat germ and WGO than while on placeboes or nothing

41. (1953-57) ... One middle-aged man, tested for 5 years, improved the Schneider index and diastolic blood pressure relatively more while on WGO than while on placeboes or nothing

42. (1954-63) ... One middle-aged man, tested for 10 years, made his fastest mile run time first with injections of vitamin C and calcium, and by taking wheat germ oil for 10 years

* For details of significance or insignificance (statistical) refer to Appendix.

NUMBER OF TIMES STATISTICAL SIGNIFICANCE OR FAVORABLE ADVANTAG
OCTACOSANOL OR WHEAT GER

Various Physiological Tests	Experiments	No. 1 Forr and Cureton	No. 2 Harrison and Cureton	No. 3 Smiley and Cureton	No. 4 Toohey and Cureton	No. 5 White and Cureton	No. 6 Ganslen and Cureton	No. 7 Storm and Cureton	No. 8 Armer and Cureton	No. 9 Constantino and Cureton	No. 10 Susic and Cureton	No. 11 Maley and Cureton	No. 12 Vohaska and Cureton
Endurance Tests	Significant												
	Favorable trend			WGO			WGO						WGO
	Not related												
"Peak" O$_2$ Intake or Net O$_2$ Debt	Significant												
	Favorable trend	WGO					WGO						
	Not related												
Total Body Reaction Time	Significant		WGO						WGO				
	Favorable trend												
	Not related												
Strength Tests	Significant												
	Favorable trend												
	Not related												
Precordial T and R Waves of ECG	Significant		WGO									WGO	WGC
	Favorable trend												
	Not related										NER		
BCG and Sphygmogram (Pulse Wave)	Significant												WGO
	Favorable trend												
	Not related									NER			
Pulse Rate, Schneider Index, Pre-ejection Intervals	Significant				WGO	WGO							WGO
	Favorable trend												
	Not related												
Basal (and Sitting) Metabolism Tests	Significant												
	Favorable trend						WGO						
	Not related												
Flicker Fusion Frequency	Significant												
	Favorable trend												
	Not related												
Composite Criterion	Significant										NER		

Key: WGO = Obtained for WGO   OCT = Obtained for OCTCNL

	No. 14 Conner and Cureton	No. 15 Hupé and Cureton	No. 16 Tillman and Cureton	No. 17 Tuma and Cureton	No. 18 Bernauer and Cureton	No. 19 Brown and Cureton	No. 20 Banister and Cureton	No. 21 Cureton, et al.	No. 22 Dempsey and Cureton	No. 23 Chen and Cureton	No. 24 Wiggett and Cureton	No. 25 Cundiff and Cureton	No. 26 Johnson and Cureton	No. 27 Franks and Cureton	No. 28 Sampson and Cureton	No. 29 Mayhew and Cureton	No. 30 Wiley and Cureton	No. 31 Milesis and Cureton
			OCT															
...GO			WGO	WGO			WGO			WGO								
	WGC								WGO									
									OCT									
						WGC												
						WGC												
		OCT									OCT							
...GO				OCT									WGO					
WGO																		
				WGO														
									NER									
				WGO														
									OCT									
...ER																		
...GO									WGO									
	WGC																	
									NER									
									WGO									
									WGO			WGO				WGO		WGO
...GO									OCT									
															WGO			
															WGO			
				OCT					WGO									
				WGO					OCT									

NER = No evidence of relationship (tried)   BLANK (no test)

SUMMARY OF THE RESULTS ACCORDING TO THE TEST CRITERIA

Endurance

Out of thirteen experiments (Table VI), there were ten (76.8%) which produced statistically significant results by the statistical methods used (usually both S.E.$_{meas.}$ and Fisher's t test). Five others made actual improvements which were in favor of the WGO or OCTCNL supplements, and combining these two sets the total in the right direction, showing some real effect of the WGO and OCTCNL were ten out of eleven (90.8%), compared to the placeboes.

In Experiments 17 and 21, carried out by Cureton and his staff at the U.S. Navy stations at Key West (Underwater Scuba School) and at Little Creek (Underwater Demolition School of the Marines) with the assistance of medical personnel at these bases who were responsible for feeding the materials in "double-blind" fashion, respectively, the WGO and OCTCNL gave very similar results, both showing advantage over the placebo groups. What does not show in the statistics is that the *placebo groups* had more difficulty in getting through these courses, both considered to be very strenuous. The Little Creek experiment was most strenuous, with an expected 65 per cent of drop-outs. There were sixteen men in each group, matched at the beginning on the composite muscular endurance index (Ave. SS of the mile run, squat jumps, push-ups, five-minute step test), and at the end of the course, thirty-five men had "washed out" to leave thirteen men at the end passing the entire course and without injury. This 73 per cent attrition upset the original matching, but of these who remained matched (only original matched 3's) the OCTCNL-fed group improved from 54.67 SS to 71.03 SS, gaining 16.36 SS; the placebo group improved from 56.32 SS to 64.30 SS, or a gain of 7.98 SS; and the WGO group improved from 59.03 to 72.15 SS, a gain of 13.12 SS. In terms of SS these gains made in the composite muscular endurance criterion can be legitimately compared. The t test was meaningless because of the losses from the groups, leaving them unmatched with uneven numbers and the data skewed. The men, considered separately as individuals or as an average, improved more taking the WGO and OCTCNL supplements than taking placeboes. The percentage of each group which successfully passed the course were, respectively, (5 taking OCTCNL, 31.3%), (2 controls, 12.4%) and (6 taking WGO, 37.6%) (Fig. 2).

Strength

It is not certain at all that WGO or OCTCNL affect strength. The three experiments gave a statistically significant result once, a trend of advantage once and no evidence once. Especially the U.S. Navy Underwater Swimmer's Study made in 1957 at Key West, Florida suggests "no relationship." Still, back and leg strength seem to show some effect in boys (Conner's Exp. No. 14) and the same type of result shows up in Tuma's study on the Underwater Demolition Navy Men at Little Creek in 1959. It must be concluded that the question is not settled.

Precordial T-Waves of the ECG

In seven experiments involving the precordial T-waves of the electrocardiogram (ECG) the results were statistically significant four times out of seven (57.1%). This evidence is graphed out in the experiments of Forr (Exp. 1), Susic (Exp. 10) and Bernauer (Exp. 18) and also shows definitely in the Vohaska experiment (Exp. 12) but is not paralleled by any appreciable advantage in the all-out treadmill run time; nor do Experiments 11 (Maley) or 13 (Cureton and Pohndorf) yield statistically significant results (NER). Once in Cureton's U.S. Navy experiment the effect of OCTCNL was favorable on the T-wave.

Brachial Pulse Waves

In six experiments involving the brachial pulse wave (BPW) or the ballistocardiogram (BCG) statistical significance was obtained three times better than the .10 level (50%), and one additional time the evidence was favorable, or a total of four out of six times (66.7%), the favorable nonsignificant effect being for wheat germ cereal, and all significant results were for WGO. In Constantino's experiment (Exp. 9) the results were NER. Both of these measures are grouped together because they reflect the *energy* of the ventricular contraction, which is unquestionably affected by a favorable nutritional state. It is probable that the nutritional substances affect the nerves which supply the heart muscle, both sympathetic and vagal nerves. In Cureton's U.S. Navy experiment (Exp. 21) the evidence was also NER, and the reason seemed to be that the men were pushed so hard that they were *always* tired, this depressed the brachial pulse wave, and the group taking placeboes did better to withstand the stress. It is certain that an overwhelmingly strong stress, as the altitude stress at 10,000 feet, can blot out the more delicate and smaller nutritional effects of a dietary supplement.

Schneider Index, Pulse Rate Tests

Nine experiments were conducted involving the pulse rates (or the Schneider index, which is predominantly a pulse rate test involving several pulse rates). The *pre-ejection intervals* are classified in this same group, as they are intervals split from the time of a single pulse beat. Although they are factorily different, as shown by the Franks and Cureton study, the pre-ejection intervals are part of a pulse beat. Four times out of nine (44.5%) these stress indicator tests gave a significant result for the effect of WGO, and five additional times gave a favorable trend in favor of WGO, one of these (Exp. 21) (Cureton, *et al.*) also showing an advantage for OCTCNL. At no time did these tests completely fail to be affected by the dietary substances, which strengthens the belief that the nervous system had been affected by the WGO and OCTCNL.

Basal Metabolic Rate

The *basal metabolic rate test* (BMR) was run only twice and Ganslen's Exp. 6 tested the men in the sitting position on the ergometer bicycle. Samson's experiment (Exp. 28) gave a statistically significant effect for WGO on BMR in terms of $D/S.E._{meas.}$, the only reliability measure which seemed to be justified. Ganslen (Exp. 6) showed a favorable trend for WGO to raise the sitting metabolic rate slightly (SMR). This is discussed more fully in the BMR Chapter.

Flicker Fusion Frequency

Only one experiment was run on flicker fusion frequency (Exp. 27) by Franks and Cureton, which demonstrated a statistically significant result in that the WGO group held their homeostasis better (more stable) in the face of stress.

Composite Muscular Endurance and Cardiovascular Condition

Composite criteria were used three times. Twice out of the three times the criterion was affected by both WGO and OCTCNL, this with the composite muscular endurance (five events); and once with the composite cardiovascular criterion in Maley's experiment, there was a NER (no evidence revealed) result.

Fat Folds

One experiment is not included in the table due to it being incommensurable, namely Experiment 7 by Storm, which demonstrated that the subjects taking WGO gained relatively less fat than the ones on placeboes.

I. RESULTS ON YOUNG MEN

A. The Original Impetus, Quite Convincing Results

Three studies caused the entire series of studies to be pursued for twenty years. The first study was by Forr (Cureton, sponsor), contract to Cureton to get the work done. So the study was planned by Cureton and Forr, with occasional advice from Mr. Levin and Dr. E. L. Sevringhaus, of the Hoffmann-La Roche Company, who furnished the vitamin E and the capsules of corn oil (refined). This study is summarized in Part Two, Exp. 1. The second study was carried out on middle-aged men (26 to 60 years of age) by Cureton and Pohndorf* (Exp. 13) and is described under section III of this chapter, it was conducted in 1953 and repeated in 1954 with a new shuffle of subjects. The

---

* Cf. Table VII.

data are given in full because of the nature of it, which stimulated many other studies. The data convinced us that WGO had
a real effect apart from exercise.

B. Ergometer Bicycle All-Out Endurance Time, Schneider Index and Pre-Ejection Intervals of the Left Ventricle of the ECG

Cureton, Ganslen, Smiley, Susic and White,[*] 1958-59, completed a controlled experiment in 1959 on the bicycle ergometer
for testing, training six experimental subjects for twenty-four
weeks. The young graduate students trained for twelve weeks
from T_1 to T_2 and the differences noted. Then a WGO feeding
was added of 10×6 minims of WGO for the last six weeks.
Three inactive controls were used. The gains were greater during
the T_2 to T_3 period when the WGO was used for six weeks compared to the twelve weeks without dietary supplementation. This
gave an unusual curve of improvement, which after plateauing
off in several measures, the Schneider index and brachial pulse
wave, improved to a new and higher level (Fig. 24). (Cf. Part
Two, Exp. 3, 5, 6, 10 and Fig. 78.)

C. Wrestling Team's Endurance on All-Out Treadmill Run

Vohaska,[†] Figure 1, completed a study on wrestlers and
showed that both WGO and cottonseed oil placeboes improved
the all-out treadmill run more than a group of controls who took
nothing. It was decided in this experiment that cottonseed oil
had some ergogenic action. The gain was also observed in the
brachial pulse wave for the WGO group over the placebo group.
The gains were relatively small because of the interference called
"competitive fatigue." This experiment was repeated with advantages showing for the WGO over placeboes in the all-out treadmill run, the T-wave of the ECG, the systolic amplitude of the
brachial pulse wave and the Schneider index.

---

[*] Published paper, Effect of physical training and a wheat germ oil dietary
supplement upon the t-wave of the ECG and the bicycle ergometer test, *Medicina
Sportiva*, 8:490-505, Oct., 1959.
[†] Vohaska, Exp. 12 in Part Two.

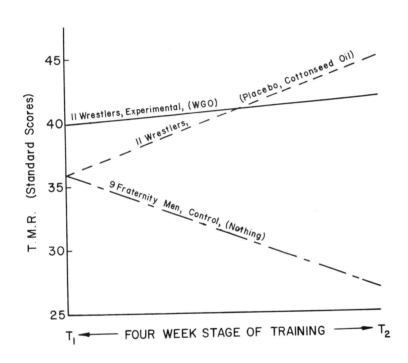

Figure 1. Improvements in treadmill run (mean SS) 7 mi/hr/8.6% grade.

D. United States Marine Demolition Swimmers

Tuma, Cureton and assistants made an evaluation of the Underwater Demolition Unit, United States Marines, in training at Little Creek, Virginia, in 1958, reported in Tuma's Ph.D. thesis at the University of Illinois in 1959.* Only two subjects remained matched, as many dropped out because of the severity of the program or because of injuries. The two experimental subjects

---

* Tuma, Cureton, *et al.*, cf. Exp. No. 17 in Part Two.

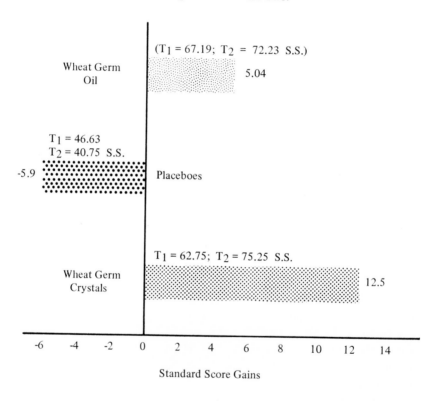

Figure 2. Advantage in gains of the UDC (Navy) WGO and OCTCNL groups (16 wks.) over the placebo group.

taking WGO, and the two matched taking octacosanol, showed significant superiority on the endurance criterion used (five muscular endurance items) and in various CV variables, over the controls on cottonseed oil. A significantly larger percentage of the men completed the course who were on WGO or octacosanol than who were on the placeboes.

In the well-designed experiment by Tuma,[13] forty-eight beginning Navy underwater demolition team candidates were given sixty-three physical fitness tests representing components of strength, physique, muscular endurance and cardiovascular fitness prior (T_1) and subsequent (T_2) in a fourteen-week intensive training course. The forty-eight candidates were divided at commencement of training into three matched groups, A (octacosanol), B (cottonseed oil placeboes), C (wheat germ oil), on the basis of a composite muscular endurance and cardiovascular test index. Each group was fed twenty 3-minim size capsules per day of its assigned dietary supplement throughout the fourteen-week training course. Again, the feeding was conducted on a double-blind basis. Fitness changes, T_2-T_1, were determined on individual survivors within each matched group, and between matched groups. Improvements within groups, averaging from fifteen tests intended to represent the four components of fitness mentioned above, revealed a mean gain of 16.36 standard scores for the octacosanol group, 13.12 SS for the wheat germ oil group, and 7.98 SS for the placebo group. Within the group *mile run time* improvements gave similar results: a mean gain of 13.6 SS for the octacosanol group, 12.3 SS for the wheat germ oil group, and 7.0 SS for the placebo group. An intra-group T_2 analysis was not possible because of the large number of men that dropped out in the placebo group, but man for man those on octacosanol or wheat germ oil did better than those on placeboes. There were eleven drop-outs in group A, fourteen in group B and ten in group C; a between-group nonparametric test gave no statistical evidence that the lesser attrition of students in groups A and C can be wholly attributed to wheat germ oil supplementation, although the fitness test results indicate that the men in groups A and C (taking octacosanol and wheat germ oil, respectively) may have acquired a tougher, more sympathetically-tuned nervous

TABLE VII

CHANGES WITHIN GROUPS*

Motor Fitness Tests	Octacosanol Raw Score	SS	Placebo Raw Score	SS	WGO Raw Score	SS	Significance A	B	C
Mile run (min.)	−1.38	17.3	−0.83	10.8	−1.14	14.8	4.06	2.96	4.77
466-yard swim (min.)	−2.67	16.0	−3.00	17.7	−1.58	9.2	4.19	2.91	4.84
Push-ups (times)	6.54	14.0	3.85	9.5	5.13	10.0	7.39	5.15	2.83
Chins (times)	0.33	1.1	0.48	2.5	0.13	1.0	0.55	1.23	0.23
Squat jumps (times) ..	10.58	14.5	8.00	11.0	19.30	25.2	5.10	2.09	5.41

* From Cureton, T. K.: *The Research Quarterly*, 34:449, Dec., 1963.

system as a result of the supplements, and this may partly explain their persistence to remain in the program.

The within-group statistical analysis revealed that in the *mile run* and muscular endurance items (except chinning), all groups made significant standard score improvement (.05 level). Refer to Table VIII for raw score changes and the *t* values. In addition, the group mean standard score improvements for the composite of the five muscular endurance tests favored octacosanol (18.40 SS) to wheat germ oil (17.98 SS) and placeboes (14.36 SS).

The between-group analysis showed a trend of advantage for the octacosanol and wheat germ oil groups but the differences between groups were not significant. In the mile run, group A (octacosanol) improved 1.59 minutes, group C (WGO) improved 1.10 minutes, and group B (placeboes) improved 0.83 minutes. These differences between the A-B and C-B groups did not quite meet the .05 level of significance but did meet the .07 level. However, group A improved the mile run significantly more than group C ($t = 2.31$, p $<$ .05), indicating the superiority of octacosanol over wheat germ oil in this study (Table VII).

E. Cross-Country Running, Split-Team

Bernauer experimented with cross-country runners* at the University of Illinois, Urbana, Illinois, in 1959, by matching men on the team, one-half on WGO and one-half on nothing. No

* Exp. 18, 1958-59.

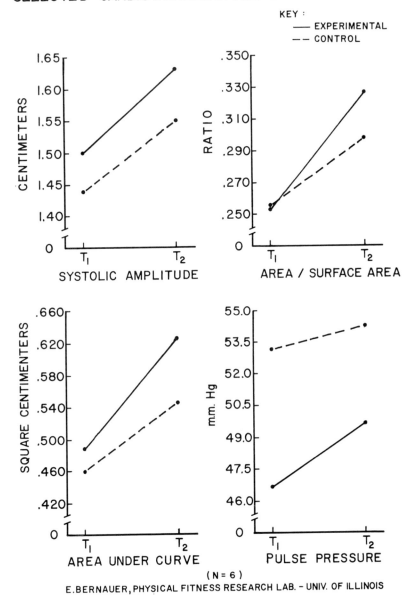

Figure 3. Effect of varsity track training upon selected cardiovascular and organic measures—A.

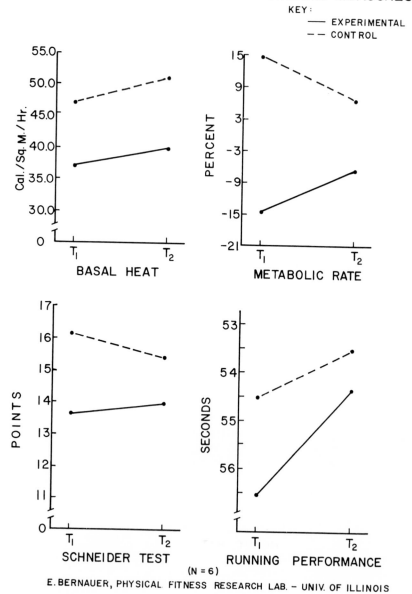

Figure 4. Effect of varsity track training upon selected cardiovascular and organic measures—B.

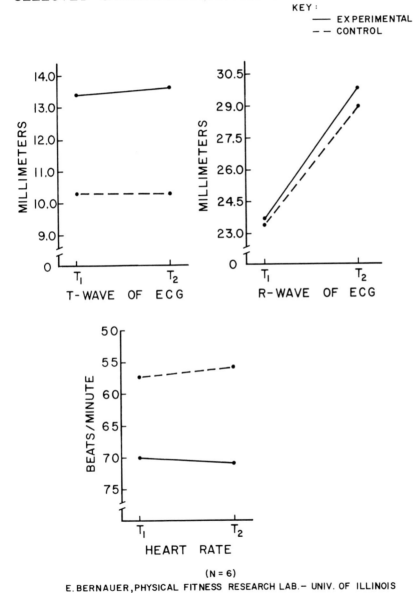

Figure 5. Effect of varsity track training upon selected cardiovascular and organic measures—C.

placeboes were used because they were not available. There were thirteen men on WGO, thirteen on nothing, and six controls who did not run or take any supplement. Advantage for the WGO group was shown in the 440-yard run time, which had also been used to match the groups, in the area/S.A. of the Cameron heartograph, and the BMR. The "t" for heartograph data was 0.254 to 0.327 sq. cm./sg. m. (t = 4.66); for per cent BMR-14% to 6.8% (t = 3.48); Schneider index 13.7 to 14.0 (t = 1.86) and the 440-yard run time 56.5 to 54.3 seconds (t = 1.69). None of these same measures were significant for the controls except BMR, 14.0% to 7.3% (t = 3.48) and area/S.A. for the heartograph, 0.256 to 0.298 (t = 1.92). While the advantages for WGO are small they seem to be present. No between group t's were computed. The T-wave of the ECG gained but the t's were equal at 2.18, and the same was true for heart rate which reduced with t's 2.06 for both groups. All other changes were insignificant.

II. RESULTS ON YOUNG BOYS

Four years of experimentation on young boys, 7-13 years of age, during 1955, 1956, 1957 and 1958 showed that a harder and longer program based upon *endurance*, more fully than upon games, improved the boys relatively more, and that boys matched in 600-yard (Cureton and Roby Exp.)[13] showed that octacosanol and WGO improved the boys over a control group taking cottonseed oil placeboes in capsules: octacosanol in refined corn oil (10.93 SS), WGO (8.72 SS), wheat germ cereal (4.58 SS) and taking cottonseed oil placeboes (3.02 SS)[13, 14, 15, 19] (Figs. 6 and 8). One year, when absolutely *fresh wheat germ* (cereal) from the Kretchmer Company was used, this gave the best results in 1958 in Hupe's experiment.[68] Wheat germ cereal, fresh from the factory, was shown to be significantly better than WGO (t = 2.06, 5% level); WGO was shown to be significantly better than the placeboes of lecithin oil (t = 2.78); and the octacosanol were better than the placeboes (t = 3.12); and wheat germ cereal was better than the placeboes (t = 3.30). The results on the brachial pulse wave were slightly different with the WGO group improving 28.03 SS in area, compared to 17.10 SS for wheat germ (fresh), octacosanol (9.74%) and lecithin oil placeboes (−19.9%). The

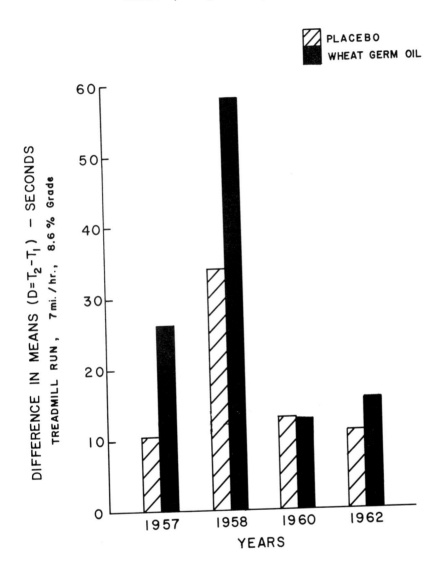

MEAN SCORES ON TREADMILL RUN TIME

UNIVERSITY OF ILLINOIS SPORTS FITNESS SCHOOL

Figure 6. Mean scores on treadmill run time, WGO versus placeboes (boys).

Treadmill all-out run gave the best improvement to the wheat germ group (14.69%), 8.76 for the placebo group, 7.89% for the WGO, and 5.70 for octacosanol. In 1961 and 1962 the capsules were washed down with a synthetic orange juice rather than milk, and this probably resulted in nullifying the effectiveness of the WGO (Fig. 9). Because of this ambiguity and lack of consistency, the work was continued in 1963 on sixty-four boys, matched on the 600-yard run in four groups, but with a change back to devitaminized lard placeboes. The WGO and octacosanol were shown to be significantly better than the placeboes ($D/S.E._{meas.} > 2.0$).

Figure 9 shows two experiments on young boys in 1961-1962 in which WGO did relatively poorly, this group improving 4.3 SS in the 600-yard run compared to 3.5 for the placebo group and 3.4 SS on the wheat germ cereal. This is the year when synthetic orange juice was used instead of milk to wash the capsules down.

In 1963 Cureton and Banister[19] completed this further experiment on young boys from the Sports Fitness School, using only one endurance program for thirty minutes of nonstop jogging and walking, followed by a free swim, and four groups were matched by the 600-yard run, using analysis of variance as a check. The supplementary feeding was fifteen of the six-minim capsules for seven days/week. By retest the 600-yard run was shown to have a reliability of 0.88, the runs were three days apart. The placebo group took the same number of devitaminized lard containing some vitamin E as in WGO. Using the $D/S.E._{meas.}$ ratio, the WGO effect on endurance was greater than the octacosanol ($T = 2.88$, one-tail significance at .05); WGO was better than the placebo group on devitaminized lard ($T = 2.88$, significance at .05, one tail). In this experiment all testing and other program interference was eliminated during the week of testing.

A report was made to the International Congress of Sport Sciences in Tokyo, 1964,* in which data from years 1957, 1958, 1960 and 1962 were combined to make seventy-four boys in all. Analysis of covariance was applied to these consolidated data by

---

* Cf. insert of article in *Sport Sciences* (Kato, Ed.), 1964.

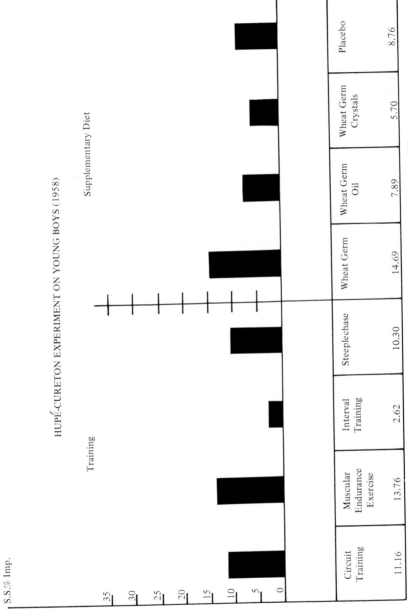

Figure 7. Hupé-Cureton experiment on young boys (1958).

IMPROVEMENTS IN 600 YARD RUN RESULTING FROM PHYSICAL TRAINING AND DIETARY SUPPLEMENTATION

BOYS, 6–13 YEARS OLD, 6 WEEKS TRAINING UNIVERSITY OF ILLINOIS SPORTS FITNESS SCHOOL

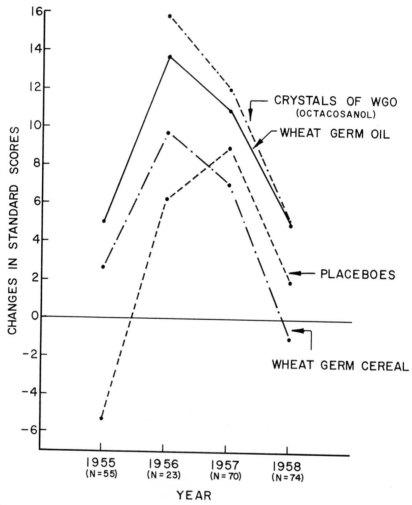

Figure 8. Improvements in 600-yard run resulting from physical training and dietary supplementation (WGO and OCTCNL versus placeboes).

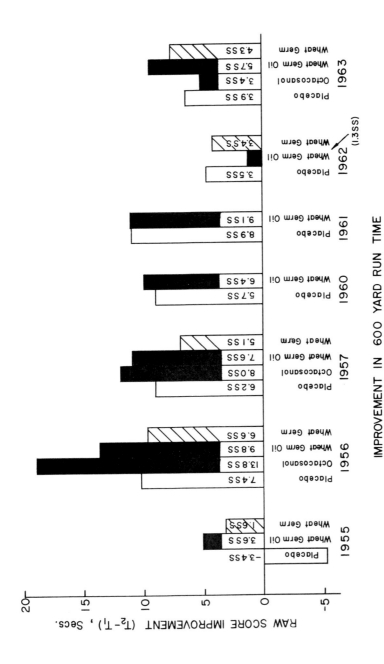

Figure 9. Improvement in 600-yard run time (boys, 1965-1963) WGO and OCTCNL and wheat germ versus placeboes.

B. Chen to give an F of 4.02, significantly better than .05 level between the WGO group and the control group.

During 1957 the improvement of the WGO group of boys over the devitaminized lard placebo group was 26.2 seconds versus 10.5 seconds; in 1958 the improvements were 58.17 seconds compared to 33.86 seconds for WGO over placeboes; during 1960 and 1961 the differences were insignificant; and in 1962 the advantage of WGO over placeboes was 15.59 versus 11.21 seconds improvement. It may be assumed that during the 1961 and 1962 years that there was some type of interference so that the usual gains did not come up between WGO and the placeboes, but real advantage is shown in the years 1955, 1956, 1957, 1960 and 1963. In 1960, 1961 and 1962 the use of synthetic orange juice may have interfered as in other years 2 per cent milk was used. The seven years of data are shown plotted in Figure 9.

Figure 6 shows the results of the supplementation (1955, 1956, 1957 and 1958) on matched groups of young boys attending the University of Illinois Sports Fitness School. The advantage of wheat germ oil, octacosanol, or wheat germ was shown in three of the four years. The endurance criteria used were 600-yard runs (unmotivated) and all-out treadmill runs (motivated); there were fewer loafers in the motivated runs, explaining the higher reliability in these treadmill runs. The results in terms of 600-yard comparisons were published in 1959 by Cureton and appear in Table IX. The average yearly improvement in standard scores clearly favors octacosanol (10.93 SS) over wheat germ oil (8.72 SS), wheat germ (4.58 SS) and placeboes (3.02 SS).

The results for the all-out treadmill run, combining the 1957 and 1958 data, have appeared in several publications. Refer to the experiment by Dempsey in Exp. 22, 1963 (cf. Figs. 6, 7, 8 and 9).

Test-retest reliability for the treadmill runs taken one week apart was 0.90. The statistical analysis shows a significant difference ($t = 2.45$, .05 level) in favor of wheat germ oil supplementary feeding over the placebo group.

Hupé[*] conducted a study in 1957 to determine the effects of

---

[*] Cf. Exp. No. 15, 1958 in Part Two.

different training methods (interval, circuit, steeplechase and muscular endurance training) and different dietary supplements (WGO, wheat germ, octacosanol and placeboes) on the physical fitness of boys participating in the University of Illinois Sports Fitness School. Within each training group there were four numerically comparable subgroups, each of which received one of the aforementioned dietary supplements; the converse was true for each of the four supplement groups. In this way, either training method or dietary supplement could be isolated as the experimental variable. The criterion for endurance was the all-out treadmill run at 7 mph, 8.6 per cent grade. Figure 7 shows that wheat germ emerged as the most advantageous supplement, improving the treadmill run by 14.69 standard scores. Standard score improvements at 8.76, 7.89 and 5.70 were observed for the placebo, WGO and octacosanol groups, respectively. Interestingly enough, "interval training" improved the treadmill run the least (cf. Table LXXV), which is consistent with the finding by Cureton that anaerobic metabolism (O_2 debt) contributes very little to the explained variance of the treadmill run. The "interval training" used consisted of short (200 yard) runs alternated with walks of about 400 yards, continued for about thirty minutes, four days per week.

Another experiment was conducted in 1963 by Banister and Cureton (Table VIII) again using the Sports Fitness School subjects. After being placed into four matched groups according to initial (T_1) 600-yard runs (having a reliability of 0.88), the boys were fed double-blind a dietary supplement depending on the group in which they were placed. The feeding was conducted seven days per week. Group I received fifteen six-minim capsules of devitaminized placeboes; group II received fifteen six-minim capsules of octacosanol; group III received fifteen six-minim capsules of whole, fresh wheat germ oil; and group IV received an ounce of wheat germ (uncamouflaged). The data and accompanying statistical analysis appear in Table VIII, and it is seen that in terms of mean raw score improvement, wheat germ oil emerged as significantly superior to octacosanol (9.50 seconds to 5.40 seconds, $t = 2.88$, significant at .05 level) or placeboes (9.50

TABLE VIII

COMPARATIVE IMPROVEMENTS IN THE 600-YARD RUN IN FOUR MATCHED GROUPS SUPPLEMENTED WITH WHEAT GERM, WHEAT GERM OIL, OCTACOSANOL VERSUS A PLACEBO

Exp. 20, Summer, 1963, Cureton and Banister
Standard Score Changes

I Control*			II Octacosanol†			III Wheat Germ Oil‡			IV Wheat Germ§		
T_1	T_2	d	T_1	T_2	d	T_1	T_2	d	T_1	T_2	d
41	57	16	55	84	29	42	56	14	38	35	– 3
56	64	8	59	66	7	56	73	17	52	69	17
77	79	2	79	78	– 1	82	84	2	78	87	9
53	65	12	69	71	2	60	69	9	59	66	7
64	70	6	59	62	3	56	71	15	59	69	10
71	82	11	62	61	– 1	71	81	10	60	68	8
64	69	– 5	63	65	2	71	71	0	70	74	4
45	42	– 3	59	63	4	47	61	14	54	70	16
74	81	7	73	74	1	73	75	2	71	69	– 2
67	71	4	66	68	2	72	75	3	54	59	5
60	54	– 6	53	56	3	61	71	10	43	44	1
41	36	– 5	71	79	8	43	62	19	43	58	15
67	77	10	71	76	5	73	81	8	73	71	– 2
70	77	7	74	71	– 3	78	82	4	69	77	8
55	63	8	35	43	8	41	38	– 3	63	64	1
78	80	2	63	67	4	75	74	– 1	76	76	0
Σ=983	1067	+98 / –14	1011	1084	78 / – 5	1001	1124	123	962	1056	101 / – 7
		84			73						94
M= 45.2	49.1	3.9	46.5	49.9	3.4	46.0	51.7	5.7	44.3	49.6	4.3
Means of RS=143.06	136.50	– 6.56	141.60	136.20	– 5.40	143.80	134.20	– 9.50	138.95	131.20	– 7.75
(secs.)											

* 15 capsules, 6 minims of devitaminized lard with ½ pint milk
† 15 capsules, 6 minims of VioBin octacosanol with ½ pint milk
‡ 15 capsules, 6 minims of VioBin whole wheat germ oil with ½ pint milk
§ 1 ounce Kretschmer's wheat germ, freshly opened, with ½ pint milk

Errors of Measurement (by retest)

$$S.E._{diff.} = \sqrt{\frac{d^2}{N(N-1)}}$$

$S.E._{diff.} = 1.09$ seconds

Significance (by ratio of D to SE$_d$)

	$D = T_1 - T_2$		r_{11} for 600 yard
	$N = 64$		Run $= 0.88$
	D	$S.E._{diff.}$	$D/S.E._{diff.}$
Wheat germ oil versus octacosanol (in favor of wheat germ oil)	4.1	1.42	2.88
Wheat germ oil versus control placeboes (on devitaminized lard)	2.94	1.37	2.14
Octacosanol versus control	-1.16	1.30	-0.79
Wheat germ versus octacosanol (in favor of wheat germ)	2.35	1.42	1.81
Wheat germ versus wheat germ oil (in favor of wheat germ oil)	-1.75	1.32	-1.29

TABLE IX

Year (n)	N	Group A (Placeboes) Greens	Group B (Wheat Germ Cereal) Reds	Group C (Wheat Germ Oil) Whites	Group D (Crystals of WGO) Blues
1955	55	− 5.2 (17)	2.6 (20)	5.1 (18)	did not use
1956	23	6.3 (6)	9.7 (5)	13.8 (6)	15.8 (6)
1957	70	9.0 (18)	7.0 (19)	11.0 (16)	12.0 (17)
1958	74	2.0 (19)	− 1.0 (18)	5.0 (18)	5.0 (19)
Total Improve. (secs.) .	222	12.0	18.3	34.9	32.8
Average Yearly Improve (secs.) .		3.02	4.58	8.72	10.93

Improvements in 600-yard run resulting from physical training and dietary supplementation in matched groups of young boys (6-13 years) in U. of Illinois Sports Fitness School. (Changes in standard scores over six weeks training, combined with basic physical education instruction.)

seconds to 6.56 seconds, $t = 2.14$, significant at the .05 level). Wheat germ exhibited an advantage over octacosanol (7.75 seconds to 5.40 seconds) or placeboes (7.75 seconds to 6.56 seconds), but neither of these differences was statistically significant at the 1 per cent level or 5 per cent level but did achieve the 10 per cent level.

PROCEEDINGS OF INTERNATIONAL CONGRESS OF SPORT SCIENCES, 1964

Edited by Kitsuo Kato[*]

Recent Findings from Dietary Supplement Studies in Relationship to the Possibility for Improving Athletic and Cardiovascular Performance

Continued research on the effects of wheat germ and its derivatives, wheat germ oil and octacosanol, *confirm earlier results*

---

[*] Proceedings committee: Shinshiro Ebashi, Michio Ikai, Toshihiro Ishiko, Kitsuo Kato, Etsuo Kurimoto, Yoshio Kuroda, Torahiko Miyahata, Reiji Natori, Mitsugu Onon and Toshio Sakai.

TABLE X

CRITERION OF THE ALL-OUT TREADMILL RUN (7 mi/hr, 8.6% Grade)

Comparison of Two Different Years of Data on Middle-Aged Men

Program of Calisthenics Plus Swimming (Five Days Per Week, One hour Per Day)

Cureton-Pohndorf Experiment

Groups	N	Age (Ave.)	T_1 (Raw Score)	(SS)	T_2 (Raw Score)	(SS)	D (Raw Score)	D (SS)
1953								
A (Exercise + WGO)	8	41.4	3.44	(51.4)	5.14	(69.4)	1.70	18.0
B (Exercise + Placeboes)	8	36.5	3.34	(50.5)	4.06	(58.0)	0.72	7.5
C (Inactive + WGO)	5	36.2	1.90	(45.0)	2.00	(47.6)	0.10	2.6
D (Inactive + Placeboes)	5	32.0	2.05	(47.4)	2.05	(48.4)	1.0	0
1954								
A (Exercise + WGO)	8	35.0	2.41	(46.6)	2.88	(54.0)	0.57	7.4
E (Exercise + Wheat Germ)	8	39.9	1.98	(41.9)	2.06	(42.8)	0.08	0.9
B (Exercise + Placeboes)	9	36.1	2.51	(52.9)	2.65	(55.3)	0.14	2.4
C (Inactive + WGO)	7	32.0	1.73	(38.1)	1.55	(34.7)	-0.18	-3.4
F (Inactive on Wheat Germ)	4	33.5	1.81	(39.2)	1.73	(38.0)	-0.08	-1.2
D (Inactive + Placeboes)	3	29.3	1.70	(40.7)	1.31	(32.4)	-0.39	-8.3

Continued—Group and Individual Statistical Significance

Groups	Group Statistical Significance (t)	Number Gained (Significant)	Number Gained (+ Trend)	Number Lost	Number No Gain
1953					
A (Exercise + WGO)	8.71	+ 4	+ 3	- 1	0
B (Exercise + Placeboes)	3.63	+ 3	+ 2	- 2	1
C (Inactive + WGO)	1.00	0	+ 4	- 1	0
D (Inactive + Placeboes)	0	0	+ 4	- 1	0
		7	12	- 5	1
1954					
A (Exercise + WGO)	3.57	+ 2	+ 5	0	1
E (Exercise + Wheat Germ)	0.42	0	+ 5	- 2	1
B (Exercise + Placeboes)	1.26	+ 1	+ 5	- 3	0
C (Inactive + WGO)	1.55	0	+ 2	- 5	0
F (Inactive on Wheat Germ)	0.43	0	0	- 3	1
D (Inactive + Placeboes)	2.47	0	+ 1	- 2	0

Individual Reliability = $\dfrac{D}{\sqrt{2}\ s}$

t for Groups = $\dfrac{\Sigma X - \Sigma Y}{\sqrt{2N}\ s}$

S = 4.13 (SS)

showing that these dietary supplements are normal foods which aid physical endurance and reaction time, and also affect the brachial pulse wave, the T-wave of the precordial leads of the ECG and stroke volume of the heart. By combining data taken on boys in the summers of 1957 and 1958, involving two groups of boys 8–12 years of age, six and seven in each group, respectively, thirteen boys in all, who were given the same sports and physical fitness program for eight weeks, were split by matched group 600-yard run method, and contrasted by one group taking wheat germ oil, a second group taking placeboes of lecithin oil (the placebo in 1957 and 1958). The results showed advantage for the experimental dietary supplements over the placebo group as follows:

		Average Gain
WGO versus placeboes of lecithin oil	t = 2.45	10.32 SS
Octacosanol versus placeboes of lecithin oil	t = 1.47	6.19 SS
Wheat germ versus placeboes of lecithin oil	t = 1.45	4.62 SS
Placebo group lost		0.22 SS

These results were further checked by analysis of covariance by combining four years of work, using seventy-four boys in all, giving significant F of 4.02, better than the 0.05 level. Reliability of the all-out treadmill run was 0.90 based upon retests, one week apart. For score, the best of two scores was used after two periods of preliminary practice.

Within the four years the WGO groups had gains distinctly greater than the placebo groups during 1957 (26.2 seconds versus 10.5 seconds), during 1958 (58.17 seconds versus 33.86 seconds), during 1960 an insignificant difference* and during 1962 (15.59 versus 11.21 seconds).

Furthermore, in the summer of 1963 Cureton and Banister ran another experiment on sixty-four boys under fourteen years of age, matched in four groups by the 600-yard run. The experimental group was fed daily for six weeks, seven days per week, fifteen capsules of the 6 minim size of VioBin whole, fresh capsu-

---

* During 1960 the main experiment was on the BCG comparison, given in the Ph.D. thesis by Cedric W. Dempsey, *A Ballistocardiographic Investigation of Cardiac Responses of Boys to Physical Training and Wheat Germ Oil*, University of Illinois, 1963, pp. 196. (Significant results were found in the basal pulse rate and IJ/t wave of the BCG$_v$.)

lated oil; whereas, one other group took 1 ounce of wheat germ, and two other groups were fed octacosanol in capsules (a derivative of WGO) and also the last group similar capsules of devitaminized lard. Performance tests and retests were given in the first and eighth week ($S.E._{meas.}=1.09$ seconds), with double-blind feeding of the capsules (except for wheat germ). The best of two 600-yard runs for time was allowed as the score each time. All boys had essentially the same exercise program of three hours of sports and endurance work per day. Results again gave the advantage to WGO over octacosanol ($D/SE_d=2.88$); WGO over the control placeboes of devitaminized lard* ($D/SE_d=2.14$); wheat germ versus control ($D/SE_d=1.81$); WGO versus wheat germ ($D/SE_d=1.29$); and wheat germ versus octacosanol ($D/SE_d=1.81$) in favor of wheat germ.

Also in the Ph.D. thesis by Dempsey (sponsored by Cureton) in the 1960 experiment on fifty-six boys, twenty-eight in each of two matched groups on the 600-yard run, the WGO experimental group was compared with the control group on devitaminized lard placeboes, over six weeks of feeding. The amount of WGO fed was ten capsules of the 6-minim size, four days per week. The work was the same for all boys over this period, three hours of sports and interval training type running (30 minutes, four days per week). Significant increase in the heartograph amplitude occurred in both of the exercised groups, whereas, a third unexercised control group did not improve significantly. The WGO group reduced the lying basal pulse rate 10–17 beats, compared to 5.82 beats on placeboes; whereas, an increase of 1.94 beats was found in the third control group. The WGO group averaged 60 seconds improvement in all-out treadmill running time, compared to 55 seconds for the lard placebo group and 25 seconds for the third control group. The advantage for the WGO group was statistically significant. The BCG test (I+J amplitude/time of I+J) also produced a significant difference in favor of the WGO over the matched exercise control group.

Dempsey's experiment (Exp. 22, 1963) compared the effects

---

* Vitamin E added to lard to equate to that in WGO; the difference then is not due to vitamin E.

of wheat germ oil (60 minims daily) versus a lard placebo (60 minims daily) on the ventricular dynamics and all-out treadmill run time in two unmatched groups of boys attending the Sports Fitness School. Analysis of covariance revealed no significant difference between groups in treadmill run time, although the wheat germ oil improved sixty seconds in running time to fifty-five seconds for the placebo group.

PRE-EJECTION INTERVAL STUDY

Linda Cundiff [*]

The boys available in the Sports Fitness School of the University of Illinois were used. These groups contained seventeen, nineteen and sixteen boys respectively, and were satisfactorily matched at T_1 on the 600-yard run and the matching proved, and with all three groups taking the full program as nearly alike as possible. They were then retested 7-8 weeks later on the pre-ejection intervals. The results are shown on Table XXXIII. By shortening relatively less in the tension period (TP) the WG (0.70 seconds) and WGO (0.07 seconds) groups appeared to show less induced stress than the P group (0.13 seconds). The inotropic (vertical energy) effect at five minutes of recovery favored a gain of 0.25 cm for the WGO group, compared to losses, particularly due to greater relative fatigue for the WG group (-0.038 seconds) and (-0.083 seconds) for P group. The pulse wave transmission time was also shortened, but there were no significant changes for any of the three groups in TP at five minutes of recovery (Figs. 66 and 67).

A comparison of the three groups (N's = 16, 19 and 19, respectively), matched by a 600-yard run, showed that all three groups shortened the pre-ejection interval of the left ventricle (TP), as in Figures 66 and 67, indicating that all were stressed by the program, thus the shortening of the Q of the ECG to G_a (G of the acceleration record, supersensitive to the beginning of the left ventricular contraction). The pulse wave transmission time was also lengthened from G_a to the beginning of the bra-

---

[*] Exp. 25, 1965-66.

chial pulse wave, this time divided into the distance from the apex of the heartbeat to the midpoint of the cuff on the arm (thus D/t = velocity). The training *lengthened* the cycle time while shortening the TP and time of the pulse wave from the apex to the brachial cuff.

The R to R' cycle time was taken from the ECG record. While the differences from T_1 to T_2 were slight, the wheat germ oil, wheat germ and placebo groups all showed stress in terms of the TP shortening and also quickening of the transmission time of the pulse wave. The WGO group was shortened least, compared to the WG and placebo groups. This, we interpret as indicating that there was a trend for the WGO to fortify the boys against the stress of the program, the WG rating next and the placebo group least fortified.

The systolic amplitude of the brachial pulse wave, the vertical inotropic (energy) dimension, was increased in the WGO group and, whereas the WG and placebo groups were diminished (there was a decrease of amplitude and energy). The increased amplitude correlated with a slight advantage in endurance in the WGO-fed group. This difference was statistically significant for the WGO group over the other two groups. The three groups (wheat germ oil, wheat germ and placebo) were fed double-blind according to the following scheme:

> Wheat germ oil — 90 minims four days per week
> Placeboes — 90 minims four days per week
> Wheat germ — 1 ounce four days per week

Analysis of the data in terms of standard score improvements in the 600-yard run gave an advantage to wheat germ oil (18 SS) over placeboes (14 SS) and wheat germ (8 SS). This experiment is further explained in Chapter III as the principal criterion was energy of the heart stroke from electronically picked-up pulse waves on multi-channel tape records in the cardiovascular laboratory.

Oxygen Intake and Debt Experiments

It was shown in the Experiment No. 19, 1960, by Brown, that the maximal oxygen intake in an all-out treadmill run could be improved as an average by the physical training program of the

Sports Fitness School, as operated at the University of Illinois, as part of the summer school for eight weeks. This program produced a temporary fatigue which caused some boys not to improve, and the heavyweight boys failed to improve. The errors in this work were relatively large, as discussed in the chapter on this work (Chap. IV). Some boys improved on WGO and some did not, compared to the placebo group, and also in comparison with case to case matched controls. No final conclusion could be reached except that it appeared that the type of testing was too crude to permit careful comparisons, there being large errors due to variable motivation and variable induced efficiency.

III. FINDINGS ON MIDDLE-AGED MEN

A. Endurance and Brachial Pulse Wave (Heartograph)

The 1953-54 experiment on middle-aged men, published in 1955, was surprising (Cureton-Pohndorf study) as eight experimental subjects taking WGO (20 of the 3-minim capsules) improved more than eight men who were matched at the start with the WGO group by all-out runs on the treadmill, seven miles per hour, 8.6 per cent grade. The exercise work was the same for six weeks in the pool, and on the deck, fifty minutes of continuous work, which was pretty hard, five days per week (Figs. 63-A and 63-B). Figure 63-A shows the advantage in the all-out treadmill run time and Figure 63-B shows the comparable advantage on the area of the brachial pulse wave, a naive test which has been shown in various studies to correlate well with the all-out treadmill run time and with endurance in swimming. The experiment was repeated the next year with similar results. (Cf. Part Two for the published write-up of this experiment.)

In the article published by Cureton and Pohndorf, *Res. Quart.,* Influence of Wheat Germ Oil as a Dietary Supplement in a Program of Conditioning Exercises with Middle-Aged Men, 26:391-407, Dec., 1955 and Cureton's report to the American Physiological Society, *Amer. J. Physiol.,* 199:628, Dec., 1954, the announcement was made of the discovery of the potency of WGO to improve human endurance. It was not known at that time if the effect was due to vitamin E or not, and the report regarding

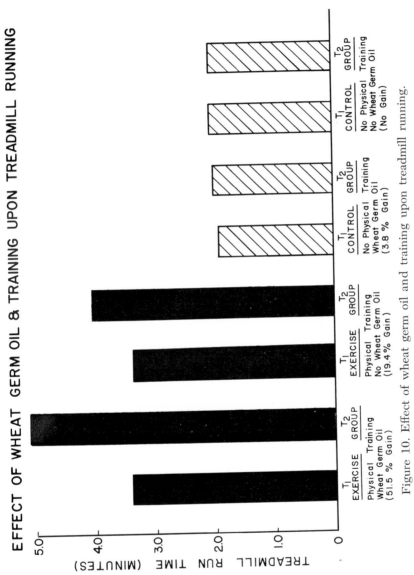

Figure 10. Effect of wheat germ oil and training upon treadmill running.

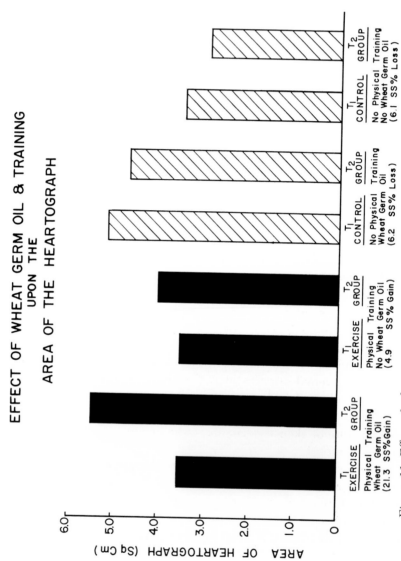

Figure 11. Effect of wheat germ oil and training upon the area of the heartograph.

physiology carried the title, The Effect of Wheat Germ Oil and Vitamin E on Normal Human Subjects in Physical Training Programs. Since this time we have concluded that it is due to octacosanol.

It is important to notice, in the data for these studies in 1953 and 1954 that the inactive subjects gained little, as shown on Figures 63-A and 63-B, whereas, the subjects on the active program who took WGO improved more than the WGO supplemented group. It is also seen that the experimental group taking WGO gained more than the placebo active group and the inactive group taking WGO combined. This was true for both of these years. This was also the major staff experiment of these two years, and they were done with care. Of course, few people believed all of what was reported, but the studies were applauded by the American Physiological Society at the University of Wisconsin, when they were reported by the author. Rather prominent notices appeared in the Associated Press and in the Champaign-Urbana papers. However, the skeptics were to be found on every hand. If the gains were only in the all-out treadmill run time, that would have been something, but the gains were just as strong in the brachial pulse wave (sphygmogram), so it was decided to continue the studies with other types of cardiovascular tests, and other kinds of subjects. The all-out treadmill run is conceivably affected by willpower, although this is probably evened out in matched groups; but the heartograph test is not affected by willpower. Getting the results clearly in both led us to believe that the influence of WGO was absolutely there, in spite of skeptics. The data are shown in Table X and in Figures 10 and 11.

Another supportive study favoring wheat germ oil or octacosanol was produced by the author (Exp. No. 21, Part Two) on the comparative effects of differential dietary supplementation on three matched groups (10 per group) of United States Navy Underwater Swimming School trainees participating in an intensive six-week physical training program at Key West, Florida, 1956. The entire squadron was tested before T_1 and after T_2, the training being standardized, six days per week, five to six hours per day, on: 17 physique tests, 13 cardiovascular tests and 13 motor fitness tests. The matching was done on the basis of the mean standard score on five muscular endurance tests: a) squat jumps; b) push-ups; c) sitting tucks; d) pull-ups; and e) mile run. The daily supplements were fed in terms of ten capsules (6-minims each); group A received octacosanol, group B received placeboes and group C received whole, fresh wheat germ oil which had been kept at a freezing temperature until used. All capsules were shipped to the base in dry ice and were kept refrigerated to prevent spoilage. Administration was by the medical doctor who instructed petty officers at the daily muster roll. This experiment was published by *Res. Quart.*, 34:440-453, Dec., 1963.

B. Effects on Basal Metabolic Rate

Experiments with middle-aged men in 1953 and 1954 (published in 1955) showed that there were statistically insignificant differences in BMR due to WGO but some positive effect was due to the exercise.

Changes in BMR

Group A: 8 middle-aged men, 6 weeks, on endurance exercise and cottonseed oil placeboes .... 10.6 SS

Group B: 5 middle-aged men, ibid., with WGO supplement, 10 × 6 minim capsules/day .... 2.0 SS
(shows oxygen conserving effect)

Group C: 4 middle-aged men, inactive but taking WGO as controls .... 3.25 SS

Group D: 2 controls, inactive on placeboes .... −5.0 SS

The *least* change was in the WGO group, which is interpreted as "holding the homeostatic state best in the face of stress." This interpretation suggests that the WGO helped the subjects to bear the stress.

C. Effects on Total Body Reaction Time

Gary A. Johnson completed a study* in 1966 on the effects of WGO on total body reaction time using nine volunteer subjects thirty to forty years of age from the University of Illinois Adult Fitness Program. The subjects followed the Cureton Progressive Exercise Program outlined in *Physical Fitness and Dynamic Health* (New York, Dial Press, 1965). The subjects were given preliminary testing for six weeks to familiarize them with the

---

* Experiment 26, Part Two.

visual, auditory and combined tests, and to establish the S.E.$_{meas.}$
This continued until the subjects had plateaued, the learning effects finished. The subjects were then matched into two groups with group means within .003 seconds of each other, equal to 1 S.E., and were considered matched closely enough. One group was given WGO capsules, 10 per day, in a double-blind experiment. The testing continued for sixteen weeks as a whole. Significance of the differences was tested by $t = D/\sqrt{2N} \times s$. The matched group experiment was terminated at the end of the sixth week and by groups using nonparametric statistics there was no advantage of one group over the other, but by computation using the formula given above for individual cases, three of the four subjects taking WGO made statistically significant improvements; the fourth subject taking WGO was very nearly made a statistical significant change; two of the control subjects failed to make a significant change, and four made changes comparable to the WGO group. The results indicated some advantage for the subjects taking WGO.

Chris Milesis, *et al.* carried out an experiment[*] in 1969 with the boys in the Sports Fitness School at the University of Illinois, 7-13 years of age, respectively. Thirty boys were matched into three groups and were tested at the beginning and at the end of the eight-week experiment on the total body reaction time. A random block design was used with the feeding of the WGO supplements on four days per week under close supervision. The changes were greater for the experimental group taking WGO after the fifth week. The S.E.$_{mean}$ was 4.70 ms.

Group A (exercised group taking WGO) raised the BMR 1.75 per cent compared to group B (exercised group taking placeboes) raising the BMR +10.62 per cent. Inactive controls raised the BMR 3.26 per cent and group D (professional men as controls taking placeboes lowered the BMR −4.82%). The effect of WGO seems to be depressive to the use of oxygen in the basal state. This effect is significant at the .10 level, a difference of 8.87 per cent. The sedentary professional group dropped in BMR after going out of training, whereas the exercised middle-aged

---

[*] Experiment 31, Part Two.

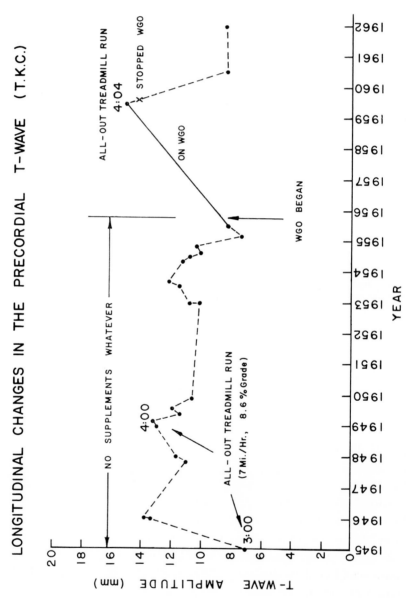

Figure 12. Longitudinal changes in the precordial T-wave (T.K.C., 1945-1962).

group raised the BMR 8.10 per cent compared to the professional group out of training. The exercised group taking placeboes had the greatest actual gain of 15.44 per cent (significant at the .05 level), this difference being due to the exercise effect. The influence of WGO to depress the rise in BMR was significant at the .20 level (cf. Exp. 31, Part Two).

Jacques Sampson (Part Two, Exp. 28) completed a follow-up study on the effect of WGO on the basal metabolic rate and selected cardiovascular measures, using middle-aged men as subjects. The group of twenty-four men were divided into two groups: one, the experimental group, taking wheat germ oil, and the other taking devitaminized lard placeboes. The groups were compared with a third group taking no supplementation but which went through the training exercises. The group taking WGO improved more than the other two groups in the R-wave of the ECG (highest precordial wave) and held the BMR more stable (less change in the face of the stress of the program). The precordial T-wave changes also favored the WGO group, the CR ratio being 1.612 for the WGO versus the placebo group; as compared with 10.43 for the placebo group versus the group on exercise but no supplementation, showing that the placeboes had an effect. The $I_{ncceleration}$ wave of the direct body albeit BCG improved 3.2 mm in the WGO group compared to the placebo group improving 0.2 mm and the group on no supplementation improving 0.6 mm. The CR ratio for the WGO group versus the placebo group was 26.25, indicating that the heart force improved the most and the most reliably in the WGO group.

D. Influence Upon Fat-Folds

Storm (Exp. 7) conducted a study in 1952 to see if feeding WGO to middle-aged men would increase their fat or weight. Three groups of men, eight in each group were used, matched in weight. One group was fed WGO, twenty capsules of the 3-minim size, five days per week. One group was fed an equivalent feeding of cottonseed oil placeboes; and the third took no capsules or exercise. The WGO group showed an insignificant group-

NORMAL, TRAINED ON WGO, DETRAINED AND RETRAINED SPHYGMOGRAMS
OF SUBJECT S.L.T., 1953-1956

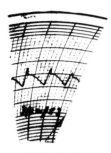

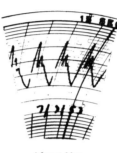

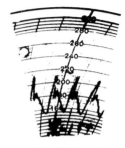

"Untrained"
at
START OF TRAINING

After 4 Mos.
of Fairly Hard
Physical Training
on WGO, daily
(10 x 3 minims)

After 10 Mos. of
Physical Training,
Calisthenics and Swimming,
on Irregular WGO
(10 x 3 minims)

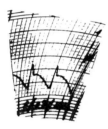

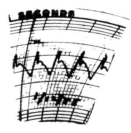

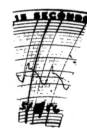

DETRAINED
(Off of WGO and
only irregular
Exercise)

IN TRAINING AGAIN
(on Lard Placeboes)

AFTER 4 MOS. TRAINING
(on Lard Placeboes)

change in weight, averaging ± 2.0 lb. On the exercise program, five days per week, the WGO group lost fat by caliper measurements from 140 mm to 124 mm (6 fat-folds, Cureton method). The group on cottonseed oil changed insignificantly, from 137 to 138 mm on the same measurements over the twelve weeks in the experiment. The control group on no exercise or capsules lost from 144 mm to 125 mm. The WGO group closely paralleled the control group.

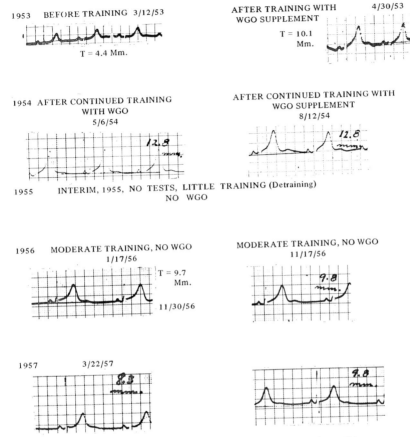

Figure 13-A. ECG training record of SLT, 1953-1957.

IV. RESULTS OF THE INDIVIDUAL LONGITUDINAL CASE STUDIES

Over a span of eighteen years, eleven of these with no supplements of any kind, Cureton reached a peak in his precordial T-wave after adding ten capsules of WGO at the end of his workouts, and also improved his all-out treadmill run slightly (Exp. 32).

In Exp. 33, subject S.T. markedly improved his amplitude of the heartograph (HGF), both systolic and diastolic aspects, and these "sluffed off" to lower levels after giving up the taking of

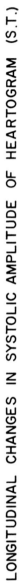
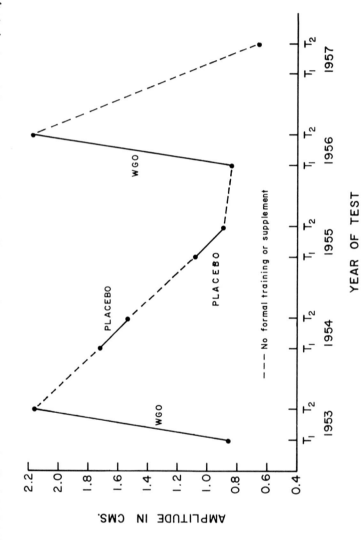

Figure 13-B. Longitudinal changes in diastolic amplitude of heartogram (S.T.).

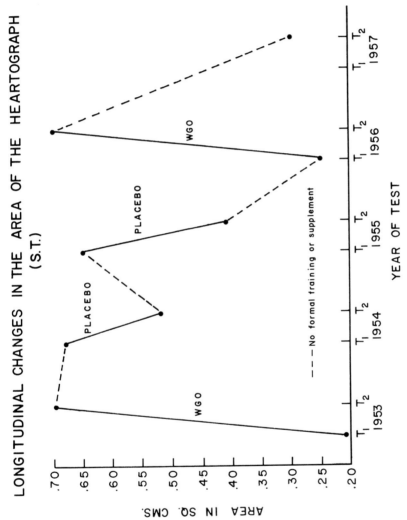

Figure 13-C. Longitudinal changes in the area of the heartograph (S.T.).

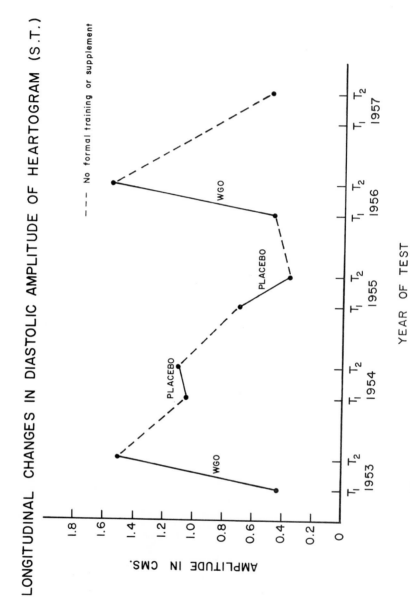

Figure 13-D. Longitudinal changes in systolic amplitude of heartogram (S.T.).

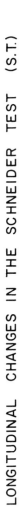
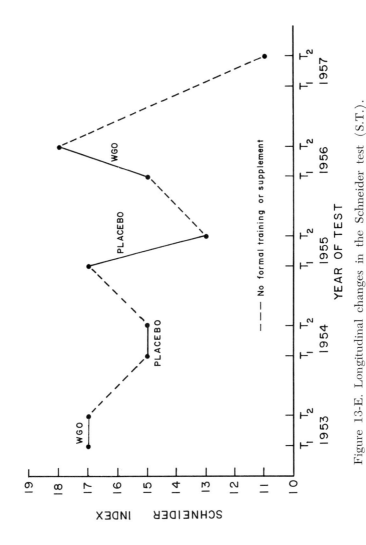

Figure 13-E. Longitudinal changes in the Schneider test (S.T.).

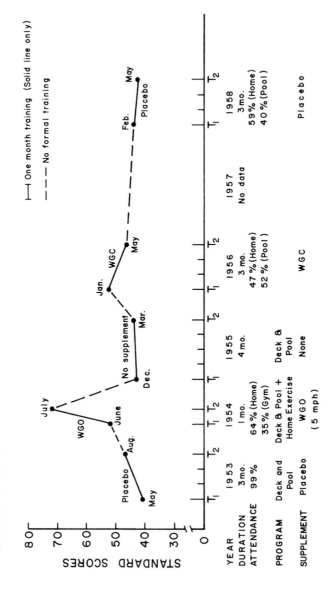

Figure 14-A. Longitudinal changes in all-out treadmill run time (D.H.).

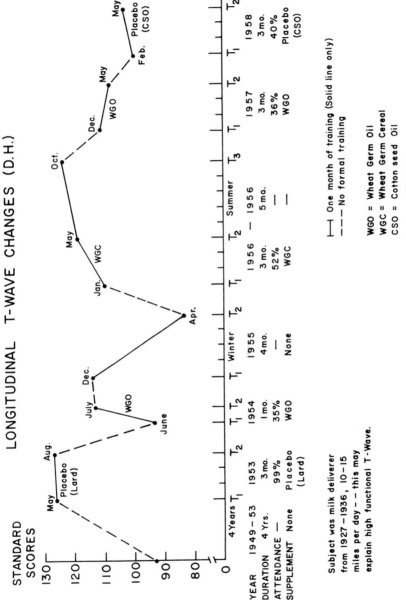

Figure 14-B. Longitudinal T-wave changes (D.H.).

WGO, or switching to placeboes. Figure 13-A shows both the amplitude of the precordial T-wave and the amplitude of the brachial pulse wave (systolic) in the different phases of Exp. 33 on S. L. T. (Tuckey), extended over two years. With the daily exercise, five days per week, continued at the same intensity level, using a mixture of calisthenics followed by swimming, the amplitudes of both tests deteriorated when WGO was discontinued. His M.D. reported a marked improvement in this subject. It is also seen that the taking of daily doses of WGO in 1953 and 1956 caused marked changes in the diastolic amplitude of the heartograph compared to placeboes, with exercise being continued on about the same level. The graphs of the area and systolic amplitude of the brachial pulse wave also show the positive effects of WGO compared to placeboes taken while the same program of exercise was being continued. The Schneider index also showed similar effects with the WGO causing marked improvements and the placeboes causing a relative deterioration (cf. Figs. 13-A, 13-B, 13-C, 13-D and 13-E for Exp. 33 on S.L.T.).

Subject D. H. (Hubbard) shows two graphs wherein the WGO made the sharpest and greatest improvements compared to the placeboes, with exercise being continued, 3-5 times per week under our supervision. Both the T-wave of the ECG (Fig. 14-A for Exp. 34) and (Fig. 14-B for Exp. 34)

The Individual Longitudinal Case Studies, Graphs

Additional evidence is shown in the case of Individual Experiments (cf. Part Two).

The subjects improved relatively more on WGO than on placeboes, nothing was displayed on wheat germ. It is convincing to see the WGO increase the gains more than once in a series on a given subject, while all subjects were on the adult exercise program as in *Physical Fitness and Dynamic Health*, or on a mixed calisthenics plus swimming program.

In this case it is best to look at the graphs, each in turn to see how much the WGO effect is compared to that of the placeboes or nothing at all, or the wheat germ effect.

EXPERIMENT NO. 32

Stage I

The ECG T-Waves of T.K.C. (Highest Precordial T-Wave)
Over Sixteen Years

Eighteen years of records on T.K.C. were available in the files of the Physical Fitness Research Laboratory of the University of Illinois, 1945 to 1950. During this period *no vitamins or supplements were taken at any time.* In 1945 the only ECG available gave a highest precordial T-wave of 6.6 mm in amplitude (Table XI) during a period when the hardest training was being done, the subject running a four-mile steeplechase almost daily, with intermittent bouts of hard running on the motor driven treadmill, 8.6 per cent grade, seven and ten miles per hour. The training was interrupted by a fall, an accident in which five ribs were broken close to the spine. This was at the end of a summer when the work was very hard, the weather extremely hot, and possibly the subject was over-working and felt tired.

Stage II

The regular and continuous physical training was interrupted by the fall, necessitating six months rest and moderate overfeeding in which the weight rose from 178 to 192. In the fall of 1946, a little over a year after the accident, with regular moderate exercise, walking and swimming, the T-wave rose to 13.3 and 13.8 mm during this period with *no vitamins or WGO supplements* of any kind. In this rest period, with regular, moderate exercise, the nutritive state of the body and heart muscle seemed to rise. The subject felt good.

Stage III

During 1946-48 the exercise was kept up regularly, with some harder exercise introduced. When the hardest training in this period was on, the T-wave was 11.0 and 11.7 in two tests taken in March of 1948, a peak for this period with *no supplements of any kind.* The T-wave fell to 8.1 mm 5 minutes after an all-out tread-

TABLE XI

RECORDS OF T.K.C. (Birthday Aug. 4, 1901)

Date	Age (Yrs.)	Maximum O₂ Intake (L./Min.)	Weight (lb.)	S.A. (M²)	R-Wave (Highest Precordial) (mm.)	T	Heart Rate (B./Min.)	Area Hgm. (Cm.²)	Sys. Amp. Hgm. (Cms.)	Ob. Ang. (Deg.)	TTM Run (Min. and Sec.)
In hardest training, no supplements											
5/8/45	44		180	1.94	16.0	6.6	52	0.85	1.83	19	6:42
Forced into inactivity by a fall, breaking five ribs—bandaged up for three months and refrained from all physical activity (Aug. 1, 1945 to Feb. 1, 1946)											
Relatively out of training at start of reconditioning experiment (no supplements)											
2/2/46	46				26	13.3					
10/10/46			186	1.98	26.8	13.8	72	0.37	1.35	23	
3/9/48	48		192	1.99		11.3	54	0.40	1.08	23	
3/24/48 .... 48 (After TM Run 4'7"/hr.)					14.6 to 7.0	11.7 / 8.1					
At the end of build-up training lasting through the summer of 1948 and into the fall of 1948 and to Jan., 1949 (no supplements)											
1/18/49		3.23 L./min.			16.2 / 32.5	12.9 / 13.1	48	0.39	1.71	19	
**											
Reduced training (no supplements)											
7/22/49					26.1	11.0		0.39	1.69	19	
In moderate training (no training)											
8/8/50			194		12.9	11.8		0.65	1.72	16	
Out of training											
6/14/52	50		186		20.1 / 21.7	10.6 / 10.1	52	0.63	1.54 / 2.59	19.5 / 17.0	3:28
2/28/53											
Experiment on Use of Wheat Germ Oil:											
5/12/53					30.6 / 29.6	10.9 / 11.6 / 12.2		0.38 / 0.87	1.24 / 2.38	19.0 / 19.0	3:28 / 4:03
7/30/53											
8/4/53 .... (after 6 weeks more on WGO)											

Then on placeboes:

Date							
6/25/54		27.9	11.3	0.50	1.46	22	4:01
7/2/54 52		27.2	10.9				3:57
8/5/54 53		21.7	10.1				
8/16/54		22.2	10.4	0.60	1.17	22	
11/13/54		13.4	7.5	0.56	1.38	19.5	
1/17/55 .... on wheat germ		15.3	8.4	0.43	1.18	24.0	4:00
5/9/55 .... on wheat germ		34.3	15.0	0.59	1.45	22	5:02
5/25/55 .... on wheat germ		9.0	6.9	0.57	1.51	20	
6/3/55 .... on WGO		22.9	14.5		1.89		
7/10/59 .... 15' after all-out TM run				0.61	1.50	21	4:04
7/11/59 .... one day after run					1.93		

mill run at 7 miles/hour, 8.6 per cent grade, time 4 minutes-seconds in this run.

Stage IV

Training in the summer of 1948 with swimming a mile per day and 4-5 miles on Saturday and Sunday in the summer, the T-wave was in January of 1949 12.9 and 13.1 mm in two tests, and a month later was 11.0, with the subject feeling fine. His "peak" O_2 intake in an all-out treadmill run was *net* 3.23 L/min (38.3 cc/min/kg). During a relative lay-off period of two months during May and June the T-wave was 11.0 mm with *no supplements of any kind.*

Stage V

During 1949 and 1950 the T-wave was 11.0, 11.8 and 10.6 mm *with no supplements of any kind.* No attempt was made to diet. Physical training was moderate and continuous. Weight was 196 lb.

Stage VI

The subject decided to add *wheat germ cereal* to his diet, taking this along with a class of middle-aged men in 1953, and at the start of the swimming experiment, the T-wave was 10.1 mm $\pm$ 0.44 mm. In the several months of this swimming experiment the T-wave increased from 10.1 to 10.9 mm on 5/12/53, to 11.6 on 7/30/53 and 12.2 mm on 8/4/53. The difference was from 10.1 to 12.2 equal to 2.1 mm, which was a gain of 4.77 times the S.E.$_{\text{meas.}}$

Stage VII

The next year, 1954, the subject switched to devitaminized lard capsules (6-minim size), ten per day, and during this period from June through August, inclusively, there was a decline in the T-wave, although the physical activity program was kept up the same as usual and the drop in the T-wave was from 11.3 (6/25/54) to 10.9 mm (7/2/54) and finally to 10.1 mm (8/5/54) at fifty-three years of age.

Stage VIII

In an informal period of vacation for a month, the T-wave, at the end of this time was 10.4 mm.

Stage IX

The subject switched from placeboes of devitaminized lard to wheat germ cereal, taking 1½ ounces daily at breakfast and another 1 ounce at night before going to bed, using milk with the cereal. The next T-waves were measured at 7.5 (1/17/55) and 8.4 (6/3/55), while keeping up regular exercise as was his habit.

Stage X

The subject then switched to taking ten capsules of VioBin WGO, 6-minim size, taking these five days per week at the end of the physical workouts, a mixture of calisthenics and swimming. On the next test (7/10/59) the T-wave was an all-time high of 15.0 (Fig. 12), which reduced to 9.0 mm at the end of an all-out treadmill run, 8.6 per cent grade, 7 miles per hour in 4:04. Twenty-four hours after this run the T-wave had recovered to 14.5 mm.

Stage XI

During 1960, *no supplements were taken,* nor during 1961, 1962 and 1963, and the T-wave declined 8.3 in this period and leveled off here. The R-wave was 34.3 mm on 7/10/59 while on WGO, whereas it averaged 17.97 during 1954 and 1955 on wheat germ cereal.

Conclusion

It was concluded that WGO helped the amplitude of the T-wave of the ECG, measuring the highest of the precordial lead. The gains of the eleven individuals reported herein, as longitudinal cases, improved relatively more while taking WGO than taking the placebo substances, or taking wheat germ cereal, the comparisons are during periods when the experimental subjects were on a steady exercise program (solid lines) compared to no regular program or supplementary feeding (dotted lines) as shown in Figures 11 through 22.

LONGITUDINAL CHANGES IN THE T-WAVE OF THE ECG (H.S.)

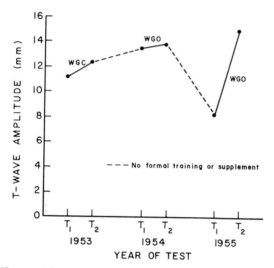

Figure 15. Longitudinal changes in the T-wave of the ECG (H.S.).

Individual H. S. (Skornia) showed moderate increases on WG and then two further improvements on WGO, taking him to a relatively higher score on the T-wave of the ECG (Fig. 15, Exp. 35).

Subject C. B. (Birkland) improved his Schneider index twice while taking WGO and reached his peak score taking WGO, but in another year also improved somewhat taking placeboes and deteriorated taking WG (Fig. 16, Exp. 36).

Subject R. D. improved most in the amplitude of the heartograph in two years taking WGO and also about the same amount taking WGC, but deteriorated while taking WG and also while taking placeboes (Fig. 17-A, Exp. 33). He also made his best improvement on the T-wave of the ECG while taking WGO the following year (Fig. 17-B, Exp. 33-B).

Subject F. K. (Kummerow) made his largest improvements on the amplitude of the heartograph while taking WGO compared to placeboes (Fig. 38, Exp. No. 38-A). These improvements were

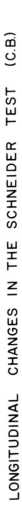

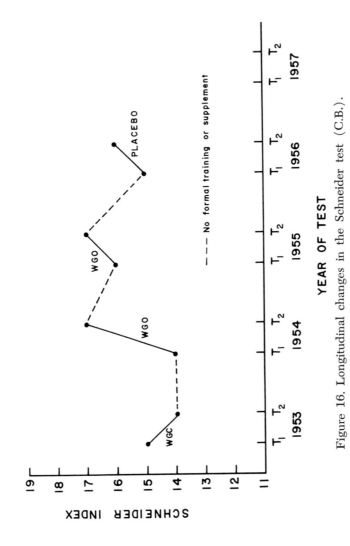

Figure 16. Longitudinal changes in the Schneider test (C.B.).

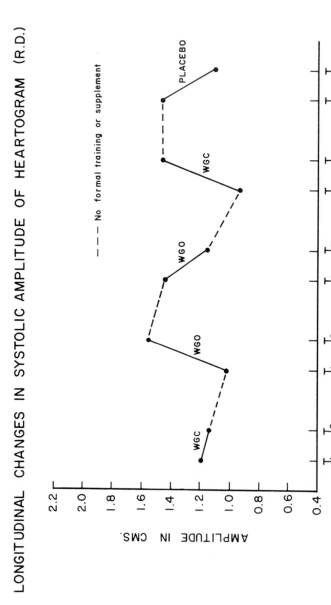

Figure 17-A. Longitudinal changes in systolic amplitude of heartogram (R.D.).

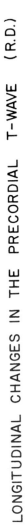
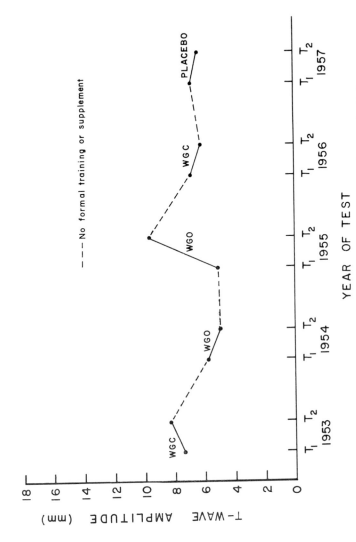

Figure 17-B. Longitudinal changes in the precordial T-wave (R.D.).

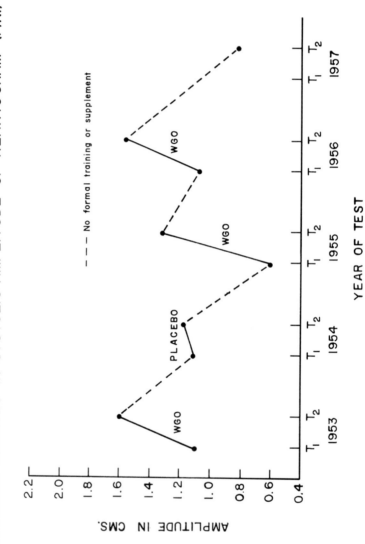

LONGITUDINAL CHANGES IN SYSTOLIC AMPLITUDE OF HEARTOGRAM (F.K.)

Figure 18-A. Longitudinal changes in systolic amplitude of heartogram (F.K.).

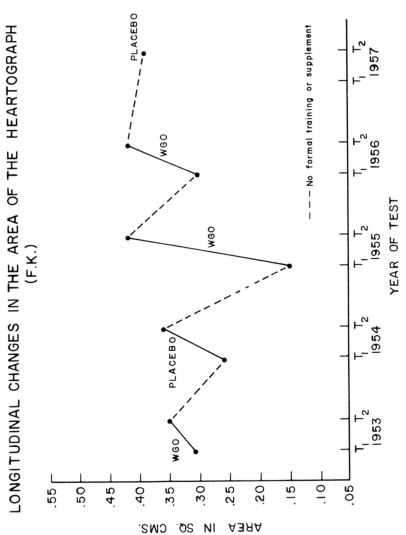

Figure 18-B. Longitudinal changes in the area of the heartograph (F.K.).

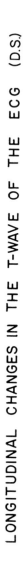

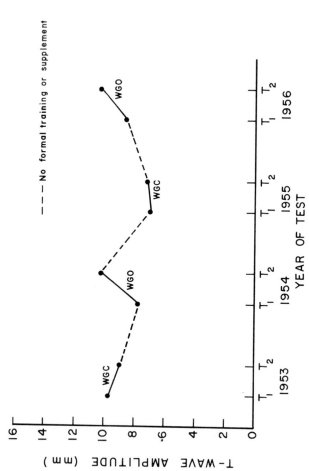

Figure 19. Longitudinal changes in the T-wave of the ECG (D.S.).

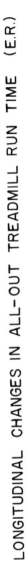
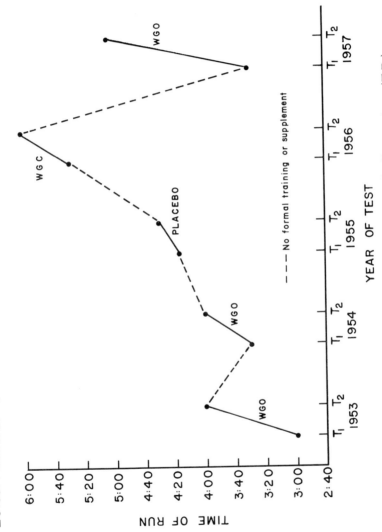

Figure 20. Longitudinal changes in all-out treadmill run time (E.R.).

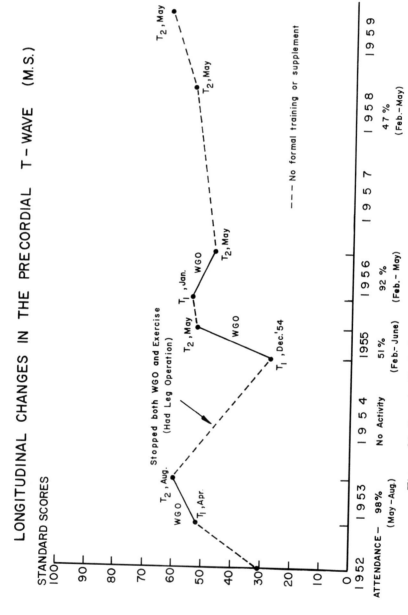

Figure 21. Longitudinal changes in the precordial T-wave (M.S.).

also shown for the area of the heartograph for 1953, 1955 and 1956, reaching his highest peak on this test after the third round of WGO. His training program was about the same, mainly calisthenics and swimming over these three years. If these improvements were due to overcoming a dietary deficiency, which the WGO remedied, then it is suggested here that considerable time is required to overcome the deficiency. The placebo also had some moderate positive effect, which suggests that none of the placeboes except devitaminized lard were really inert in their biological effect.

Subject D. S. (Smythe) improved more while taking WGO than he did while taking WGC, two different yearly comparisons, the precordial T-wave of the ECG being the variable. When such improvements are repeated in such a series of alternations, the author believes that the effect of WGO is certainly there (Fig. 19, Exp. 39).

Subject E. R. (Rae) demonstrated marked improvements in three different years, on WGO compared to placeboes, although slight improvements were made on placeboes and somewhat greater improvement was made on WGC (Fig. 20, Exp. 40).

Subject M. S. (Steidner) made definite changes for the better on WGO twice, and then on the third round on WGO dropped a slight bit during the January to May period, when such precordial T-wave measurements are usually a bit lower anyway. When he stopped both exercise and WGO his record reached its lowest point, December 1954 (Fig. 21, Exp. 41).

Subject J. R. (Ray) (Exp. 42) trained for ten years, taking WGO throughout except for two small breaks when he ran out of it. There were steady improvements in his mile run time, and many other measurements, but in 1958 Dr. Ramsdall, Joie's physician, injected calcium shots into his veins, and in this year he improved the most. Except for this "dip" in his mile performance times, he improved steadily for ten years after he was fifty-nine years of age. His experiment is a remarkable one in several ways, so it is reprinted in full.* (refer to Chapter XII for Summary of Conclusions and Discussion).

---

* Cf. *Ass. Phys. Ment. Rehab.*: 18:No. 3, 64-80, May-June, 1964.

INDIVIDUAL CASES OF OLYMPIC SWIMMERS

Cureton's observations on the 1956 Olympic Games swimming at Melbourne, Australia° pointed out that four American swimmers were taking WGO for six months prior to the start of the games: Bill Yorzyk, George Breen, Nancy Ramey and Shelly Mann, and no others on the American team. Bill Yorzyk established a new Olympic record for the 200 meter butterfly stroke to win; George Breen established a new world's record for the 1500 meter swim in the trials, and was defeated by Murray Rose two days later in the finals (without any WGO between); Shelly Mann and Nancy Ramey won first and second place in the 100 meter butterfly race. The rest of the American team, except divers, were without a win, and did poorly. It is believed that the WGO taken for six months helped the swimmers.

° T. K. Cureton: Science Aids Australian Swimmers, *Ath. J.*, 38:40, Sept., 1957.

TABLE XII

PERCENTAGE OF ATHLETES AND COACHES SUPPORTING (AND USING) DIETARY SUPPLEMENTATION, 1959-60, INCLUDING ROME OLYMPICS°

(Sample Obtained by Cureton-Boehm-Bosco-Liverman-Skinner)

Group	N	Wheat Germ Per Cent	Wheat Germ Oil Per Cent	Vitamins Per Cent
U.S.A. Olympic Games Athletes	56	87.6	85.7	84.3
U.S.A. Coaches and Trainers	22	54.7	50.2	72.9
Foreign Olympic Games Athletes	50	16.0	26.1	68.1
Foreign Coaches and Trainers	37	13.5	18.9	59.6

° From: reference 14.

Chapter III

Muscular Endurance: Its Interpretation, Methods of Testing and Effects of Wheat Germ Oil, Octacosanol and Wheat Germ

THE NATURE OF MUSCULAR ENDURANCE

THERE are several types of endurance, each being fairly specific and responsive to a particular type of training. Cureton[1] demonstrated by factor analysis of twenty-eight muscular endurance events that four principal factors emerged from the matrix of intercorrelations of the twenty-eight events, using Thurstone's multiple factor analysis with rotation. Each principal type of endurance is considered to be quite specific and is responsive to a particular type of training: a) the locomotive muscles (leg and thigh extensors) and arm flexors, b) the lateral muscles, c) the arm extensors and d) long running endurance (circulatory-respiratory, O_2 intake capacity). McCloy[2] also demonstrated by the same factor analysis methods that "strength-endurance" stands apart from circulatory-respiratory endurance. Neither holding out the arms as long as possible, nor chinning the bar, nor pushing up to the toes as long as the muscles last, as examples, are particularly correlated with maximal O_2 intake. Patt[3] reported the correlations between a 23.5 mile run, done in the evening, by 105 Navy and Marine recruits and several of the traditional physical fitness tests (AAF tests: chinning, vertical jumps, dips ($r = 0.01$); dynamometer fatigue tests ($r = 0.06$); blood pressures and heart rate on a tilt table ($r = 0.01$ and $.06$); body sway ($r = 0.43$); medical officers rating ($r = 0.37$); steps completed in step-up test ($r = 0.32$); blood ray reduction test ($r = 0.30$ and 0.05). The multiple R was 0.51. Such results only illustrate that most short-time, so-called endurance tests do not carry on long enough to test the nutritive reserves. The outstanding thing about endurance tests of the muscular type (not O_2 intake type tests) is that they are *very* improvable with training. The oxygen intake tests are very difficult to improve. Recent studies suggest that inheritance is a predominant factor. (Klissouras, *J. App. Physiol.*, 31:338-344 (Sept.), 1971.)

From various books on physiology of exercise the following principal variables are involved in endurance, more or less, according to the type of endurance:

1. The effectiveness of the pulmonary circulation to take in sufficient oxygen and to remove carbon dioxide in the internal respiration, and the total amount of air breathed in hard work.

2. The stroke volume of the heart (or indirectly vigor, by either ballistocardiograph or heartograph on the per beat basis, i.e. determining the anacrotic slope of the wave, the velocity and the acceleration, or proportionate measures).[5, 6, 7, 8]

3. The extent of capillarization in the skeletal muscles and heart muscle, permitting the delivery of available fuel, oxygen, enzymes, hormones, vitamins, minerals, coenzymes and other substances to the working tissues.[9, 10, 11]

4. The ability of the muscle cells to exchange oxygen and carbon dioxide with the capillary blood, as a result of proper imbalance in osmotic and hydrostatic pressures. This internal respiration is reflected in the arteriovenous oxygen difference ($O_{2A-V \text{ diff.}}$).

5. The effectiveness of the sympathoadrenergic system and corticoid (adrenal cortex) system to govern the exchange between the arterioles and venules (where the bottle neck is) and to adjust during endurance efforts. This involves to some extent cardiac stimulation through the accelerator (sympathetic) nerves and the prying open of the precapillary sphincter valves at the terminal ends of the meta-arterioles in the body (muscles doing the work), the heart, motor brain and brain stem. The blood flow, and inversely, the total peripheral resistance (TPR) may be regulated by the constriction or dilation of these small valves which are under autonomic nervous control. When a person exercises and the diastolic pressure and TPR drop during the exercise, it is largely due to whether the individual has a "trained" response of the nerves which open

these small valves and drain the blood off from the large arteries. If this did not happen, the blood pressure would mount to intolerable levels.[12]

6. The training of the motor nerve endings in the muscles, and the relative (alkalinity-acidity) pH of the blood perfusing them, may explain why endurance is very specific to particular parts of the body.

7. A relatively high body density, or lean body mass (the maximum O_2 intake, which correlates highly with the 2-mile or 12-minute run depends upon it) and relatively less fat, and small bones.

8. The rhythmic pulsations of the walls of the vessels, i.e. vascular tone and suppleness, and a relatively low diastolic blood pressure and low total peripheral resistance, influence circulation, and this varies as their fitness—the more venous return circulation, the greater the stroke output of the heart (the heart cannot eject what it cannot get). Thus, circulation has much to do with endurance but it is not all, as the fatigability of the neuromuscular junctions (synapses), the quality of the blood, the Hb reserves in the myoglobin all play a part. The rhythmic movements of the muscles, contracting and relaxing, also influence circulation, and hence, endurance.

9. The efficiency of the metabolic engine (Krebs cycle) in the muscle cells to use oxygen and burn the nutrient material, to make ATP. The mitochrondria use O_2.

10. The extent of the glycogen stores in the muscles, and blood, liver and various organs.

11. The level of motivation, and conversely, the degree of inhibition.

12. The body build of the subject, i.e. a lean frame and great strength per pound of body weight favors long distance running ability; but the fat storage may be a factor in long swims.

Hence, endurance is a complicated matter to explain, and the practical aspect is to demonstrate its presence by appropriate endurance performances. The performance can be affected without understanding just how it comes about. The *fact* may be the actual improvement of endurance, and the full explanation is desirable but may never be exactly known for certainty. The use of matched groups rules out the possibility of one's psychological mental-drive being the cause, if the groups are matched at the beginning, this is excluded.

CONTRACTION AND RECOVERY OF MUSCLE

Needham[4] gives a good review of modern developments in muscle physiology. It was shown in Myerhoff's laboratory that in thirty seconds after contraction and relaxation there was resynthesis of about 30 per cent of the creatine phosphate. Basically, ATP (adenosine-tri-phosphate) is used up. Each ATP "high energy" bond yields 10.54 calories of energy but must be split by an enzyme. In the inner chemistry Mg and Ca provide the bridge to form actomyosin which makes muscles contract. Ionized calcium is essential. If blood calcium falls, muscles may cramp up. Beyond ATP the creatine phosphate is called upon as exhaustion nears. But even in exhaustion there is about 20 per cent of ATP left as a safety margin. Why this much is always left is not fully understood.

Myoglobin is heavily concentrated in the red fibers of muscle and combines with oxygen to make a reservoir over and above the O_2 intake, and recent estimates of this suggest about 30 per cent of the energy in hard work can come from this source, associated with the net oxygen debt.

Muscles do not function well when excessively chilled, and function more efficiently when "warmed up." In short physical "bursts" of energy are not so apparent but in longer duration events, this additional efficiency becomes more apparent, and yet *excessive* heat can cause a man to fail sooner than he otherwise would.

There is a delicate balance between blood calcium and phosphate if striated muscles are to function properly. The regulation is partly by the parathyroid glands. High function is associated with a fall in calcium and potassium, a rise in phosphorus, good function of the thyroid and adrenal glands, central nervous system, heart and avoidance of tension (to cramp). As exhaustion approaches, a depletion of the adrenal corticoids may be shown to occur. They buffer fatigue.

Good circulation is essential to the relatively fast recovery of muscle. In the heart, for instance, as the training of men proceeds on a systematically progressive basis, the *rest* part of the heart cycle gets relatively longer as compared with the systole. This is probably associated with development of many more minute blood vessels to supply the heart musculature in the left ventricle. The energy of muscle comes from a chemical reaction, as creatine phosphate, carbohydrate and fresh polyunsaturated fatty acids may be broken down to supply the energy. In the physiologies it has mainly been given that adenosine-tri-phosphate (ATP) hydrolyzes and yields energy as it breaks down to adenosine-di-phosphate (ADP) and inorganic phosphate.

The sequence of events for developing energy for contraction is as follows: a) dephosphorylation of ATP, b) immediate rephosphorylation of ADP by reaction with creatine phosphate and c) rephosphorylation of ADP by phosphopyruvate and diphosphyoglycerate formed as carbohydrate breaks down.

It has been shown that the ratio of phosphate esterified to oxy-

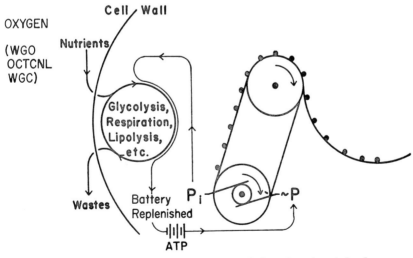

Figure 22. The biologic engine to catabolize (combust) food.

gen consumed (P:O ratio) may be as high as 3 or 4, then 36-48 energy-rich phosphate bonds are developed. The resynthesis of ATP is much more important than the anerobic resynthesis. But as training proceeds the "training effect" is to lower the respiratory quotient (RQ) and the energy is derived somewhat more aerobically than anaerobically, with a gain in metabolic efficiency.

Lipman conceived the storage of energy in phosphate bonds, coining the terms "energy rich" and "energy poor" phosphate bonds in 1941. Szent-Györgyi developed the idea of the tricarboxylic acid cycle (Krebs) with the view that oxygen and sodium phosphate are needed to run the Krebs cycle, which burns glycogen in the muscle (Fig. 22). Energy dynamics, therefore, come from chemical reactions within the muscle cell.

Before Lundsgaard's work of 1930 it was sufficient to say that carbohydrate food broke down and formed lactic acid. Lundsgaard added that creatine phosphate (phosphagen) was used up by muscle contractions.

Other Limiting Factors

The surface membrane of muscle cells limits the rapid exchange of ions between cells and their surrounding media. The main function of the muscle membrane is to receive the motor impulse, distribute it over the whole length of the muscle fiber and pass it on to the contractile material in the interior of the fiber. It is recognized that there are "slow" and "fast" muscle fibers, due to the varying speed with which the nerve impulse is propagated along the nerve fiber. The larger the nerve fiber the faster is the passage. This can be improved by repetitious "fast-reaction" training.

The source of energy for the propagation of the impulse is the relative concentration gradients of Na and K ions across the filament membrane. The conduction of an impulse involves the entry of a minute amount of sodium into the fiber (4×10^{-12} equivalent per cm^2) and an equivalent leakage of K into the surrounding fluid. An "enzymic pump" is responsible for continuous extrusion of Na and accumulation of K in the nerve fiber.

The end-plate potential changes are inhibited by curare and enhanced by anticholinesterases. The synovial junctional region is bombarded by minute quantities of acetylcholine which are released spontaneously, at random moments, from the nerve endings. This results in the appearance of "miniature end-plate potentials."

The Krebs (citric acid) Cycle grinds up glucose (carbohydrate, *et al.*) to produce acids and glycogen. Dr. Fritz Lipman was awarded the Nobel Prize in 1953 for working out the chemistry of the Krebs Cycle. The Krebs Cycle is regulated by oxygen availability and ATP, so physical training of the endurance type has a compound effect of increasing the vascularization in muscle and burning up relatively more foodstuffs than would ordinarily be consumed. Great interest now attaches to the improvement of circulatory-respiratory fitness by means of endurance exercise, and using up the polyunsaturated fatty acid fats by exercise. It would appear logical that such exercise would guarantee the full use of any added supplement, such as WGO. But the ready use of WGO might also depend upon the availability of the calcium and potassium to phyophorolyze (break down) the complex molecules of WGO so that it can be used. Its effect appears to be very slow, not quick like aspirin, and both the animal studies and the human reaction studies (Farrell's animal study) and Exp. 31, the Milesis-Cureton reaction time study; take about 4-5 weeks to bring up significant differences. Exercise brings out enzymes from within the muscle cells, which help to further "digest" the oil, so that it can go through the cell wall.

NUTRITIONAL SUPPLY TO MUSCLE

Dr. Fred Kummerow, of the Burnsides laboratory (lipids) was asked to state the biochemical implications of improving the nutritive state in a way which might help athletic performances. He thought that it would be primarily a matter of supplying additional energy to athletes in the form of materials which would help the formation of high energy bonds. The reactions are as follows:

1. The overall pathway of glycolysis in muscle tissue—

$$\text{GLYCOGEN} + 3\,\text{ADP} + 3\,\text{PO}_4 \longrightarrow 2\,\text{LACTIC ACID} + 3\,\text{ATP} \quad (1)$$

2. Muscle functions under anaerobic conditions and the redox system available for the continuation of the cycle is as follows—

D GLYCERALDEHYDE 3-PHOSPHATE ⟶ ⟍ ⟋DPNH⟍ ⟋LACTIC
    1, 3 DIPHOSPHORYL D GLYCERIC ACID⟵ (+H +) (
                                          ⟍DPN ⟋ ⟍PYRUVATE (2)

3. When actomyosin in muscle fibers is treated with ATP, the fibers contract. ATP is simultaneously split to *ADP + inorganic phosphate*. The energy is used in muscular contraction comes from the conversion of glycogen to lactic acid (reaction 1 above). However, the source of energy is obtained from the breakdown of creatine phosphate—

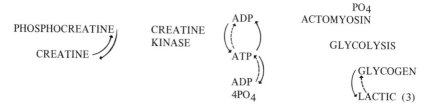

Hence, the major limiting factors include the following:
1. An adequate caloric intake to maintain glycogen supply— easily provided.
2. An available supply of organic phosphate. This could be supplied in the forms of a *calcium phosphate* similar to those used for pregnant women.
3. Creatine supply is needed, an end-product of glycine, arginine and methionine metabolism.
4. Adenosine supply, involving *aspartic acid* and *glutamic acid* and *glycine*. The metabolism of the purines is so interlinked that this becomes very complicated and is not considered in detail.
5. Involved as various co-factors would be most of the B-vitamins (thiamine, nicotinic acid, pantothenic acid). These would have to be added as supplements above the normal requirement. It may also be necessary to provide small

additional mineral supplements such as iron, magnesium, manganese and molybdenum in particular.

The recommendation would include (daily) the intake of vitamin-mineral capsules (fat and B-vitamins) by using a commercial preparation at the level suggested for pregnant women, something like Unicap M® (Upjohn). Argenine and methionine can be provided by a gelatin fruit salad supplemented by cottage cheese. Aspartic acid and glutamate would also be provided in this salad. "I would not recommend *large* dosages of wheat germ oil." I still believe the best trained athletes win, regardless of diets.

Case Studies and Testimonials

There are hundreds of testimonials to the presumed effectiveness of WGO but these have been ruled out of this report, but the fact that experienced coaches, after years of trial, with and without, generally stand behind the use of WGO and dietary supplements, and support mainly the vitamin C, B-complex, and E (in wheat germ oil). A canvas of Olympic athletes at the Olympic Games by Dr. Wilbur Bohm and the author demonstrated that the top coaches strongly favored such supplementation, in spite of doubts by some of the medical attending doctors.[13, 14, 15] We do have some faith in the results of several years of *longitudinal trial and error*, systematically rotated, on WGO and then off for a period, then on placeboes, and then on octacosanol, off again and on placeboes, on nothing, and then on wheat germ cereal. With tests taken concurrently with these trials, the data are valuable (cf. 11 case studies in Chapter II and Figs. 12 to 21).

THE ENDURANCE TESTS USED IN THE EXPERIMENTS

The thirteen experiments involving *endurance* (events lasting more than one full minute) used certain standardized tests, described as follows:

A. 600-Yard Run

This test is performed on a track, outdoors, in reasonably dry weather, with young boys. The event has been shown to correlate well with "Peak" O_2 Intake,[16] this correlation being 0.733. It was practiced at about two thirds speed with an instructor setting the pace, at least once before taking the time. Then on another occasion, when the boys were rested, it was run for time to count, then after a day or two it was run again, and the best of the two trials was used to represent the ability in this event. It is one of the official American Association for Health, Physical Education and Recreation Tests, run by boys and girls all over the United States. In our work the r_{11} ranged from 0.86 to 0.98, the better results made after several practices. In a factor analysis study the endurance was unique.[17]

B. All-Out Treadmill Run

This test is performed on a motor driven treadmill, with adjustable speed control, in the Physical Fitness Research Laboratory. Usually tests were taken at 7 mi/hr and 8.6 per cent grade but if a boy could not handle this pace for at least one minute, the speed was dropped to 5 mi/hr so that he could run for at least a minute. Warm-up was always practiced for 15-20 minutes by walking and jogging around an indoor gym floor, then taking a 30 second practice run; then more warm-up and a run for one minute; then a walk and about 10 minutes later the all-out run test was given. The r_{11} was 0.86 to 0.94 (cf. *Improving the Physical Fitness of Youth* (1964) by Cureton and Barry).[19] The same run is used with the O_2 Intake and Debt Equipment. A boy was told, "Run just fast enough to keep up with the treadmill belt, toward the front of the treadmill. If you feel that you cannot do any more, then raise your elbows up to the horizontal (like this—demonstration) and we will then catch you under the armpits and lift you off, and stop the treadmill. Then stand right there until we check your heart rate, and while we are doing this we will have you sit down to recover, and you will keep the mouthpiece in your mouth and breathe as well as you can, throughout the entire test, standing, running and sitting." By having a serial-bag rack of Douglas bags, the switch from the O_2 intake (exhaust gas during the run) bag to the O_2 debt bag (used during recovery) was made by a valve with no need to remove the mouthpiece at any time. Needless to say, this mouthpiece and noseclip had to be watched every second to see that *all* of the gas went into the bags. The run was timed.

C. All-Out Muscular Endurance Tests

These tests were given after some practice on another day. Some preliminary walking and jogging was given as a warm-up, usually ten to fifteen minutes, then under close supervision for "form" each boy was counted in what he could do, or was timed. The tests were as follows: (cf. specifications in *Endurance of Young Men* by Cureton).[20]

1. *Push-ups.* Done with back as straight as possible, and only the chin or chest touching, never the abdomen. Hands were straight forward from the shoulders. The number is counted for those done right.

2. *Side Leg-Raisings.* Performed from the side, leaning-rest position, right hand and then the left hand to the floor, and the upper leg raised to the horizontal. The number is counted for those done right.

3. *Chinning the Bar.* Reverse grip recommended, full let down. Total number counted, even to the half chin.

4. *Sit-ups.* Performed with feet held by a partner, fingers laced behind the neck. Number completed is counted.

5. *Sitting Tucks.* Performed with hands on hips or on the floor at the sides of the hips, heels off of the floor at all times after starting. The heels are thrust forward until the legs are straight, then retracted until close to the buttocks. The number done is counted.

6. *Squat Jumps.* Performed from a standing position, and upon "Go!" the fingers are touched to the floor and then a vertical jump of about four inches is made, and the whole movement rapidly repeated for count.

7. *Dips on Parallel Bars.* Done by giving one count for springing up onto the bars at shoulder height. Bars are at a width just equal to overall shoulder width (it is a great handicap to have the bars too far apart). The number one is counted to the nearest half count. During the dip, the shoulder tip is checked with the fist when the upper arm becomes horizontal, otherwise the subject may go down too far.

The tables for these muscular endurance events, along with tables for physique and cardiovascular measures and additional motor events (strength, agility, balance, flexibility) are in the monograph, *Improving the Physical Fitness of Youth* (Cureton) and Barry, 1964).*

Precautions

Some rules were instituted to prevent undue interference with the testing. No strenuous activities were permitted, other than ordinary class instructional work, in the two day period before a test was to be taken. If competitions were scheduled individually or between sides, they were spaced a week ahead or a week after the tests of physical fitness. This was done to eliminate fatigue affecting the scores. The boys were always told when a test was to be held and advised to abstain from all very strenuous work until the tests were over. They were told to report any sickness at once to their instructor, and to avoid taking any medicines or pills unless their instructor knew of it. Their parents were asked not to feed the boys any wheat germ or wheat germ oil at home during the span of the Sports Fitness School, but they were not told what each boy was taking at the Sports Fitness School as part of the experimental program until after it was over.

Referring to Table XIII which summarizes and compares the gains made by all groups, thirteen experiments, it was possible to convert the raw score gains into standard (60 range) scores which would make comparisons possible, otherwise tests made on the ergometer bicycle, 440-yard run, 600-yard run and treadmill run could not be compared. The overall results show that the WGO groups have made an average improvement of 12.51 SS, the OCTCNL groups 8.41 SS, the placebo training groups 6.77 SS the WGC training group 5.71 SS, the sedentary WGO group 2.6 SS and the sedentary on nothing group lost (−9.22 SS) as they were told to do no physical activity. These are appreciable differences showing that WGO and octacosanol groups outdid the others.

---

* This monograph gives illustrations of the treadmills used with the boys. It discusses the data obtained in the all-out treadmill run and 600-yard run in detail, and the prediction of the times made and standard score tables for all events used with the boys.

SUMMARY TABLE OF THE IMPROVEMENTS IN THE ENDURANCE STUDIES COMPARING THE POSSIBLE EFFECTS OF WGO, OCTACOSANOL AND WHEAT GERM VERSUS PLACEBOES (in Standard Scores) FOR SIXTEEN WEEKS

Test Method	Studies	Training Program +WGO	Training Program +OCTCNL	Training Program +WGC	Training and Placeboes	Training and WGO	Sedentary and Placeboes	Sedentary and Nothing
Ergometer bicycle .... No. 3—	Smiley and Cureton	18.0			-1.14			
Ergometer bicycle .... No. 6—	Ganslen and Cureton	18.0			6.0	2.6		
Treadmill run 7 mi/hr/8.6% .... No. 12—	Vohaska and Cureton	2.46			6.24			-9.22
Treadmill run 7 mi/hr/8.6% .... No. 13—	Cureton and Pohndorf	15.35 (1953) 18.0 (1954)			7.50		1.0	
440 yard run .... No. 18—	Bernauer and Cureton	11.0			5.0			
600 yard run .... No. 15—	Hupé and Cureton	7.89	5.70	14.69	8.76			
Composite score (SS) 4 tests .... No. 17—	Tuma and Cureton	12.3	13.6		7.0			
600-yard run (summation 4 yrs.) ...	Cureton, 1955-58	8.72	10.93	4.58	3.02			
Treadmill run 5 mi/hr/8.6 .... No. 19—	Brown and Cureton			9.0 / -6.3	12.0			
No. 20—	Banister and Cureton	5.7	3.4	4.3	3.9			
Treadmill run .... No. 23—	Chen and Cureton	12.38			9.75			
Treadmill run .... No. 23—	Dempsey and Cureton	23.0			6.0			
600-yard run .... No. 25—	Cundiff and Cureton			8.0	14.0			
Averages		12.51 SS	8.41 SS	5.71 SS	6.77 SS	2.6 SS	1.0 SS	-9.22 SS

Note: The WGO and OCTCNL groups have produced results fairly alike, but the other groups are far below in improvement. The advantage of the WGO group over the placebo group, both in the same physical training program was 5.74 SS and the OCTCNL group over the placebo group was 1.64 SS.

TABLE XIV
RELIABILITY RESULTS OF THE ENDURANCE EXPERIMENTS

Number of Experiment	Experimenters	Statistical Significance <.10 (nature of units) in result	Favorable results for supplements listed	No evidence revealed to favor supplements	Name of supplement used
1					
2					
3	Smiley and Cureton	* (Ground level time)	* (altitude time)		WGO
4					
5					
6	Ganslen and Cureton	* (Time)	* (O_2 debt)		WGO
7					
8					
9					
10					
11					
12	Vohaska and Cureton	* (Time)			WGO
†13 (2 yrs.)	Cureton and Pohndorf	* (Time)	* (repeated, 1953 and 1964)		WGO
14	Conner and Cureton				
15	Hupé and Cureton	* (Time)			WGC
16					
17	Tuma and Cureton, et al.	* (SS average)			OCTCNL and WGO
18	Bernauer and Cureton		* (Time)		WGO
19	Brown and Cureton			*	WGC
20	Banister and Cureton	* (Time)			WGO
21	Cureton, et al.	* (SS average)			OCTCNL and WGO
22					
23	Chen and Cureton	* (Time)			WGO
24	Cureton and Wiggett	* (Time)			WGO
25	Cundiff and Cureton		* (Time)		WGO
26					
27					
28					
29					
30					
31					

Out of thirteen experiments completed in which endurance was the principal criterion, the WGO has made more improvement in the experimental subjects ten times out of thirteen; the OCTCNL has twice been clearly superior to the placeboes out of four times tried; and WGC has had an advantage three times out of six times used.

With WGO and OCTCNL being considered identical substances, the advantage seems definite for these dietary supplements.

Eleven out of thirteen times, the WGO has shown an advantage larger than two times the S.E.$_{meas.}$ and, similarly, OCTCNL has twice shown the same type of advantage. Once the WGC has been best when compared with WGO and OCTCNL.

REFERENCES

1. Cureton, T. K.: *Endurance of Young Men*, Washington, D. C., Society for Research in Child Development, National Research Council, Research Monograph No. 1, Vol. X, 1945, p. 284.

2. McCloy, C. H.: A factory analysis of endurance, *Res. Quart.*, 27:213-216, May, 1956.

3. Patt, H. M.: Evaluation of certain tests of physical fitness, *J. Aviat. Med.*, April 18, 1947, pp. 169-175.

4. Needham, D. M.: The physiology of muscle contraction, *Brit. Med. Bull.*, 12:No. 3, Sept., 1956.

5. Jokl, E. and Wells, J. B.: Exercise training and cardiac force, in Raab, W. (Ed.): *Prevention of Ischemic Heart Disease.* Springfield, Illinois: Thomas, 1966, pp. 135-146.

6. Cureton, T. K.: Validity of testing the cardiovascular fitness by the sphygmograph (external cuff, heartograph) method, pp. 118-191 in *The Physiological Effects of Exercise Programs on Adults.* Springfield, Illinois, Thomas, 1949.

7. Wiggers, C. J.: *Circulatory Dynamics*, New York, Grune, 1952, p. 38.

8. Kroeker, E. J. and Wood, E. H.: Comparison of simultaneously recorded

---

← ∰

* A blank line means that no endurance was involved that could be measured on a continuous basis. While endurance is usually measured in time units on an ergometer bicycle or on a motor driven treadmill (at 7 mi/hr, 8.6 per cent grade) experiments 17 and 21 involved composite muscular endurance criteria of events such as the mile run, sitting pucks, chins, push-ups and squat jumps, these were scored both by each event and by the composite SS (standard score) average of all five events. One experiment by Marx was dropped as explained elsewhere because of drop-outs which unbalanced the two matched groups.

† There were two experiments, one in 1953-54 and a second one in 1954-55. The first was significant and the second one was "near significant" in reliability.

intra-arterial and extra-arterial pressure pulse in man, *Circ. Res.*, 3:623, 1955.

9. Petren, T. Sjöstrand and Sylvan, B.: "Der Einfluss des Trainings aufdie Haufigkeit der Capillaren in Herz und Skelmuskulatur," *Arbeitsphysiologie*, 9:376, 1936.

10. Uvnas, B.: Sympathetic vasodilator outflow, *Physiol. Rev.*, 34:608-618, July, 1954.

11. Keul, J. and Doll, E.: The Substrate-Supply of Human Skeletal Muscle During Physical Labor, in XVI. Weltkongress für Sportmedicin in Hannover (12-16, June, 1966, *Kongressbericht*, Koln-Berlin: Deutsche Arzte-Verlag, pp. 135-144).

12. Cureton, T. K.: Post-exercise blood pressures in maximum exertion tests and relationships to performance time, oxygen intake, oxygen debt and peripheral resistance, *J. Lancet*, 77:81-82, 1957.

13. Cureton, T. K.: Science aids Australian swimmers, *Ath. J.*, 38:40, March, 1957.

14. Cureton, T. K.: New dietary methods and dietary supplements are responsible for many of the new records, *Ath. J.*, 42:12-14, 1962.

15. Cureton, T. K.: Diet related to athletics and physical fitness, *J. Phys. Ed.*, 57:Nos. 2, 3, 4, 5, 1959-60.

16. Corroll, V. A.: AAHPER Youth Fitness Test Items and Maximum Oxygen Intake, Urbana, Ph.D. thesis, Physical Education, University of Illinois, 1967, p. 123.

17. Olree, H., Stevens, C., and Macleod, P. F.: Estimation of maximum oxygen intake from AAHPER test, *J. Sports Med. Phys. Fitness*, 5:67, June, 1965.

18. Falls, H. B., Ismail, A. H., and Macleod: Estimation of the maximum oxygen intake from AAHPER test items, *Res. Quart.*, 37:192-201, 5:67, June, 1900.

19. Cureton, T. K. and Barry, A. J.: Performance prediction and improvement in the all-out treadmill run and the 600-yard run, in *Improving the Physical Fitness of Youth*, Chicago, University of Chicago Press, Child Development Research Society, Monograph Serial No. 95, 1964, Vol. 29, No. 4, pp. 113-126.

Chapter IV

The Measured Effects of Wheat Germ Oil, Wheat Germ and Octacosanol on the "Peak" Oxygen Intake, Oxygen Debt and Breath Holding

INTRODUCTION

THE studies described in this chapter do not indicate that WGO indicates a consistent positive influence on "peak" oxygen intake, as the study of Brown (Exp. 19) showed a gain of 9 SS for the WGC group and 12 SS for the control group, with boys eleven and twelve years of age, with nine in each group. This was the only study made with WGC in this area. The oxygen debt was not measured. While the trend favors WGC over controls, the difference is statistically insignificant.

The experiment of Ganslen (Exp. 6) produced a slight favorable effect on both oxygen intake (L/min) and net oxygen debt (L) but both of these changes were statistically insignificant. The gain in the net O_2 debt of the six graduate students in this experiment was impressive (from 5.718 L to 6.372 L), a gain of 12.92 per cent but the errors in determining O_2 debt are notorious. They were too large to suggest that this gain could be predicted by statistical inference at a satisfactory level of reliability, i.e. $<.10$ level. The oxygen intake in this experiment increased from 2.166 to 2.571 L/min in twelve weeks of training without any supplement, then in a six-week period, on the same intensity and duration of training and from the plateau established in the twelve-week period, the average O_2 intake rose from the T_2 level of 2.571 L/min to 2.681 L/min, a gain of 4.26 per cent *may* have been due to the use of WGO by the subjects, but the gain was not statistically significant. During this period there was also a very favorable and significant increase in the precordial T-wave, which strengthens the belief that the gain was related to the use of WGO. It is posted as a favorable trend but not statistically significant.

It is also true that the Harvison experiment (Exp. 2) on breath holding and anoxic breath holding (on the anoxia photometer for oxygen percentage depletion during a standard exercise) resulted in the same kind of slight favorable trend (7.75% at ground level, and 3.0% at 10,000 feet of simulated altitude). The gain attributable to the WGO on breath holding was only 1.48 per cent. This may be considered a slight trend, along with favorable T-wave changes and an economical down-turn in BMR from 0.265 L/min to 0.235 (11.7%). All of these changes are statistically insignificant.

MAXIMAL O_2 INTAKE AND PHYSICAL FITNESS

Numerous investigators have reported a rather high correlation between maximal O_2 intake and endurance performances.[1, 2, 3, 4] Still others have reported that physical training produces an increase in aerobic capacity.[5, 6, 7, 8, 9, 10] These findings encourage an increased acceptance of aerobic capacity as a criterion of physical fitness. To quote Åstrand,[11] ". . . the aerobic capacity probably is the best measure of a person's physical endurance." He further states that, ". . . the individual's capacity for O_2 intake should be decisive in determining his ability to sustain heavy, prolonged work." In this statement Åstrand infers that aerobic capacity is the direct cause of endurance, when actually there are no studies on intact humans that demonstrate that a high maximal O_2 intake *causes* good endurance. The studies have shown only that high aerobic capacity is *related* to good endurance, and may not necessarily be the direct cause of it; indeed, there is evidence[12] that as training continues, the maximal O_2 intake may actually decline while the time of the all-out TMR may increase! It is quite possible that both aerobic capacity and endurance are dominated by a single common factor such as the efficacy of the muscles to develop force and simultaneously "pump" venous blood to the heart, or the state of training of the sympathetic nervous system, or the action of hormones on muscles and blood vessels. Many other mechanisms of control could be listed. An outline of the specific factors that determine the limits of O_2 intake will help in understanding that the maximal O_2 intake is not an independent process, but rather is regulated by numerous factors and mechanisms, partly independent and partly intercorrelated.

FACTORS LIMITING THE MAXIMAL O_2 INTAKE

There is considerable difference of opinion among investigators regarding the factors limiting aerobic capacity. Part of the confusion stems from differing techniques of research, i.e. nature and duration of the exercise used to elicit maximal O_2 intake, types of variables used in experiments, characteristics of the subject used (including their state of training) and type of laboratory equipment.

The literature contains several factors that bear evidence of limiting the O_2 intake:

1. *Pulmonary ventilation and respiratory gas exchange.* Authors point up the importance of distributing inspired gas uniformly to the terminal units of the lungs, keeping the O_2 requirement of the respiratory muscles low so that more O_2 can be delivered to exercising limb muscles, the area of the lung surface, the diffusion capacity of the lung tissues, the rate at which hemoglobin is carried by the blood past the lung surface and the completeness with which the blood is exposed to the lung gases. Taylor[14] discounts respiratory factors as being important to O_2 intake, concluding that ". . . the diffusion capacity of the lungs is adequate to oxygenate the arterial blood at high levels of performance." Åstrand does not consider that pulmonary ventilation is a limiting factor, although he recognizes the work of Otis, who found that at high pulmonary ventilations, the respiratory muscles consume disproportionate amounts of O_2, thus allowing less for other working muscles. Nevertheless, there is a high relationship in hard exercise between the total volume of air breathed and the level of the maximal O_2 intake achieved. Moreover, the practical experience has revealed that as much as 30 per cent more O_2 intake is possible (T.K.C. at Illinois) in all-out treadmill runs by subjects who take long deep breaths and force them out, rather than breathe normally in an un-

instructed way. Less distress is felt by the subjects who *force* their breath out in such a run.

2. *Stroke volume.* Taylor[15] regards stroke volume as important on the grounds that the well-trained man can increase his stroke volume more than the untrained man and that the higher the cardiac output, the larger the maximal O_2 intake. On the other hand, Åstrand points out that the minute volume of the heart seems to be primarily determined by the number of muscles at work. Others state that ". . . neither the heart nor the lungs is the limiting factor in the healthy well-trained person."

3. *Peripheral vascularity.* This factor is becoming increasingly recognized by noted authorities as possibly being the most crucial determinant of maximal O_2 intake. It is interesting that the decline in circulation through the leg muscles with age, as found by Hardin Jones (1952), roughly parallels the decline with age of aerobic capacity as found by Robinson.[17]

4. *Hemoglobin.* Although Åstrand[16] reported an r of 0.980 ± 0.004 between total circulating hemoglobin and maximal O_2 intake, this was probably a reflection of body weight, *as the body weight correlates 0.98 with maximal O_2 intake in males irrespective of age.* Moreover, Åstrand found a very high correlation between body weight and circulating hemoglobin.

It is probable that no single factor alone limits aerobic capacity, but that the limit is set by multiple factors, some of which may not have yet been discovered. Henry, *et al.*,[18] offers a somewhat different explanation for the limitation of aerobic capacity, at least in terms of aging.

If it be assumed that the limiting factor in supplying the working cell with oxygen in moderate work is between the capillary and the cell, one cause of the decline in the speed of gas exchange with age can be looked for in this region. Probably the most fundamental changes in the aging process take place in the tissues which intervene between the capillaries and the cells which they nourish. With age, the muco-polysaccharides of the amorphous intercellular substance are gradually displaced by more fibrous intercellular substance. As a result of this, the diffusion of oxygen and food from the capillaries to the cells and the return of the products of cellular metabolism, are retarded.

Moreover, the regulation of the circulation is by a complex interplay of endocrine, nervous, circulatory, respiratory and hemodynamic regulatory mechanisms, and probably by the ability of the muscular movements to move the venous blood. Margaria[13] has outlined the energy processes in muscle activity pointing out that the 100 meter sprint race is run at the expense of phosphagen breakdown, the promptest and most powerful source of energy, providing here about 120-150 cal/kg, an additional 40-50 cal/kg provided by lactic acid formation from glycogen, and about 10 cal/kg from oxidative processes. This could leave the individual quite exhausted.

The relationship of gross oxygen intake in liters is fairly linear, (Fig. 24) and even more so in L/kg. But the L/min relationship is curvilinear, but dividing by kilogram of body weight makes it more linear, so L/min/kg are the units usually used.

The limitations of using O_2 intake in this research to discover the possible effect of WGO and octacosanol on this measure are to be shown. It is better to use the actual measures of performance, as both the all-out treadmill run to exhaustion and the 600-yard run are more reliable as test measures. The "peak" O_2 intake is fairly unreliable, especially with young boys, and very clearly does *not* account closely for the actual performance in terms of time. This has been carefully investigated with the data corrected for curvilinearity (using the log form).* The aerobic intake is only part of the oxygen required for the energy, as about one-third of the oxygen is related to the anaerobic process, these reserves being larger than formerly believed. The amount of oxygen reserve in the myoglobin, as oxymyoglobin having been generally underestimated. The failure in performance is usually psychological, in that the subject just gives up; and in any case as Kaijser[19] has shown in his researches, the limitation is *not* in oxygen intake but is in factors at the site of the used muscles, in the

---

* Cf. figures 24-28 and Cureton and Barry, pp. 113-126 in *Improving the Physical Fitness of Youth*, Dec., 1964.

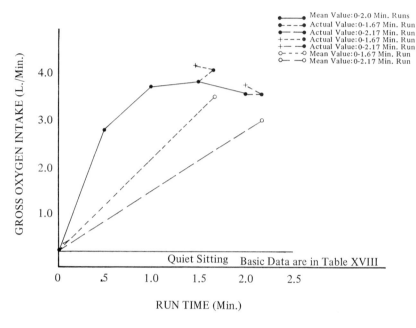

EXERCISE GROSS OXYGEN INTAKES (SUBJECT F.L.)
10 M.P.H., 8.6% Grade

Figure 23. Exercise gross oxygen intake, serial observations (10 mi/hr/8.6% grade).

specific location. So, the greatest limitation is the lack of specificity of oxygen intake. No one can say at this stage of knowledge just what it means but mitochrondria drink up O_2.

PEAK OXYGEN INTAKE

The serial Douglas bag rig in our laboratory[*] enabled the gas samples to be taken each minute of the run, with one minute of gas in each bag. The type of plotted record is shown in Figure 23.

OXYGEN ARTERIOVENOUS DIFFERENCE AS A LIMITING FACTOR

The arteriovenous difference ($O_{2A\text{-}V\ diff.}$) is perhaps the closest measure to approximate the ability of the tissues to take up the oxygen which is delivered to the muscular cells in work. When

---

[*] Physical Fitness Research Laboratory, Urbana, Illinois.

this measure levels off, the limit is fixed for the oxygen intake, and this coincides with a pulse rate of about 130 for young men and 180 for boys. But it is known that with oxygen intake on a plateau or even turning downward, the work performance can go on for some time. This would belie the fact that the O_2 intake is the absolute limiting factor for performance. In aerobic oxygen intake, the $O_{2A-V \text{ diff.}}$ is frequently ignored. This is also supported in a report by Kaijser[19] who found that with the oxygen intake constant that the arterial blood could be varied as much as 3 to 10 per cent without affecting the oxygen intake.* This would suggest that the oxygen intake measure is a crude and rather insensitive measure, and possibly not sensitive enough for our purposes in this research. Kaijser also concluded that the lactate could not be taken as a close reflection of the lack of oxygen at the cellular level, but the point of exhaustion was pin-pointed at the pH level in the cellular area affected, and not as close in the venous blood. He also discussed motivational factors and relative tolerance of distress and pain; and the excitation-contraction coupling, the energy yielding of the contractile elements in the muscle, the substrate supply or metabolite concentration. He emphasized that the lactate in the blood is not the same as the lactate at the loaded muscle. *His major observation as related to this study was that there were very large individual variations, differences in the oxygen utilization and transport systems.* In the course of physical training, the first change is usually an increase in aerobic capacity via autonomic nervous regulation, then later, after many bouts of work and rest, there are moderate developmental changes, but heredity is also conceded to be a great factor. Dill[19] also discussed these limiting factors which determine oxygen intake capacity, indicating that inadequacy with the fuel (carbohydrate or fat) supply, or oxygen supply or heat elimination would limit the performance.

THE CAUSAL ANALYSIS OF NET OXYGEN INTAKE AND THE TREADMILL ALL-OUT RUN

It may be seen by looking closely at the causal analysis data in Table XV that there is a real difference between the variables

---

* Since from the Fick equation, O_2 intake = circulation (L/min) × stroke volume, this would be suspected.

which account for the principal variances in the net oxygen intake from which the "net contribution" of each variable can be computed as proportionate by the Sewell Wright path coefficient system.[21] Each of the percentages given in Table XV is independent of the others. The total accounted for is indicated in the summation of the B² values for the *net* total, and the R² indicates the total on a gross correlational basis.[21]

From a study by Sloninger[22] made in our laboratory we derived the following contributions of several variables to oxygen intake in all-out work.

Holmgren[23] also has presented an elaborate analysis of oxygen intake, using correlations on a small number of cases to show that it is affected by diffusion in the lungs, oxygen transport, diffusion at the cellular level, and also by the "built-in" constitutional type, the latter being relatively unchangeable after being grown physically; and also affected by the total Hb levels, respiratory capacity and other factors. The trouble with this is, that it is impossible to say exactly what $\dot{V}O_2$ is and the analysis is almost a guess, and cannot be made exactly. So, oxygen intake defies exact analysis. Many physical performances do not last long enough to measure $\dot{V}$ but instead "peak" O_2 is used.

Another study was made in our laboratory by Mayfield,[24] who derived the weightings (betas) for predicting peak oxygen intake in 1968. The results of this study are shown in Table XVI.

TABLE XV

CONTRIBUTION OF TEST VARIABLES TO PEAK OXYGEN
INTAKE IN ALL-OUT WORK

Test Item	Net Beta Weight	Net Contribution (Per Cent)
1. Oxygen intake (L/min) at 1½ minutes after the all-out ergometer ride	0.482	32.9
2. Eosinopenia (per cent reduction in all-out ride)	0.447	28.3
3. Area under the brachial pulse wave (by planimeter) sq. cm.	0.287	12.0
4. Net oxygen debt (L/kg)	0.267	10.1
5. Anacrotic slope angle of brachial pulse wave	−.255	9.2
6. Amplitude of the brachial pulse wave (cm.)	0.111	7.5

TABLE XVI

NET CAUSAL COEFFICIENTS (B^2) FOR CONTRIBUTIONS TO
PEAK OXYGEN INTAKE

Test Item	Beta Squared	Net Percentage Contribution
Mile run time	0.632	56.6
Iliac fat fold	0.179	16.02
Brachial pulse wave systolic amplitude	0.019	1.70
Fat free weight	0.179	16.02
Body weight	0.108	9.66
Total net variance	1.117	100.00

Faulkner, *et al.*,[25] reported that all-out performance on the bicycle ergometer that the "peak" O_2 intake was reached at a later time than cardiac output and $O_{2A\text{-}V\ diff.}$ the conclusion was that the maximum $\dot{V}O_2$ was attained through an increase of the $O_{2A\text{-}V\ diff.}$ when cardiac output was declining, and that the *limitation of oxygen intake was due to the heart failing to maintain maximum cardiac output* (stroke). There was a lesser stroke volume in cycling (128 ml/b) compared to running (141 ml/b) at a heart rate of 177/min and an $O_{2A\text{-}V\ diff.}$ of 160 ml/liter for eight men. The error of the latter was estimated at $\pm$ 10 cc/liter.

The amount of blood flow is, of course, related to the type of movements made, and different amounts of tension affect the blood flow. At the end of a hard run, or cycle ride against resistance, there is unusual tensing on the part of the subject, which hurts the blood flow. It may be noticed that the oxygen intake curve turns downward.[26] Åstrand and Saltin[27] also show differences in different events, depending upon the speed and also upon the position of the subject. In our own work we have seen a top swimmer make a high O_2 intake test in the pool but, who tensed up early on the treadmill, and had a low "peak" O_2 intake in this test. We demonstrated a difference between flat and grade running.

It is known that in the face of progressive acute physical stress, neural and hormonal mechanisms within the trained individual may enable him to tolerate (or resist) the stress even *after* the maximal O_2 intake has been reached. The role of the nervous system, as Steggerda[38] has expertly described, and of the endocrine system, as Selye[39] has long documented, seem to fit the above concept most interestingly. In addition, Zimkin and Korobkov[40] reported the superiority of trained animals over untrained animals in surviving longer under unfavorable environmental conditions (hyperthermia, irradiation, high pressure, etc.) that do not demand high O_2 intake. Thus, the superiority of the trained animals could not have been due to their O_2 transport mechanisms, and especially in the situation wherein trained rats, held under water (with no oxygen intake) survived longer than untrained animals.[42] Since they had no oxygen intake, their survival must have been due to other factors (total hemoglobin and tough, resistant C.N.S.).

BIOLOGICAL INDIVIDUALITY IN OXYGEN INTAKE CAPACITY

In laboratory work, spread through two summers, 1964 and 1965, young boys were tested on "peak" oxygen intake and oxygen debt, in the all-out treadmill run test, at 7 miles/hour, 8.6 per cent grade, in the Physical Fitness Research Laboratory in Urbana. Careful retesting was done to establish the errors of measurement, using eighteen boys. The results were just the same as had been previously determined by Orban[43] and Brown[44] who used this same test with young boys. The reliability of the 600-yard run was established as 0.821 in 1964 and 0.969 in 1965. But the reliability of the all-out treadmill run with the young boys was poorer, although once it was as high as 0.91. Inspection of Figures 31, 34 and 35 should convince anyone that great individual variation exists, both intravariation and intervariation.

ORBAN'S STUDY

An experiment was run by William A. R. Orban[43] to determine if ice skating would improve the maximum oxygen intake ($\dot{V}O_2$). To determine the reliability of the measures, he tested a group of thirty-two boys, 7-13 years of age, on four successive days. He also tested seven of these boys before and after a winter season of ice skating (three months). The standard errors of measurement are given in Table XXI for all tests used. Satisfactory reliability was obtained for lying and standing blood pressures,

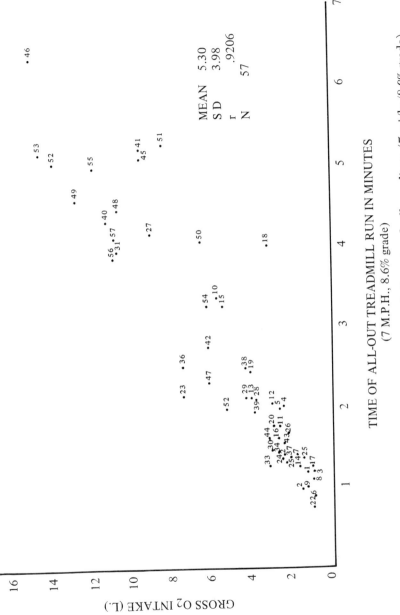

TIME OF ALL-OUT TREADMILL RUN IN MINUTES
(7 M.P.H., 8.6% grade)

Figure 24. Relation of gross oxygen intake to time of all-out treadmill run, liters (7 mi/hr/8.6% grade).

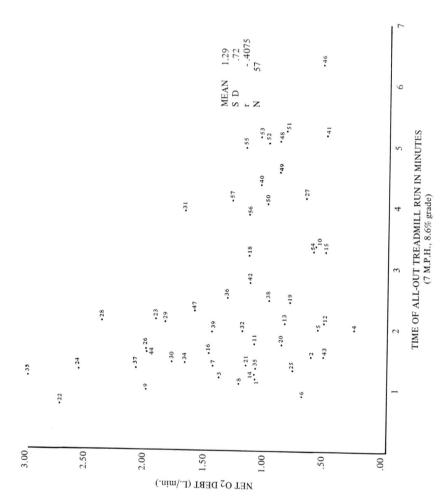

Figure 25. Relation of net oxygen debt to time of all-out treadmill run (L/min) (7 mi/hr/8.6%grade).

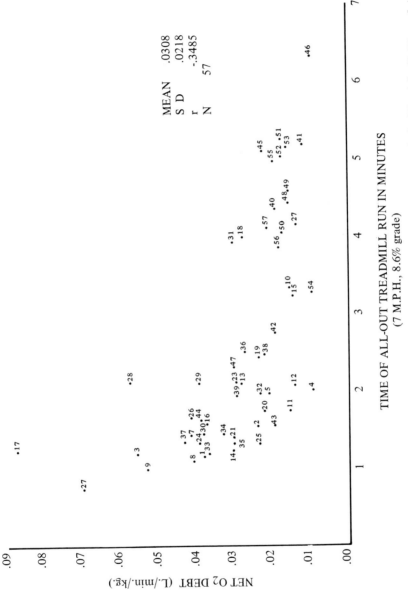

Figure 26. Relation of net oxygen debt to time of all-out treadmill run (L/min/kg) (7 mi/hr/8.6% grade).

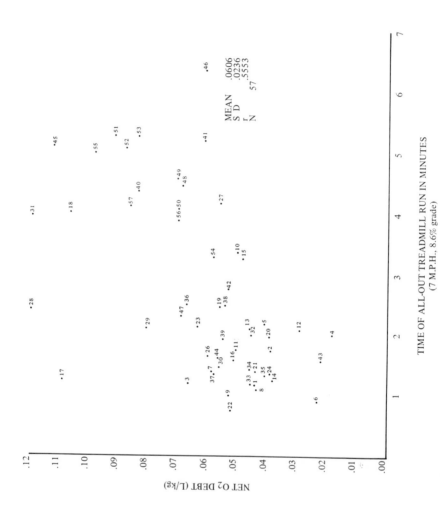

Figure 27. Relation of net oxygen debt to time of all-out treadmill run (L/kg).

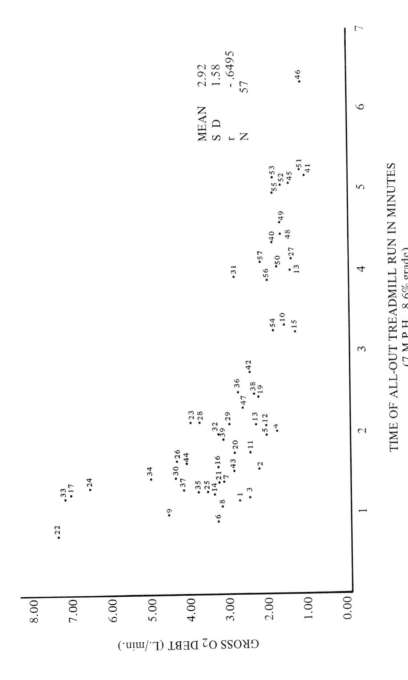

TIME OF ALL-OUT TREADMILL RUN IN MINUTES
(7 M.P.H., 8.6% grade)

Figure 28. Relation of gross oxygen debt to time of all-out treadmill run (L/min).

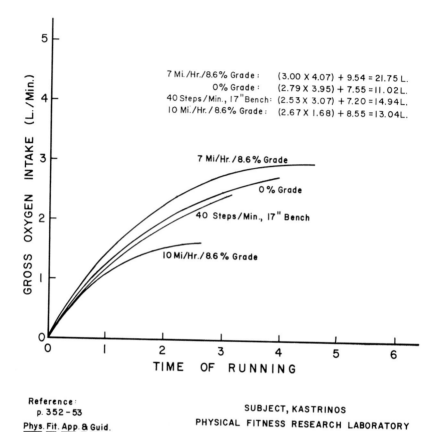

Figure 29. Variation in all-out metabolic tests, rates of work, grades.

lying and sitting heart rates, the total recuperation count after the five-minute step test, the systolic amplitude of the brachial pulse wave on the heartometer, the S-wave of the electrocardiogram, the total of the two minute heartbeat count, taken after different types of stepping exercises, the O_2 intake measures in the quiet state, and during submaximal and maximal exercise.

The standard error of measurement for collecting expired air, metering and analyzing the gas in forty-one paired observations was ± 0.09 cc.

There was no relationship between the O_2 debt measures in a

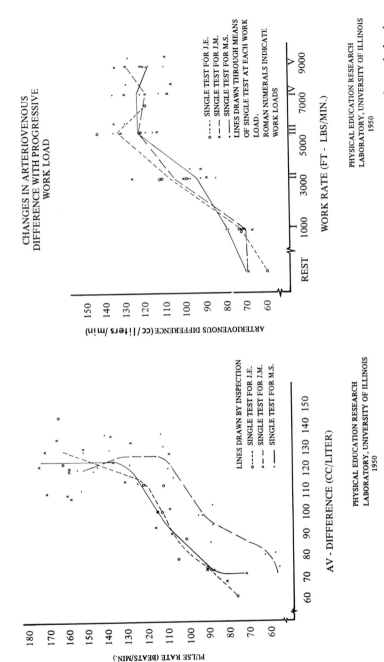

Figure 30. Arteriovenous difference related to pulse rate; changes in arteriovenous differences with work load.

15-minute recovery period and the time of the all-out treadmill run. The O_2 debt was smaller for the longer runs and greater for the shorter runs.

The maximal O_2 intake in one experimental subject increased progressively throughout the training and then regressed immediately after the cessation of the training.

The results are shown in Figures 24, 25, 26, 27 and 28. Subject B. O. was an experienced skater, who improved from a peak O_2 intake of 1.79 L/min to 2.53 L/min while extending his all-out treadmill run, 7 mi./hr./8.6 per cent grade from 2.85 minutes to 5 minutes (Fig. 31). But Figure 31 shows that three boys improved and three did not, units in L/min/kg. In the Net O_2 Debt, three reduced and three did not change significantly.

There were improvements in the Tigerstedt Index, the Stone Index, the Erlanger-Hooker Index and also the maximal oxygen intake in an all-out run, 7 miles/hour, 8.6 per cent grade. Each boy was affected in a unique way. Some improved and some did not in the maximal O_2 intake test. One boy got sick during the training while he was skating about fifteen miles per day, and during this time his maximal O_2 intake decreased. Steggerda[39] gives the central nervous system much credit for a good physical performance, and also Dr. Roger Bannister commented after observing that maximal O_2 intake did not explain some types of physical performances, or oxygen debt either, "As a neurological surgeon, I think I see the great part that the brain stem may play in these endurance performances, not accounted for fully by the oxygen measurements." (Int. Cong. Sports Med., Oxford, Sept., 1970.)

GREAT VARIABILITY (INDIVIDUAL DIFFERENCES IN THE IMPROVEMENT OF O_2 INTAKE IN A COURSE OF PHYSICAL CONDITIONING)

The great variability of individuals in a course of training with respect to the oxygen intake measure is illustrated by an example from Orban's study, shown in Figure 31, wherein six boys engaged in the same program of hockey training. Three improved and three did not.

Behnke[28] relates the maximal O_2 intake to the number of active

AVERAGE OF FRACTIONATED RATES
OF GROSS OXYGEN INTAKE DURING ALL OUT TMR AT 7 MPH

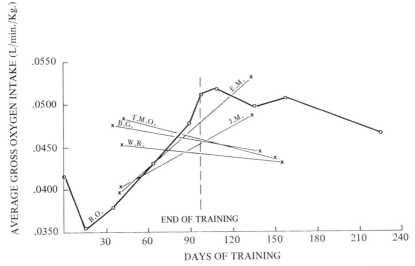

Figure 31. Some boys improve and some do not, 5-6 months in hockey training (no supplements).

muscle cells in use, and has shown high relations between maximum oxygen intake and lean body mass. Various authors have confirmed this.[29] Cotes, Davies and Healy[30] state, "maximal O_2 intake is determined mainly by the amount of skeletal muscle and the ability of the cardiovascular system to perfuse the system with blood. Other relative attributes are the ventilatory and gas transfer properties of the lungs, the blood concentration and the total amount of hemoglobin."

OTHER FACTORS THAN OXYGEN INTAKE

Much evidence has accumulated lately to suggest that endurance is caused as much or more by neuromuscular and cardiovascular factors as by oxygen transport factors. Sherman[31] discovered that in the latter stages of his endurance training program the maximal O_2 intake of his subjects reached a plateau and eventually decreased slightly, while their endurance performance (all-out treadmill run) continued to improve. This same study turned up an r of only 0.23 between gains in endurance running and gains in aerobic capacity. Adams[32] found that although "peak" O_2 intake (ml/min/kg) correlated 0.637 with all-out treadmill running (log base e form), it contributed only 3.68 per cent to the explained variance, owing to the fact that it correlated highly with most other variables, thus making its own unique contribution very small. Doroschuk[33] found that of the total explained variance to predict the 600-yard run time, neuromuscular variable contributed 42 per cent, while O_2 transport variables contributed 36 per cent. Of the total explained variance to predict all-out treadmill run time, neuromuscular variables contributed 38 per cent while O_2 transport variables contributed 43 per cent. *These studies provide clear evidence that factors other than O_2 intake must certainly be considered when attempting to explain endurance.* In this regard, it is quite logical to present the multivariate evidence to show that many factors are involved in trying to use the "peak" O_2 intake tests and net O_2 debt tests. At the same time some of these factors help to show what is reflected in the practical endurance tests, the 600-yard run time and all-out treadmill run.

Saltin[34] concluded that the physiological effects of regular physical conditioning are many, and not only is the maximal O_2 intake affected but total hemoglobin, the buffering capacity of the blood, the myoglobin and ventilatory capacity are also affected. No *net* causal coefficients were computed, and final estimates are not possible from the raw correlations (rank order method) shown on a few cases.

Buskirk and Taylor[35] studied the maximal O_2 intake with reference to body composition using forty-six healthy male college students and thirteen soldiers, by using immersion densiometry. The correlations obtained in this study were as follows: a) active tissue (0.85), b) body weight (0.91) and c) cell mass (0.45). The maximal O_2 intake was related to blood volume (0.78) and to red cell volume (0.69). It was concluded here again that the maximal O_2 intake should be expressed in kilograms of body weight. But here again the figures quoted are only raw correlations and the unique effect of each is not shown. To some extent the physical conditioning probably affects the aerobic O_2 intake but just how much this is so, independently from the lean body mass and other factors is not proved by this study.

Doroschuk[36] comes closer to this solution, following the method recommended to him by Cureton, this being the Sewall Wright causal (net) coefficient system, in which each variable is computed for its *net* (unique) effect. The results were published by Doroschuk and Cureton, Bernauer and Bosco[2] and Doroschuk[33] but perhaps few understand this multivariate system and therefore do not know what to make of it. The results are shown in Table XVII, including forty-nine boys, 10-14 years of age.

It may be noticed in Table XVIII that the peak O_2 intake accounts for only 16.7 per cent of the 600-yard run performance and only 11.7 per cent of the treadmill run time. Many other items contribute to the performance, such as age, weight, pulse rate recovery, agility run time and standing broad jump, also back and leg strength. The same generalization is true for the prediction of the all-out treatmill run time, such as back strength 26 per cent, agility run 36 per cent, standing broad jump 45 per cent, compared to peak O_2 intake 11.7 per cent.

Weber[37] made a similar solution in our laboratory for predic-

TABLE XVII

NET (CAUSAL) STATISTICAL VALUES, RELATIVELY OF TESTS
USED TO PREDICT THE 600-YARD RUN and ALL-OUT
TREADMILL RUN TIME

Test Item	Beta Weight Squared to Predict the 600-Yard Run	Beta Weight Squared to the All-out Treadmill Run
Age	0.036	0.002
Weight	0.024	0.081
Peak oxygen intake	0.167	0.117
Net oxygen debt	0.007	0.072
Leg strength	0.020	0.005
Back strength	0.029	0.026
Total strength/weight	0.001	0.018
Total body reaction time	0.006	0.004
Endurance hops	0.004	0.013
Agility run time	0.065	0.036
Standing broad jump	0.057	0.045
60-yard dash	0.012	0.023
Breath holding time after 1-minute step-test on 17-inch bench	0.014	0.011

TABLE XVIII

NET PER CENT CONTRIBUTIONS OF VARIABLES TO
ALL-OUT TREADMILL RUN TIME

Test Variable	Net Per Cent Contribution (by Beta^2 system)
Weight	51.73 of the net explained variance
Strength/weight	3.47 of the net explained variance
Chinning the bar	0.19 of the net explained variance
Dipping on the parallels	7.48 of the net explained variance
Vertical jump	12.64 of the net explained variance
Agility run (Illinois)	1.39 of the net explained variance
Balance beam score	2.55 of the net explained variance
Standing broad jump	0.54 of the net explained variance

tion of peak O_2 intake with young men and obtained the following per cent *net* contributions. The results are shown in Table XVIII.

It is significant to note that after all of these variables are "taken out" first before peak O_2 intake, there is nothing left to the peak O_2 intake contribution. This indicates that in an event of such limited time duration that the performance is due to other factors than peak O_2 intake.

LONG DISTANCE RUNNING TIME IS RELATED TO OXYGEN INTAKE

It has been shown that long distance running time is related to oxygen intake capacity.[45] Such events have also been related highly to a cardiovascular condition in terms of rather simple cardiovascular tests, used to predict the times in the long runs. More recently, Ribisl and Kachadorian,[46] working in our laboratory, and Cooper[45] have shown high relationships between running time for the two-mile run, and the distance run in twelve minutes, respectively. These are only gross associations and do not represent the critical *net* contribution of aerobic oxygen intake. More exact analyses are typified by the work of Adams[32] who has shown that running all-out time on the treadmill (7 mi/hr/8.6% grade) may be accounted for as shown in Table XIX.

The study by Adams shows that with the various tests accounted for and taken out of the matrix values by statistically eliminating the intercorrelations once the first five items are accounted for, there is little left for the peak oxygen intake or oxygen debt. It also indicates that the real basic values are in the first five test variables and in the agility run. It is clear that the time on the all-out treadmill run is dependent upon many abilities, which are coordinated with each other in the actual performance. This looks at the problem in a multivariate way instead of as if peak O_2 intake were the all-important variable. It is obvious that this is not so.

Long distance running, as long as two miles or thereabouts, such as the twelve-minute run for distance advocated by Cooper,[45] is apparently highly correlated with maximal O_2 intake (measured in a series of work-loads until a plateau, usually by the Balke test, a series of two-minute bouts as the treadmill is gradually increased in slope 1 degree for each bout), provided that the group is young enough and relatively homogenous in body build.[45, 46] Lower predictions are obtained when there are "overweight" people in the group, or many of extreme endomorphic or ectomorphic build. A group of lean medial mesomorphs, this ruling out the other disturbing factors, would give most consistent results on a straight-line relationship. Seasonal variations, altitude and motivation also affect these results. The relationship is not as good in women or fat people.

TABLE XIX

NET PERCENTAGE CONTRIBUTION OF TEST ITEMS TO
THE ALL-OUT TREADMILL RUN TIME

Test Item	Net Percentage Contribution from Beta Square
Sum of six fat-folds	2.58
Five-minute step test, 30/minute terminal pulse rate	32.63
Vital capacity residual	11.97
Systolic amplitude of the brachial pulse wave	10.33
Peak run pulmonary ventilation	9.39
Net oxygen debt	1.64
Net peak oxygen intake in all-out run	1.64
Illinois agility run	24.41
Full squat jumps	3.76
Bar hang for time	1.64
	99.99

TABLE XX

REPEAT TRIALS ON TWO BOYS SHOWING MOTIVATIONAL AND
EDUCATIONAL EFFECTS (7 mi/hr/8.6% grade)

Trials (*K Ran, then W*)	*All-out Treadmill Run Time* (*minutes and seconds*)		*Peak Intake* *cc/min/kg*		*Net Oxygen Debt* (*Liters*)	
Subjects	K	W	K	W	K	W
1	5:00	7:00	46.6	63.3	0.12	0.12
2	7:00	8:05	60.5	55.0	3.60	2.75
3	8:30	9:00	43.3	42.5	2.11	0.11
S.E.$_{meas.}$	± 0.868 (mins.)		± 5.028		± 0.789	

From Doroschuk's[33] study the following results are shown for two 14-year-old boys who competed with each other in an all-out treadmill run test, each knowing what the other did, and alternately tested:

It is shown in Table XX that on trial 1, neither boy went really all out, as there was virtually no oxygen debt (0.12 L). Subject K ran before W each round of repeats. K ran 5:00 minutes, then W ran 7:00 minutes (first round), then K ran 7:00 minutes and W ran 8:05, then K ran 8:30 and W ran 9:00. One boy was trying to beat the other. K improved his peak O_2 intake on the second trial, but W ran longer with progressively lower O_2 intake.

Different laboratories have shown different results due to technological differences in equipment and procedures. Using the apparatus at Indiana University, Newton[49] compared the Balke Method (successively elevating the treadmill) with Cureton's "single bag method" (at the Illinois Laboratory) in which the treadmill is not changed but kept at 8.6 per cent grade, 7 mi/hr throughout the test. On the submaximal tests, the results were very different with the Balke method giving higher results but in the all-out test they were closely alike.

EXPERIMENT ON THE EFFECT OF WGO AND OCTACOSANOL ON OXYGEN INTAKE AND DEBT

The Group Experiment, 1964 and 1965

On the basis of the 600-yard run, eighteen of the Sports Fitness School boys, after summer school was over, during August and the first two weeks in September, were tested for peak oxygen intake and net oxygen debt. They were then matched by the 600-yard run, and proved to be satisfactorily matched (cf. Table XXI). The means for the peak O_2 intake were 49.58 and 48.91 cc/min/kg at the start and finish, respectively, of the experiment, corresponding to treadmill run times of 245.67 seconds and 256.33 seconds, respectively; and corresponding to 142 and 138 seconds in the 600-yard run on the track. The standard errors of the two groups were, in the same order: (S.E._{mean diff.}) 1.41 and 1.30 cc/min/kg for peak O_2 intake; 26.58 and 50.72 seconds for the all-out treadmill run; 5.00 and 3.26 seconds for the 600-yard run. The computed t's between the WGO group and the placebo group were all insignificant. The changes in both of the peak O_2 intake groups were also insignificant, namely (-0.38 cc/min/kg), for the WGO group and 1.63 cc/min/kg for the placebo group. But in the 600-yard run the WGO group lost thirteen seconds and also the placebo group lost eight seconds. It is probable that fear of the treadmill complicated this test for the young boys. Since both groups lost, and there was an insignificant difference

TABLE XXI

OXYGEN INTAKE AND ENDURANCE WITHIN GROUP CHANGES
(T_1 to T_2) OVER SIX WEEKS (YOUNG BOYS)

	"Peak" O_2 Intake (ml/min/kg)	Total Energy (Liters of O_2)	Treadmill Time (seconds)	600-yd. Run (seconds)
WGO Group				
T_1 Mean	49.58	7.760	245.67	142
T_2 Mean	49.20	7.762	239.89	129
Mean Diff. (T_2-T_1) .	$-$ 0.38	.002	$-$ 5.78	$-$ 13
S_d	3.98	2.065	75.16	14.15
S.E._{Mean Diff.}	1.41	0.780	26.58	5.00
t	0.27 (N.S.)	0.003 (N.S.)	0.22 (N.S.)	2.60 (.05)
Placebo Group				
T_1 Mean	48.91	11.807	256.33	138
T_2 Mean	50.54	10.025	313.00	130
Mean Diff. (T_2-T_1) .	1.63	$-$ 1.782	56.67	$-$ 8
S_d	3.68	4.864	143.43	9.23
S.E._{Mean Diff.}	1.30	1.838	50.72	3.26
t	1.25 (N.S.)	0.970 (N.S.)	1.12 (N.S.)	2.45 (.05)

N.S. equals not significant
.05 equals significant at the .05 level

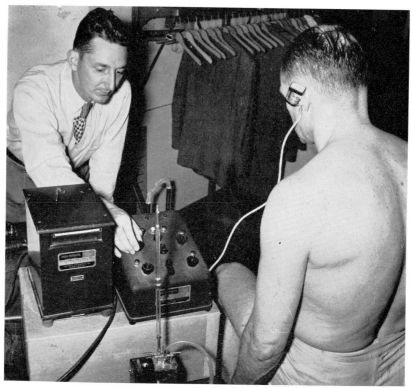

Figure 32. The anoxia photometer equipment for oxygen depletion of ear blood during breath holding.

between the groups ($D = 5$ seconds, the root mean square S.E.$_{\text{mean diff.}}$ was 3.34 cc/min/kg), it was decided to disqualify this experiment for reasons now to be described:

1. The O_2 intake test is not very improvable and some researches have proved it to be dominated by the lean body mass, which is an inherited characteristic, mainly the research of Dr. Vassilis Klissouras, of McGill University reported it to be 86 per cent inherited (at International Sports-Medicine Congress, at Oxford, Sept., 1970).*

2. Unusual errors of fear in some boys complicated the measurement, and some boys ran well, the smaller boys did not.

* *J. App. Physiol.*, 31:338-344 (Sept.), 1971.

Errors of Measurement

Whether the peak oxygen intake test is suitable for measuring the marginal influence of WGO over and above the physical training effect is partly answerable by taking a look at the standard errors of measurement (S.E.$_{meas.}$) obtained from retesting of young boys. Craig Taylor[14] reported the reliability of the O_2 intake test in a hard treadmill run to be 0.70 for L/min, and an average test-retest difference in L/min of 0.264, with S.E.$_{meas.}$ ± 0.013 L/min (this was obtained on thirty-one college age males at Stanford University).

From T_1 to T_2, over the six-weeks period in the summer Sports Fitness School, the means for the peak O_2 intake were 49.58 and 49.20 cc/min/kg, a difference of (−0.38 cc/min/kg), whereas, the S.E.$_{M\ diff.}$ was 1.41, which is larger in itself than the obtained difference, this from the entire program plus the WGO effect. The placebo group was in a similar situation with the T_1 to T_2 means of 48.91 to 50.54, a difference of 1.63 cc/min/kg, respectively. The S.E.$_{meas.}$ was ± 1.30. Both changes were statistically insignificant. The magnitude of these *changes* show in raw score units that neither the boys in our summer Sports Fitness School program, nor the boys in Orban's program changed the peak O_2 intake very much, nor in our controlled experiment in either the WGO or placebo groups, so that is the main difficulty. A case by case analysis shows that some boys improved and some did not (fatigued) and the average change was slight, not beyond the size of 2 S.E.$_{meas.}$ The "sluggishness" of the change is indicated, but the time of the all-out treadmill run lost 5.78 seconds in the WGO group and gained 56.67 seconds in the placebo group, both being statistically insignificant. The fact that some boys went "stale" overwhelmed any possible contribution of WGO. This was likewise the same in the instance of Ganslen's experiment, when the subjects were tested at 10,000 feet of simulated altitude in the decompression chamber. The influence of this stress overwhelmed the subjects and overshadowed the possible effects of the WGO to such an extent that it was indiscernable.

Henry[18] reported the reliability of the O_2 debt test to be only

0.41 (on twenty-five college students) in slow movements and
0.45 in fast movements. Taylor reported the reliability of the
maximal O_2 intake test to be 0.59 with open circuit, whereas,
Mitchell reported 0.88 and Taylor 0.70. Our subjects were worse.

SOME RESULTS COMPARED BEFORE AND AFTER THE SAME PHYSICAL TRAINING PROGRAM ON MAXIMAL O_2 INTAKE AND ON THE ALL-OUT TREADMILL RUN FOR TIME

The group data do not show consistent results in favor of
wheat germ oil over the matched groups on placeboes. This is,
of course, by comparing the means of the groups and testing the
statistical significance between the groups. Nevertheless, a study
of four sets of pairs who went through the testing together show
the nature of the discrepancies—to indicate why the errors of
measurement are so large.

It is clear that the reliability of the maximal O_2 intake work is
not as good as the reliability of the all-out runs on the treadmill,
computed from retest data. H. L. Taylor[48] reported the rather low
reliabilities of 0.59 for O_2 intake retests in the submaximal work
and 0.70 in the maximal work tests. The r_{11} data for the 600-yard
run for time on a flat, circular track are much better, and also the
all-out treadmill r_{11} data are about 0.90 as an average. Various
other limitations of the maximal O_2 intake test are given. Such
poor reliability in the peak O_2 intake test would cause large
standard errors of measurement.

There is a wide discrepancy in the comparison of the maximal
O_2 intake results and the all-out treadmill run results in these
four cases, and in a cross-sectional study the prediction of all-out
run time was as high as 0.319 in a study reported by Doroschuk,
Bernauer, Bosco and Cureton[2] made in the Physical Fitness Research Laboratory with the same equipment. The prediction in
terms for liters/min was better, 0.508 and liters/kg 0.935. The
liters/min/kg or cc/min/kg is considered the best measure to determine the relative value of the aerobic O_2 intake. The results
are disappointing and show that the test is too crude to be ex-

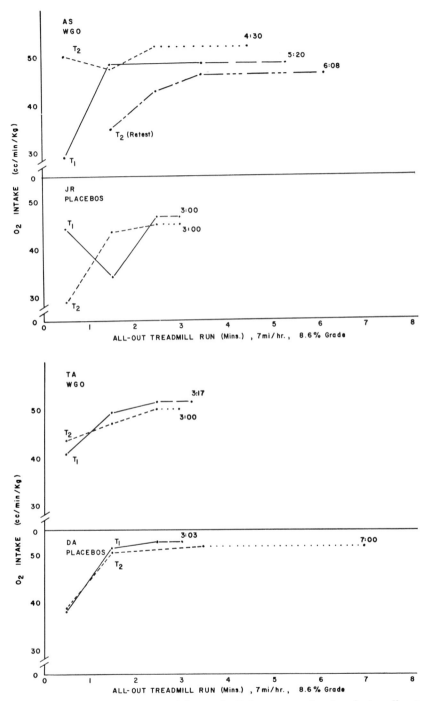

Figure 33. Matched pairs of boys (WGO versus placeboes) in all-out treadmill runs (7 mi/hr/8.6% grade) A.S. versus J.R. and T.A. versus D.A.

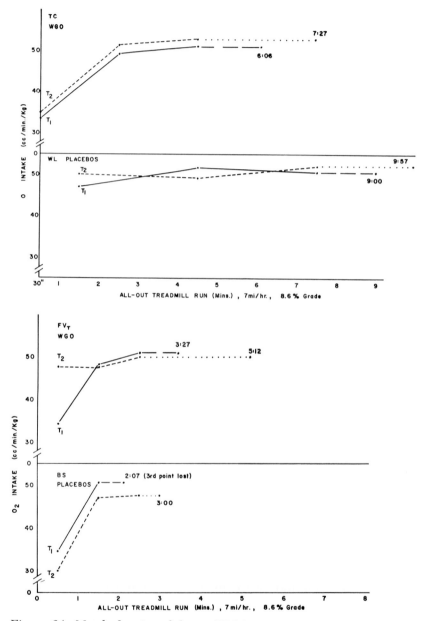

Figure 34. Matched pairs of boys (WGO versus placeboes) in all-out treadmill runs (7 mi/hr/8.6% grade) T.C. versus W.L. and F.V. versus B.S.

pected to measure the difference due to the effect of the wheat germ oil, the changes being from T_1 (49.58 seconds to 49.20 at T_2), and the difference (−0.38) was insignificant.

However, to complete the record the data of these experiments are given as a guide for what they are worth to further investigators. It can only be said that the test was too crude to measure the result expected.

The Evidence of Paired Cases

Four pairs of subjects are represented on the graphs 33a, 33b, 34a and 34b matched by preliminary all-out treadmill run times.

Pair I—A.S. (on WGO capsules versus J.R. on placebo capsules).

A.S. (experimental). 9 yrs., 76 lb. (34.5 kg.), 55.25 inches tall.

Subject A.S. ran 5:20 on WGO at T_1 and on T_2 ran 4:30 but with an improvement in Maximal O_2 Intake from 48.5 to 52 cc/min/kg in the All-Out Treadmill Run, 8.6 per cent grade, 7 mi/hr. In a second try he ran 6:08 on a Maximal O_2 Intake of 46.5 cc/min/kg.

J.R. (control), 11 yrs., 120 lb. (54 kg.), 61.25 inches tall.

The control subject, J.R., on T_1 ran 3:00 on 46.7 cc/min/kg of oxygen supply. In the retest (T_2) he ran 3:00 on 45.7 cc/min/kg of oxygen.

There is lack of agreement between maximal O_2 intake and the all-out run time. In the retest he ran better but did not develop as high maximal O_2 intake. Other factors, perhaps mental attitude or perhaps being a bit more rested the second time, might explain the discrepancy. Obviously other factors than O_2 intake are operating. Subject J.R. was visibly exhausted after 1:30 minutes on the treadmill. By encouragement he went on 3:00 minutes. Both boys had the same terminal heart rate of 210 b/min. at T_1 and had the terminal blood pressures of 143/59 and 175/78 on T_1; at T_2 the corresponding pulse rates were 210 for A.S. and 192 for J.R.; blood pressures were 144/68 for A.S. and 140/70 for J.R.

Subject A.S. on WGO capsules for the eight weeks did better in the all-out run and also gained 3.5 cc/min/kg compared to a loss of 1.5 cc/min/kg for subject J.R. who ran 3:00 both times, being on placeboes.

Pair II—T.A. is compared with D.A. T.A. took WGO capsules, while D.A. took placebo capsules, same amount and same size. Both took the same physical training program for eight weeks.

T.A. (experimental), 8 yrs., 59 lb. (27 kg.), 53 ins. tall.

T.A. (on WGO) ran 3:17 on T_1 and 3:00 on T_2, the Maximal O_2 Intake being 51.6 cc/min/kg for T.A. and 52.7 for D.A. at the beginning T_1 trials. The corresponding run times were 3:17 for T.A. and 3:03 for D.A. Over the eight-week period with both boys on the same training program, T.A. lost a bit on his T_2 All-Out Run and dropped from 3:17 to 3:00, and the Maximal O_2 Intake dropped from 51.6 to 50.1 cc/min/kg. Weight change was from 59 to 60.5 lb.

D.A. (control), 8 yrs., 52.0 lb. (27 kg.), 52 ins. tall.

D.A. (on placeboes) dropped from 52.7 to 51.6, but the T_2 Run Time was 7:00 a great improvement from 3:03 on his first official run (T_1). The body weight of D.A. elevated from 59 to 59.5 lb.

Both boys appeared to be a bit tired, as the retests in August were made in very hot weather. It is very interesting that with subject D.A. there appears to be no agreement at all between the improvement in maximal O_2 intake and the improvement in all-out run time. Actually, the maximal O_2 intake was lower on the second run (at T_2) than at T_1 but the time of the run was just the opposite, being a very great improvement from 3:03 to 7:00 without the corresponding improvement in maximal O_2 intake. This would suggest that other factors were operating to make possible the performance, whereas, willpower, fitness in the central nervous system and reduction in weight could have explained a longer run in the face of a lowered cc/min/kg of maximal O_2 intake. This should certainly make anyone wary of saying that the run time could be exactly accounted for by the maximal O_2 intake. Both boys carried out the same program together under the same instructor.

Pair III—T.C. is compared with W.L. T.A. took WGO capsules and W.L. took placebo capsules. Both boys took the same program under the same instructor for eight weeks.

T.C. (experimental), 11 yrs., 84 lb. (38 kg.), 57.75 ins. tall.

T.C. improved from 51.6 cc/min/kg to 53.2 cc/min/kg in the eight weeks, and the corresponding improvement in the All-Out Treadmill Run Time was from 6:00 to 7:27.

W.L. (control), 13 yrs.,

W.L. improved from 52.2 cc/min/kg at T_1 to

106 lb. (48 kg.), 63.75 ins. tall.

60.7 cc/min/kg at T_2 on Maximal O_2 Intake, and the corresponding improvement was from 9:00 to 9:57 in the All-Out Treadmill Run.

The improvement was greater for T.C. on WGO compared to W.L. on placeboes but the boys were not well matched in either maximal O_2 intake nor on the treadmill all-out run time. The program appeared to improve both boys a bit in both maximal O_2 intake and all-out treadmill run time.

Pair IV—Comparison of F.V. and B.S. F.V. was on WGO capsules and B.S. was on placebo capsules.

F.V. 9 yrs., 61 lb. (28 kg.), 54.25 ins. tall versus B.S. (control).

F.V. began (T_1) with Maximal O_2 Intake at 34.5 cc/min/kg compared to B.S. at 34.6 cc/min/kg. On the T_1 tests, F.V. ran 3:27 and B.S. ran 2:07 in the All-Out Treadmill Run. In the retests at T_2 after eight weeks of training as nearly the same as could be arranged under the same instructor at the same time, F.V. improved from 3:27 to 5:12 while taking WGO, whereas, B.S. improved from 2:07 to 3:00 on placeboes. The starting level of Maximal O_2 Intake was very nearly the same, which was the basis of matching. The advantage in the running test was very much with the boy who took the WGO throughout the training. However, in the Maximal O_2 Intake Test, F.V. deteriorated from 50.7 cc/min/kg to 50.0 cc/min/kg, actually remaining just about the same in spite of approximately three hours of calisthenics, games and running per day, five days per week. B.S. also lost in Maximal O_2 Intake status but lost more relatively than F.V. B.S. deteriorated from 50.7 to 47.6 cc/min/kg in spite of running somewhat longer, 3:07, compared to the T_1 time of 2:07.

Again it is clear that there is a wide discrepancy between the maximal O_2 intake status and the corresponding all-out run time. The run test was quite reliable ($r_{11} = 0.90$) and the 600-yard run for time was similarly checked as 0.821 in 1964 and 0.979 in 1965. Taylor's[48] results show 0.70 for the maximal O_2 intake from retests on the same subjects. The exact source of the difficulty is not known except that it is not in the analysis of the gases or the collection technique, as the apparatus and methodology was the same. It is apparent that the subjects are different, either physiologically (more or less glycogen loading) or are differently motivated from time to time. In retesting one boy several times, wide discrepancies were found with motivational levels.

THE FARRELL-GIER STUDY AT KANSAS STATE UNIVERSITY (1965)

Farrell[11] studied the effect of octacosanol on the swimming time of rats in a thirty-minute swim to near exhaustion and carefully measured O_2 debt for sixty minutes after each swim. The rats were divided into five groups according to the amount of octacosanol in the diets: Controls, .0001% and Experimentals, .001% and .01% of octacosanol. The hypothesis was that the animals who had relatively more of the octacosanol in their diets would have less O_2 debt in the exhaustion tests. The results showed that these octacosanol animals consumed relatively less oxygen (significant at .01) during the sixty minutes of recovery time used for all animals after the thirty-minute swim (Fig. 36). It is interesting that the octacosanol required 3-4 weeks to begin

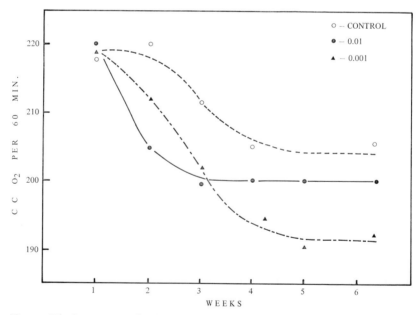

Figure 35. Oxygen uptake by mice in recovery, octacosanol versus control diet (Farrell-Gier Experiment).

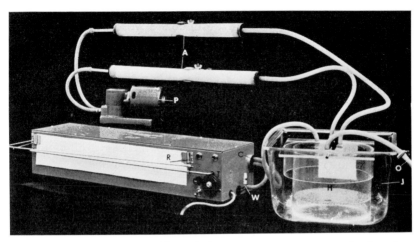

Figure 36. Apparatus (Farrell-Gier) for measuring oxygen uptake in mice.

to show a difference and 4-5 weeks to develop a significant difference. There was an insignificant difference in swimming time between the groups. The .001 level of octacosanol was more economical than for a .01 level (Fig. 35).

Oxygen Debt Capacity as Affected by Octacosanol and Wheat Germ Oil

Farrell[41] studied the effects of differential octacosanol on the O_2 consumed during sixty minutes of recovery after a thirty-minute swim to near exhaustion, using rats and mice as subjects. The rats were divided into five groups according to the percentage of octacosanol in their diet: control, .0001 per cent; .001 per cent; .01 per cent; and .1 per cent; similarly, the mice were placed into three groups: control, .0001 per cent, .001 per cent and .01 per cent. The hypothesis was that animals receiving higher proportions of octacosanol in their diet would incur less of an O_2 debt from the standardized thirty-minute swim. The findings indicated no significant differences in the swimming time among the five groups of rats; however, Farrell reported that, "Adult rats that received 0.01 and 0.001 per cent octacosanol in the feed required consistently less oxygen during the recovery period than animals of the same weight on control feed." This suggests an induced factor of oxygen economy attributable to octacosanol.

The results of the mice experiments revealed that the two groups on .01 per cent and .001 per cent octacosanol body consumed significantly less oxygen (p. .01) than the control group during the sixty minutes of recovery after the standard thirty-minute swim. This is graphically shown in Figure 35. It is interesting that with successive swim tests an adaptation apparently took place such that the O_2 debt became less as the animals became increasingly adapted. Farrell sums up her results thusly: "Octacosanol, as a good additive, provided results equal or superior to those obtained from comparable animals maintained on the same food without octacosanol."

CONCLUSIONS OF THE EFFECTS OF OCTACOSANOL AND WHEAT GERM ON THE "PEAK" OXYGEN INTAKE TEST AND NET O_2 DEBT

The "peak" O_2 intake test with humans is too crude a test (sluggish) to show the changes due to the possible effects of the dietary supplements. It is shown that the test is too variable, especially with small boys, who become overtrained easily and otherwise react adversely to the all-out run test on the treadmill.

In the paired cases, shown graphically, some boys respond very definitely to wheat germ oil and others do not. This may be simply a reflection of the severity of the training through which they were going. But the inconsistency of the results are noted, in that the Placebo group improved in the 600-yard run but did not improve in the "peak" O_2 intake test in anything like the same proportion. In the WGO group there was actually a loss in "peak" O_2 intake and a slight loss in both the "peak" O_2 intake group and in the 600-yard run time.

Consideration of the S.E.$_{meas.}$ from other experiments also show that these errors are also too large to permit the detection of small differences, and in many subjects there is a great inconsistency between the performance time becoming longer without a parallel increase in "peak" O_2 intake, with some subjects running longer on relatively less "peak" O_2 intake.

The O_2 debt test was even worse, as other experimenters have testified. Consideration of the reliability of the coefficients as determined in our own experiment and also by other experimenters shows that this test is too unreliable to use in this type of experiment.

The results of this section are inconclusive, and mainly due to the crudeness of the tests of this type with humans. There is also great difficulty interpreting the "peak" O_2 intake test, as the lengthy presentation of the many factors supposedly in it shows.

In some of the individual "paired" cases, with one boy on WGO and the other on placeboes, some respond to WGO and some do not.

REFERENCES

1. Adams, William C.: Relationship and possible cause effect of selected variables to treadmill endurance running performance, *Res. Quart.*, 38:515-526, Dec., 1967.
2. Doroschuk, E., Bernauer, E., Bosco, J. and Cureton, T. K.: Prediction of all-out treadmill running time in young boys in the sports-fitness school, University of Illinois, *Aust. J. Phys. Ed.*, No. 29, 36-40, 1963.
3. Haskell, W. L.: The Relationships Between Certain Objective Tests of Motivation, Motor Performance Measures, Highest Oxygen Intake, Oxygen Debt and All-Out Treadmill Run Time, Urbana, M.S. in Physical Education, University of Illinois, 1963.
4. Cureton, T. K.: Treadmill tests of maximum physical efficiency, pp. 314-350 in *Physical Fitness of Champion Athletes.* Urbana, Ill., University Press, 1951.
5. Cureton, T. K.: Improvements in oxygen intake capacity resulting from sports and exercise training programs: A review, *Amer. Corrective Ther. J.*, 23:144-147, Sept.-Oct., 1969.
6. Robinson, S.: Metabolic adaptations to exhaustive work as affected by training, *Amer. J. Physiol.*, 133:428, 1941.
7. Ganslen, R. V.: The Influence of Training Upon Aerobic and Anaerobic Metabolic Variables, Urbana, Ill., Ph.D. thesis, University of Illinois, 1953, p. 135.
8. Huesner, W. W.: Progressive Changes in the Physical Fitness of an Adult Male During a Season of Training for Competitive Swimming, Urbana, Ph.D. thesis, Physical Education, Urbana, University of Illinois, 1955; and pp. 80-82 in Cureton, *The Physiological Effects of Exercise Programs on Adults*, Springfield, Ill., Thomas, 1969.
9. Cureton, T. K. and Phillips, E. E.: Changes Induced in Eight Weeks of Training, Non-Training and Re-Training, Urbana, Ph.D. thesis, Physical Education, University of Illinois, 1960; and in *J. Sports Med.*, 4:87, 1964.
10. Pollock, M. L., Cureton, T. K. and Greninger, L.: Effects of frequency

of training on working capacity, cardiovascular function and body composition of adult man, *Med. Sci. Sports*, 70-74, June, 1969.

11. Åstrand, P-O and Christensen, E. H.: Aerobic work capacity, reprint from *The Animal Organism*. London, Symposium Report, Pergamon Press, 1964.

12. Orban, William A. R.: An Analysis of Measurement of Organic Efficiency of Boys, Urbana, Ph.D. in Physical Education, University of Illinois, 1957, p. 199.

13. Margaria, R.: Capacity and power of the energy processes in muscle activity: Their practical relevance in athletics, *Int. Z. Angew. Physiol.*, 25:352-360, 1968.

14. Taylor, C.: Some properties of maximal and sub-maximal exercise with reference to physiological variation and measurement of exercise tolerance, *Amer. J. Physiol.*, 142:200-212, 1944.

15. Taylor, H. L., Buskirk, E. and Henschel, A.: Maximal oxygen intake as an objective measure of cardio-respiratory performance, 8:73-80, 1955.

16. Åstrand, P-O.: *Experimental Studies of Physical Working Capacity in Relation to Sex and Age*. Copenhagen, Munksgaard, 1952, p. 171.

17. Robinson, S.: Experimental studies of physical fitness in relation to age, *Arbeitsphysiologie*, 10:251, 1958.

18. Henry, F. M. and J. de Moor: Metabolic efficiency of exercise in relation to work load at constant speed, *J. Appl. Physiol.*, 2:481, 1950.

19. Kaijser, Lennart: Limiting factors for aerobic muscle performance, *Acta Physiol. Scand.*, 346, 1970, p. 96.

20. Dill, D. B., Edwards, H. T. and Talbott, J. H.: Factors limiting the capacity for work, *J. Physiol.*, 77:49, 1932.

21. Wright, S.: Correlation and causation, *J. Ag. Res.*, 20:562-98, 1921, and also, see Abelson, H. H.: *The Art of Educational Research*, Yonkers, N. Y., World Book Co., 1933; and Cureton, T. K.: *Endurance of Young Men*, 1945; Adams, W. C.: *Res. Quart.*, 38:515-527, 1965.

22. Sloninger, E. L.: The Relationship of Stress Indicators to Pre-Ejection Cardiac Intervals, Urbana, Ph.D. in Physical Education, University of Illinois, 1966.

23. Holmgren, A.: The oxygen conduction line of the human body, pp. 391-400 in *Karger's Symposium on Cardiovascular Fitness*. Kingston, Ontario, 1966.

24. Mayfield, Gail E.: Prediction of Maximal Oxygen Intake from Selected Fitness Variables, Urbana, Ill., M.S. thesis, Phys. Ed., University of Illinois, 1968.

25. Faulkner, J. A., *et al.*: Maximum cardiovascular responses to bicycling and running, *The Physiologist* (University of Michigan's Medical School), Ann Arbor, Michigan, No. 3, April, 1970, p. 195.

26. Cureton, T. K.: In *Physical Fitness of Champion Athletes*, 1951, p. 356.

27. Åstrand, P-O and Saltin, B.: *J. Appl. Physiol.*, 17:487-491, 1962; and 16:977, 1961.

28. Behnkee, A. H.: *Human Biol.*, 31:295-315, 1959; *ibid.*, 31:213-234, 1959.

29. Taylor, H. L. and Buskirk, E.: Maximal O₂ intake as an objective measure of cardio-respiratory performance, *Amer. J. Physiol.*, 8:73-80, 1955; and *Amer. J. Physiol.*, 11:72-78, 1957.

30. Cotes, J. E., Davies, C. M. T. and Healy, M. J. R.: Factors relating to maximal oxygen intake in young adult male and female subjects, *Proc. Physiol. Soc.*, Jan., 1967; *J. Physiol. (London)*, 189:79-80, 1967.

31. Sherman, M. A.: Maximal Oxygen Intake Changes of Experimentally Exercised Junior High Boys, Urbana, Ph.D. thesis, Physical Education, University of Illinois, 1967, p. 223.

32. Adama, W. C.: Relationship and Possible Causal Effect of Selected Variables to Treadmill Endurance Running Performance, *Res. Quart.*, 38:515-527, Dec., 1967.

33. Doroschuk, E.: The Prediction of All-Out Treadmill Running of Young Boys from Oxygen Utilization Measures, Urbana, M.S. thesis, Physical Education, University of Illinois, 1957, p. 51.

34. Saltin, B.: Physiological effects of physical conditioning, *Med. Sci. Sports*, 1:50-56, March, 1969.

35. Buskirk, E. R. and Taylor, H. L.: Maximal oxygen intake and its relation to body composition with special reference to chronic physical capacity and obesity, *J. Appl. Physiol.*, 11:72-78, 1957.

36. Doroschuk, E.: *op. cit.*, ref. 33.

37. Weber, H.: A Quantitative Study of Eosinopenia and Other Stress Indices, Urbana, Ph.D. thesis, Physical Education, University of Illinois, 1965, p. 321.

38. Steggerda, F. R.: The role of the nervous system in fitness, pp. 68-72 in *Exercise and Fitness* (Stanley, Cureton, Barry and Huelster), Chicago, The Athletic Institute, 1960.

39. Selye, Hans: The physiology and pathology of exposure to stress, Montreal, Canada, Acta, Inc., 1951-56; and in Raab: *The Prevention of Ischemic Heart Disease*, Springfield, Ill., Thomas, 1966.

40. Zimkin, N. V. and Korobokov, A. V.: The importance of physical exercise as a factor of increasing resistance of the body to unfavorable influence under conditions of modern civilization, pp. 63-68 in *XVI Weltkongress für Sportmedicin*, 1966 (Hannover).

41. Farrell, P. R.: The Effects of Octacosanol on Conception and Reproduction on Maintenance and Growth of Young, and on Oxygen Uptake in the White Rat, Manhattan, Kansas, M.S. thesis, Kansas State University, 1965.

42. Karpovich, P. V.: *Arch. Path.* (Chicago), 15:828, 1933.

43. Orban, Wm. A. R.: An Analysis of Measurements of Organic Efficiency of Boys, p. 59, Urbana, Ph.D. thesis, Physical Education, University of Illinois, 1957.

44. Brown, Stanley R.: Factors Influencing Improvement in the Oxygen Intake of Young Boys, Urbana, Illinois, Ph.D. thesis, Physical Education, University of Illinois, 1960, p. 170.

45. Cooper, K. H.: A means of assessing maximal oxygen intake, *J.A.M.A.,* 203:201-204, Jan. 15, 1968.

46. Ribisl, P. M. and Kachidorian, W. M.: Maximal oxygen intake prediction in young and middle-aged males, *J. Sports Med.,* 2:17-22, March, 1969.

47. Faulkner, J. A.: New perspectives in training for maximal performance, *J.A.M.A.,* 205:741-746, Sept. 9, 1968; and in *The Physiologist,* p. 195, No. 3, April, 1970.

48. Moncrief, J.: Individual differences, reliabilities and intercorrelations of oxygen intake measures, *J. Sports Med.,* 8:153-157, Sept., 1968.

49. Newton, J. L.: The assessment of maximal oxygen intake, *J. Sports Med.,* 3:164-169, June-Sept., 1963.

Chapter V

The Effect of Wheat Germ, Wheat Germ Oil and Octacosanol on Total Body Reaction Time (The Garrett-Cureton Test)

THE NERVOUS BASIS OF PHYSICAL FITNESS

IT is well known that the mobility of the human body slows with age. This is especially so with respect to reaction time. Pierson and Montoye[1] have reported on such slowing with age. This slowing up of the mind-body (neuromuscular) reactions to sound and visual stimuli is synonymous with unfitness, and has long been represented by speed and agility tests in physical education programs. Sluggishness of these *total-body* speed and agility reactions is to be expected with aging, although they can be improved to a certain extent by practice of fast reactions, as is shown in many studies. Perhaps most of the decline is due to default.

The slowing of the reactions has also been related to poor nutrition, and to the slowing of the ability of the kidneys to clear the wastes from the system.[2, 3] Possibly sweating through physical labor has some cleaning effect. By regular agility exercises and by the intake of somewhat more vitamin B₁ and C and rather large dosages of vitamin E, as claimed by Dr. Shute,[4] the reactions of the body may be improved. In the slowing up of the reaction responses, the mind-body coordinations seem to become impaired. Brozek[6] has reviewed a number of Pavlonian type experiments which show that *any* principal nutritive deficiency will cause a slowing of the mind-body conditioned reflexes. Improvement is logically related to removing any such deficiency.

This study explores the possible effects of wheat germ, wheat germ oil (VioBin, low temperature extracted brand) and its derivative, octacosanol, on the Total Body Reaction Time Test of Garrett-Cureton, in use at the University of Illinois Physical Fitness Laboratory since about 1947. While called Total Body Reaction Time Test (TBRT) it is both a reaction time test and a response of movement test. These factors usually not being separated. Some considerable experimentation has been done with this test at the Illinois laboratory,* therefore it was chosen for this part of the investigation of the possible effect of such nutritional supplements as mentioned. After certain preliminary data began to show a possible relationship (Experiments 1, 8 and 13, Part Two) other experiments were added, which are described because the preliminary experiments did not require matching of the initial parallel comparative groups, it was reasonably certain that these experiments would be more meaningful if run on the matched group pattern, with concentration upon the Total Body Reaction Time. The added experiments were conducted by Cureton and Wiggett (No. 24, 1965), Johnson and Cureton (No. 26, 1966), Milesis and Cureton and Richter (No. 31, 1968). These are all described in Part Two but need to be collated and compared in this brief review.

In preliminary learning for five weeks, with an eight-minute long bicycle ride with light resistance, it was shown that this type of warm-up helped a bit (.01 second of Total Body Reaction Time). It was also shown that the TBRT test improved from 0.200 seconds to an average of 0.160 seconds with warm-up and repetitious testing. As a result, in Experiment 25 it was decided to use the eight-minute warm-up with each subject, then give the TBRT test. This experiment demonstrated that the reaction times averaged 0.030 seconds slower at the start of the experiment than for the control; this was reversed after five months so that the experimental subject taking WGO averaged 0.010 seconds faster than the control who did not take the WGO supplements. The test was given for every subject after the eight minute warm-up on the standardized ergometer bicycle. The other standards for administration are also described later, and also the equipment used. In order to properly interpret the results it is better to review briefly what research has revealed about such reaction time tests. If a nutrient could systematically improve the TBRT test, it might be generalized that a basic deficiency exists in the diet of the subjects used in these experiments. If

---

* See references 7, 8, 9, 10, 11, 12, 13, 14, 15.

the deficiency is removed by WGO or octacosanol, it would seem clear that not enough of such fresh, natural (uncooked) oils are available in the diet and that WGO or octacosanol are basic in their aid to the mind-body reactions.

THE RELATED LITERATURE OF HUMAN REACTION TIME

Definition of Terms

Reaction time is defined by *Taber's Cyclopedic Medical Dictionary* as "The time elapsing between giving a stimulus . . . and the response to it." *Gould and Dye Medical Dictionary* define reaction time as:

> A certain interval necessarily elapses between the time of application of the stimulus and the moment at which the resulting action takes place, say muscular response. . . . For voluntary response a somewhat similar reaction is required from the time one wills to do a certain act before the impulse can be set up, transmitted to the part involved, and the elicitation of the response within it.

Griffith[16] defines reaction time through the nervous system, stating that it is due to the inertia of the nervous system and the time it takes for the nervous impulse to pass from one part of the system to another. Thus, he says, "the time will be longest when the path to be traversed is the most complex." In these terms the response used is a complex one, since it involves the response of the whole body to the stimuli involved, thus making the transversion of the nervous response comparably complex.

Woodworth and Scholsberg[17] define reaction time as the time necessary to get a response started. The reaction time is thus a *stimulus-response time interval.* The response cannot come out of the organism until it reaches the muscles and produces an observable effect on the environment. The sense organs must be aroused to activity and the nerves must conduct to the brain, and from the brain to the muscles, and the muscles must contract. All these steps in the process take some time, but the most time is taken in the brain where the work must be done. Even in the simplest possible reaction the nerve impulses coming in from the sense organ have to accumulate and build up enough excitation to arouse the motor areas of the brain and set up a discharge towards the muscles.

Nature of Reaction Time

Garrett[18] lists the following factors as influences of reaction time:

1. Complexity of stimulus situation.
2. Particular sense organ stimulated.
3. Part of sense organ stimulated.
4. Intensity, size and duration of stimulus.
5. Fore-period (time interval between the signal "ready" and the presentation of the stimulus).
6. Practice attention, distraction and fatigue.
7. Incentives, punishment, drugs and age.

Teichner[19] makes the following generalizations about simple reaction time, which he states has been reasonably well established (the author, as a result of this study, does not agree with all of these generalizations implicitly—the reasons will be given in a later part of this chapter).

1. There is a positive correlation between visual and auditory reaction times.
2. Simultaneous stimulation of more than one sense modality produces faster reaction time than stimulation of just one. On the other hand, successive stimulation of different senses produces slower reaction time than stimulation of a single sensory channel.
3. For visual and thermal reaction times the greater the extent of the stimulus in space, i.e. the greater the number of reactors stimulated, the faster the speed of reaction up to some limit.
4. Under daylight or illuminated conditions the visual reaction time becomes longer the greater the distance of the stimulation from the fovea.
5. In the case of each receptor system, reaction time is a negatively accelerated decreasing function of intensity up to a maximum intensity value, after which, reaction time either becomes suddenly lengthened, the function at this

point being discontinuous, or asymptotic to a physiological limit.

6. Reaction time is a slowly falling function of growth with chronological age, until about thirty years after which it is a slowly rising function.

7. In general, the reaction time of the human male is faster than that of the female.

8. The optimum fore-period of reaction time may be thought of as lying in a range of 1.5 and 8 seconds. Its position in this range is determined by a large number of factors including duration and intensity of the warning signal and of the stimulus, and the amount, locus and time of production of muscular tension.

9. Reaction time is related to the length, direction or speed of movement of the responding member.

10. Under vigilance conditions, the longer the period under which the subject must respond, the longer the reaction time.

Kleitman and Jackson[20] found that reaction time varied directly with temperature during daytime hours.

Relationship Between Speed of Movement (MT) and Reaction Time (RT)

Westerlund and Tuttle[21] used twenty-two University of Iowa track men in an investigation of the relationship between speed of running events in track and reaction time. The speed of movement measure involved was a 75-yard sprint and the reaction time recorded was a single response to a light stimulus. The results revealed that the champion athletes reacted faster than all the other groups. This was also the case in Cureton's[22] results, i.e. that champion athletes reacted faster than any other group.

Beise and Peasely[23] measured the RT and MT of forty-seven women skilled in golf, tennis and archery, and fourteen unskilled performers. The authors found the skilled performers to be significantly faster in both RT and MT, when they were compared with the unskilled group.

As a summary to the relationship between reaction time and movement time, Henry[24] writes:

> Current theories on reaction latency and movement speed suggest that individual differences in these two phases of neuromotor responses should be essentially uncorrelated. It has been held that response latency is determined by the nature and complexity of the stored neuromotor "program," or motor memory, that requires time to be selected and read out to the motor nerves. The speed of movement is theoretically determined by the difference factor, namely, strength of act, which is controlled by the effectiveness of the program in causing the appropriate muscles to create or apply force to the limbs and thus cause movement.

De May[25] indicated that either visual, auditory, visual and auditory, or total average reaction time of the former three would give an adequate relative index of a person's ability to react quickly when using the Garrett-Cureton TBRT Test.

From Von Ebers[26] study, it is obvious that the athletic type of student reacts faster than other types of students tested. Kastrinos[22] further developed this by establishing that mesomorphs react faster than any of the other body type classifications; combinations of mesomorphs and medials were above the average, or average, in reaction time, but the endomorphs and ectomorphs, particularly, were distinctly poorer than average. Olympic candidates and physical education majors were significantly faster than any of the five groups Kastrinos tested.

Moore[27] found the total body reaction time to be a definite factor in fitness, and noted that it was subject to change following a conditioning program and that it had a significant correlation with strength per pound of body weight. Elbel[28] found response time also shortened by athletic competition. Landry[29] from a study of the boys in the Illinois University Summer Sports-Fitness School of 1953 and 1954 found there was a significant increase in combined visual-auditory reaction time; this was traceable to an induced transient fatigue.

Westerlund and Tuttle[30] found the mean reaction time of track men to be distinctly different among the various participants. The short-distance men responded fastest, the middle-distance men were next, while of three groups the long-distance men had the slowest reaction time.

Thompson[31] from an analysis of her results makes the following conclusions:

1. Significant differences existed between women who are skilled volleyball players and women who were beginning volleyball players in their ability to perform the total body reaction time, total body movement time, directional response and decision response times. The skilled players react more quickly in all tests.

2. There is a significant relationship between simple reaction time and total body reaction time.

3. A significant relationship also exists between total body reaction time and total body movement time.

4. The ability to perform the wall volley, in volleyball, is significantly related to total body movement time, directional response time, and decision response time.

5. Volleyball playing ability, as rated by judges, was significantly related to total body reaction time, total body movement time, directional response time and decision response time.

THE EFFECTS OF DIETARY SUPPLEMENTS ON TOTAL BODY REACTION TIMES AND MUSCULAR TONE

The Effects of Dietary Supplement and Warm-Up On the Vertical Jump Reaction Time

In this study, reaction time was measured by the time it takes to respond to a stimulus with a vertical jump. The coordinating mechanism of this movement is comprised of the following factors:

1. Sensory perception—visual sensibility, auditory sensibility and equilibratory sensibility.

2. Startle reaction—temporary inhibition of movement.

3. Chemical state of the neuromuscular junctions—end plates.

4. Strength of the responding muscles.

5. Tone of the responding muscles.

6. Viscosity of the responding muscles.

Insofar as the literature seemed to indicate that training, warm-up and dietary supplement did effect the reaction time of an individual, the authors of this study sought to substantiate or refute these findings by further experiments.

The dietary supplement used in this study was whole, fresh wheat germ oil or a derivative containing a long-chain alcohol extract from VioBin wheat germ oil (octacosanol) or wheat germ itself (Kretchmer brand). Octacosanol is derived from WGO.

Of the eight reaction time studies, seven showed an advantage for the wheat germ-related dietary supplement (WGO, octacosanol or wheat germ) over the placeboes in improving the total body reaction time. Marx'[32] study was the only one to show a negative result, i.e. no advantage for either the dietary supplement or the placebo. Although this type of analysis does not indicate the relative magnitude of the changes, it nonetheless points to the consistent trend in favor of the wheat germ-related dietary supplement in improving reaction time. That these improvements were evidenced seems to agree with other evidence (studies on brachial pulse wave, T-wave of ECG, etc.) that the dietary supplements exert their favorable influence on endurance via an improved functioning of the nervous system rather than changes in the oxygen transport system.

Work on muscle dystrophy and atrophy and vitamins (notably vitamin E and B-complex[33]) has been conducted in the past without any definite conclusions, since most of this work contradicts itself from one study to the next, or the sampling methods used were too scant to draw any valid conclusions. A generous conclusion by Wechsler, Mayer and Sobotka's[34] work serves as a summary for the work done on dietary supplement in this direction. They give us a fairly-substantiated result which seems to indicate that there is a definite correlation between tocopherol level and muscular dystrophies. But this extreme dystrophy state is not the focus of the present experiments, which are limited to normal human male subjects.

The Vertical Jump Reaction Timer
Reliability

De May[15] states that the reliability of the Illinois Reaction Timer Test has been established by both the split-halves and also

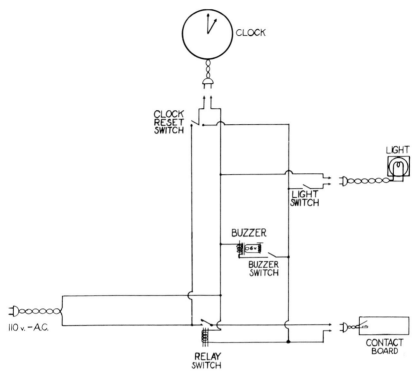

Figure 37. Circuit diagram for Garrett-Cureton total body reaction timer.

the test retest procedure. Both methods produced correlation co-efficients which are sufficiently high to assure the reliability of testing procedure (i.e. greater than 0.80 with men).*

Cureton[22] describes the reaction timer used in this study. The apparatus consists of the following: (Figs. 37, 38, 39, 40)

1. Stimulus unit.
2. Response unit.
3. Recording device.

An auditory, visual and a visual-auditory stimulus together are presented to the subject by an operator. The presentation of the stimulus and starting of the clock are synchronized. The

---

* The correlation coefficients are lower with small boys (Cureton and Barry's *Improving the Physical Fitness of Youth*, 1964).

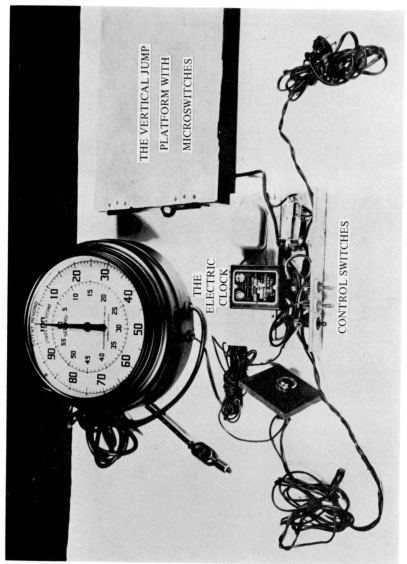

Figure 38. Equipment used in the Garrett-Cureton total body reaction timer.

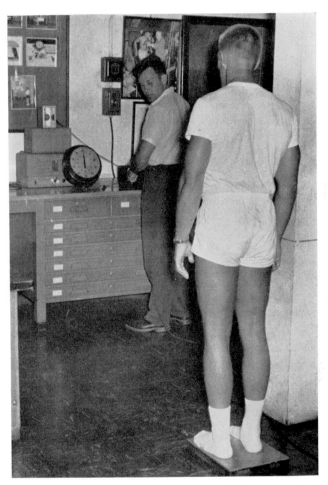

Figure 39. The subject on the vertical jump platform, ready for signal (visual, auditory or combined).

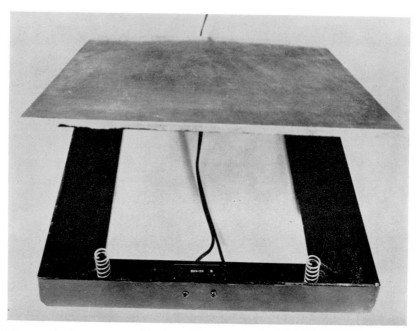

Figure 40. The contact block with microswitches and powerful springs.

stimulus unit consists of the platform, switch, and light or buzzer in series with an electric clock. With the "light" switch on, pressure on the stimulus button on the top of the box produces the electric light stimulus—similarly with the buzzer or with the light and buzzer together.

1. The Stimulus Unit

The unit is so constructed that it operates only when the subject is on the platform—toes even with the narrow unhinged side. Movement of the platform, by as little as $\frac{1}{32}$ inch, breaks the contact and stops the clock, which has been set in motion by the stimulus from the operator given from the control box. The light stimulus is directly before the subject, about waist level; when the stimulus button is pressed instantaneously the auditory stimulus buzzer sounds, or the light flashes on, or both of the stimuli go on as a unit, until contact is broken by the small vertical jump on the platform by the subject. The subjects jump as quickly as they could after perceiving or hearing the stimulus.

2. The Response Unit

The response unit consists of a platform of sheet aluminum one-fourth inch thick with an angle iron base. This platform is connected to the electrical circuit common to the entire apparatus. The top part of the platform is elevated at a very slight angle, when no one is standing on it. When the subject assumes a starting position with both feet on the platform, the platform is depressed and the circuit closed. If a stimulus is presented and the subject is maintaining contact with the platform, the stimulus continues until contact with the platform is broken. The vertical jump breaks the circuit, simultaneously stopping the recording device. Responses to all stimuli are recorded in the same manner.

3. The Recording Device

The recording device used is the Standard Electric Time Company's clock, model SW-L, D. C. Clutch. This electric stop clock starts simultaneously with the stimulus and stops the instant the circuit is broken by the jump. The finest division of the instrument is 1/100th second, but the recordings were made to the nearest 1/1000th second by estimation in the space. After each response, the clock is returned to zero so that a consecutive reading can be taken with facility. Reactions may be timed in rapid sequence, with a minimum of manipulation. The reaction timer is easily understood by the subjects, thus simplifying instruction and aiding in securing good motivation.

The operator and the subject were separated by an improvised screen so that the subject could not see the operator. For the control and experimental subject, each stimulus was preceded by five "warm-up" trials before actual recording began. No "warm-up" preceded the subject who rode the bicycle as a warm-up.

Before starting the recording the operator gave the instruction "light-ready," or whatever stimulus was applicable, and then proceeded to collect the data in the manner described above. The operator was the same wherever possible throughout the experiment, for each subject.

Cureton[22] performed a calibration check by direct and simultaneous timing using the Illinois Reaction Timer and the much more sensitive American Chronoscope. The average error in one hundred trials was 0.00571 seconds; P.E.Meas. ±0.00287 seconds. The Chronoscope in turn was checked against a Geiger-Muller Scaler and the mean difference was found to be 0.000048 ± 0.00003 seconds.

Procedure Preceding Total Body Reaction Time Tests

The subjects were separated from the operator by a cloth screen. The operator could see the subject being tested by looking at the mirror, which reflected the legs of the subject on the re-action time response unit. Hence, there was no way that the subject could anticipate any of the stimuli. Also the subject could not take up a position other than the erect position with arms at the sides without the operator knowing this.

Before recording each stimulus was preceded by five warm-up trials. Each separate stimulus was preceded by the warning "ready" by the operator. When the trials were over, the subject was told. For example, the operator might say, "Light, to record— ready." This was the procedure followed by each subject prior to each testing session. Throughout the seventeen weeks of test-ing, each subject was tested by the same operator.

The light stimulus of the Illinois Reaction Timer was admin-istered first, followed by the "buzzer," and then the light and the "buzzer" together. In recording the results, the stimuli were called visual, auditory, and visual and auditory, respectively. This was always the pattern, without exception.

The light stimuli results were added and averaged similarly for the other two stimuli. The means were then added and aver-aged, giving a mean of the means. This was called the TBRT *mean score*. The deviations from the mean score by the individual stimuli means were calculated.

Series of Studies Relating Wheat Germ, WGO and Octacosanol to Total Body Reaction Time

Four preliminary studies and three more recent studies have been completed in this area. The three more recent studies have permitted the matching of the subjects in a more precise way than the preliminary studies. They are all shown in Table XXII along with a tabulation to show a) if statistical significance was

TABLE XXII

EXPERIMENTAL STUDIES OF THE EFFECTS OF WHEAT GERM,
WGO AND OCTACOSANOL ON TOTAL BODY REACTION TIME
(Garrett-Cureton Test)

Number of Experiment	Authors	Statistically Significant Results	Trends to Shorten the Reaction Times	No Experimental Result
1	Forr and Cureton	WGO (with physical education)		—with swimming
8	Armer and Cureton	WGO (Av. and visual)	WGO Auditory RT	
13	Cureton and Pohndorf	WGO		
16	Tillman and Cureton	OCT and WG (Visual RT)	Visual RT (WGO)	
26	Johnson and Cureton		OCTCNL	
31	Milesis and Cureton	WGO (Av. of 3 tests)		

obtained (t<.10), b) definite trends to improve (shorten) the reaction times and c) no experimental result of value.

From the above table it is shown that it is generally true that the total body reaction times are affected by the supplements of WGO, OCTCNL and WGC. Of the six experiments (three preliminary and three planned for themselves) five of the six have turned up significant differences, four times for WGO and once for OCTCNL and once for wheat germ cereal (WGC). Only when the training included swimming were the results overshadowed so completely that the reaction times were reversed, as has been observed in two other experiments. Swimming seems to greatly increase the flexibility and slow the reaction times.[35, 36]

A. PRELIMINARY EXPERIMENTS WITH WGO ON TOTAL BODY REACTION TIME

No. 1, Forr-Cureton's Experiment

This experiment demonstrated that the men's swimming group reacted adversely with respect to total body reaction time, whereas, in the other half of the experiment wherein the men partici-

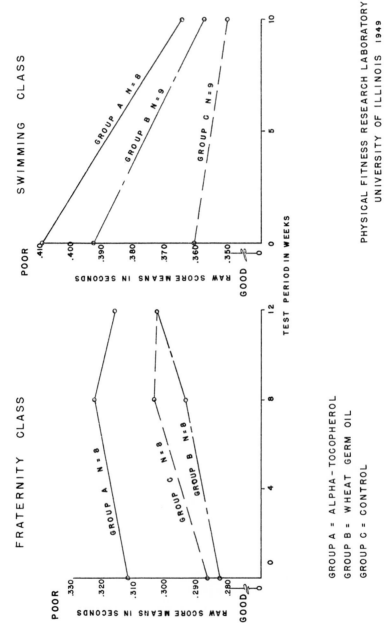

Figure 41. Changes in reaction time-visual mean scores, alpha tocopherol groups versus wheat germ oil versus controls on placeboes.

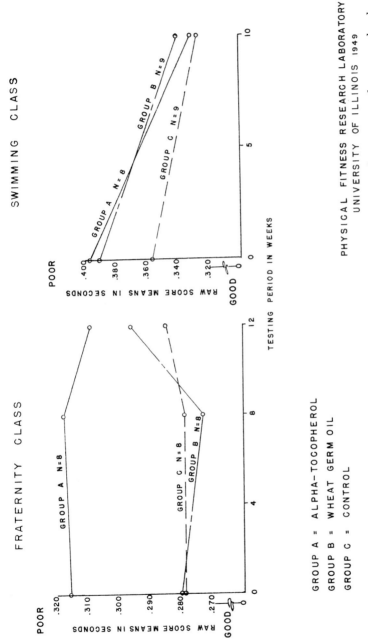

Figure 42. Changes in reaction time-auditory mean scores, alpha tocopherol versus wheat germ oil versus placeboes.

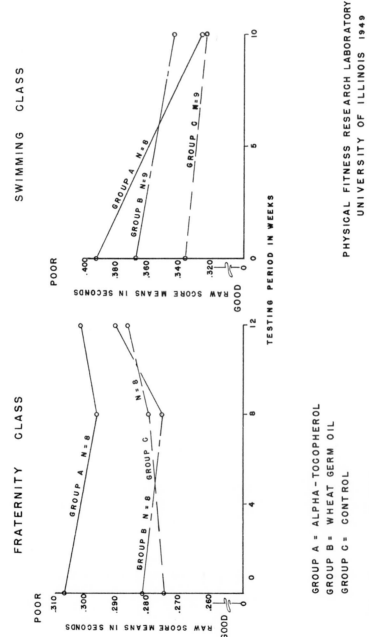

Figure 43. Changes in reaction time-visual and auditory mean scores, alpha tocopherol versus wheat germ oil versus placeboes.

pated in required physical education courses (not any swimming) the total body reaction times improved, although there was a slight regression in the 8-12 week period, but still leaving improvements (Figs. 41, 42 and 43). It may be seen in the figures that the total body reaction times (all three) have worsened in the swimming group but have improved in the fraternity group on required physical education. Such an effect is also known from other studies done on TBRT in our laboratory, with swimmers having much slower total body reaction times than other types of athletes (cf. Chapter VII in Cureton's *Physical Fitness of Champion Athletes,* 1951). Here it is shown that top gymnasts averaged 0.281 seconds; top track and field athletes averaged 0.259 seconds and swimming and diving champions averaged 0.303 seconds.

No. 13, Cureton-Pohndorf Experiment

The results of this experiment are explained in Part Two. The *combined light and sound reaction time test* changed significantly 8.9 SS (t = 2.60, significant <.05) compared to the matched group, which exercised in the same work, the same amount of time and under the same instructors, which improved 2.6 SS (t = 0.69, insignificant). The data are shown in Table XIV (groups A and B were proved to be matched by proving t = statistically insignificant between means).

The statistical significance between these groups is as follows:

$t_{AB} = 0.40$ (p<.40) insignificant
$t_{AC} = 1.200$ (p<.30) insignificant
$t_{BD} = 0.296$ (p<.08) insignificant
$t_{CD} = 0.083$ (p<.95) insignificant

In spite of not being able to guarantee a satisfactory replication for further samples out of one hundred, the trend in terms of standard scores (SS) is in favor of the WGO group improving 8.93 SS, and the Placebo Group improving only 2.6 SS, the two groups were satisfactorily matched on the initial tests.

However, if we use the S.E.$_{meas.}$ ± 0.003 as reference in the denominator, then S.E.$_{diff.}$ is estimated from $\sqrt{.003^2 + .003^2} = 0.00424$, then $D/.00424 = 4.64$. So, for the groups at hand, WGO and on placeboes, the ratio is 4.64 times the size of the root, mean

TABLE XXIII

EFFECT OF TRAINING AND WHEAT GERM OIL ON COMBINED
REACTION TIME COMPARED WITH A MATCHED GROUP ON
PLACEBOES AND TWO OTHER INACTIVE GROUPS, ONE ON
WGO AND ONE ON PLACEBOES

(Each entry is the mean of fifteen practice trials and five counting trials)

	Age (Yrs.)	T_1 (sec.) (May)	T_2 (sec.) (Aug.)	D (in sec.)	Difference in SS
A. On WGO: Active Subjects					
Cu	52	.319	.309	−.010	2
Du	30	.356	.359	.003	− 1
Ku	38	.345	.334	−.011	4
Me	35	.355	.337	−.018	5
St	39	.354	.360	.006	− 2
Tu	47	.323	.324	.001	− 1
Dun	47	.421	.366	−.055	19
Sw	41	.405	.279	−.126	45.5
Average	41.1	.3598	.3335	−.0263	+ 8.93
B. On Placeboes: Inactive Subjects					
Ra	47	.320	.315	−.005	2
Lo	24	.440	.321	−.119	40
Fe	31	.328	.341	.013	− 7
Hu	38	.311	.319	.008	− 2
Tob	32	.287	.262	−.025	10
Tam	31	.293	.281	−.012	6
Co	43	.370	.419	.049	−18
Le	46	.335	.371	.036	− 9.5
Sm	46	.339	.335	−.004	2.5
Average	37.6	.3359	.3293	−.0066	+ 2.6
C. Inactive on WGO					
Bl	30	.281	.304	.023	−11
Lu	26	.224	.190	−.034	12
Van H	35	.304	.326	.022	− 7
Wi	59	.363	.362	−.001	0.5
Average	37.5	.293	.2955	.0025	− 1.38
D. Inactives on Placeboes					
Ba	27	.297	.269	−.028	15.0
He	26	.312	.313	.001	0
Re	29	.280	.279	−.001	0
Ro	34	.321	.383	.062	−20.0
St	53	.347	.374	.027	− 6.5
Ti	25	.392	.334	−.058	23.0
Average	32.3	.3249	.3254	.0005	1.91

square error, therefore it is reliable enough to be tabulated as a favorable trend in the summary table. But, nothing can be guaranteed about the reliability of future samples.

No. 8, Armer's Experiment

Armer[7] compared the physical fitness improvements made by two groups of adult men in a voluntary participation program; the experimental group was fed WGO while the placebo group was fed cottonseed oil containing an amount of vitamin E equivalent to that found in wheat germ oil. A control group of five subjects was also used as a check on environmental changes during the course of the experiment. His results are shown in Figures 2, 3, 4 and 5. Taking into consideration all of the physical fitness tests (chins, dips, grip strength, back lift, leg lift, speed agility run, vertical jump and T.B. reaction times), the only ones that resulted in significant differences between the WGO and placebo groups were *average reaction time* ($t = 2.641$, $p < .05$) and *visual reaction time* ($t = 3.199$, $p < .01$). In the average reaction time test, the WGO group improved from 54.8 to 63.7 S.S., while the placebo group improved from 48 to 53.7 S.S. In the visual reaction time test, the WGO group improved from 54.3 to 60.4 S.S., while the placebo group improved from 48.1 to 49.7 S.S.

No. 16, Tillman's Experiment (1958)

The experimental design used by Tillman[37] permitted the determination of the effects of different training methods and different dietary supplements on the reaction time of seventy-one boys attending the University of Illinois Sports-Fitness School in 1957. The boys were placed into matched groups initially on the basis of T_1, 600-yard runs. Statistical treatment consisted of between group analyses based on mean changes for each group from T_1 to T_2.

The training methods that were used were circuit, muscular endurance, interval and steeple chase. The dietary supplements were wheat germ oil, octacosanol, wheat germ and placeboes. All boys participated in the same activities at the Sports-Fitness School except for thirty minutes each day when the differential training was conducted. During the "feeding break" the boys

TABLE XXIV

TOTAL BODY REACTION TIME IMPROVEMENT

(Garrett-Cureton Test)
(in Standard Scores)

Group	Visual	Auditory	Combined	X
Octacosanol	14.26	15.05	10.77	13.36
Wheat germ	12.36	11.63	9.26	11.08
Wheat germ oil	6.66	7.13	10.20	8.00
Placeboes	7.76	7.58	5.52	6.95

were fed the differential supplements with milk. In this manner, approximately one fourth of the boys in each training group received WGO, one fourth octacosanol, one fourth wheat germ and one fourth placeboes. Each dietary supplement group was similarly subdivided into four training groups. All boys took milk.

The results revealed that no training method was found significantly better than any one of the other training methods for improving reaction times; the same was true for the dietary supplement groups. However, every group improved in all three of the reaction time tests over the eight-week period, a trend that may have been due to motor learning. Table XV permits comparisons between the different dietary supplement groups in terms of standard score improvement for each of the three types of reaction time tests. The octacosanol group had the largest mean gain in all three forms of the reaction time test. The mean of all three test forms at the extreme right of the table shows the groups in ranked order.

In conclusion—there is a trend of advantage for the octacosanol and wheat germ supplements but by the usual t-test method, the differences were not significant.

No. 24, Cureton and Wiggett's Experiment

In another study by Cureton and Wiggett (No. 23, 1964) octacosanol was administered to a male subject for five months to determine if this substance favorably influenced reaction time tests taken in a series. A control subject who did not receive the supplement was also used. Both subjects were trained athletes.

Prior to the start of the experiment, a month of preliminary testing was conducted for stabilization, elimination of motor educability and standardization, until a plateau had been reached in both subjects. The experiment lasted six months, during which time 231 tests were made on the experimental subject and 471 tests were made on the control subject. Tests were given on seventy-seven different days. The standard error, thusly calculated:

$$\text{S.E.} = \frac{s}{\sqrt{\text{N-1}}} \quad (\text{N} = 20 \text{ trials})$$
$$\text{(Meas.)}$$

Neither subject on any form of reaction time test was higher than 0.004 seconds, nor lower than 0.002 seconds. The results of the experiment are presented in Table XXV.

The advantage is decidedly in favor of the octacosanol supplemented subject. The sharpest difference was manifested in the combined visual and auditory reaction time where the gain was 14 S.S. for the experimental subject compared to a gain of 3 S.S. for the nonsupplemented control subject (cf. Figs. 44, 45 and 46).

No. 26, Johnson's Longitudinal Study

The experimental design was similar to Wiggett's, except that the visual, auditory and combined visual-auditory scores were

TABLE XXV

TOTAL BODY REACTION TIMES FOR THE OCTACOSANOL SUBJECT
VERSUS THE CONTROL SUBJECT

(Raw Scores in Seconds)

	T_1 Raw Score	T_1 SS	T_2 Raw Score	T_2 SS	Raw Score Diff.	SS Diff.
Experimental Subject						
Visual	0.243	76	0.198	83	0.045	7
Auditory	0.233	76	0.190	82	0.043	6
Combined ...	0.244	69	0.199	83	0.045	14
Control Subject						
Visual	0.215	79	0.196	83	0.019	4
Auditory	0.208	78	0.199	80	0.009	2
Combined ...	0.210	80	0.197	83	0.013	3

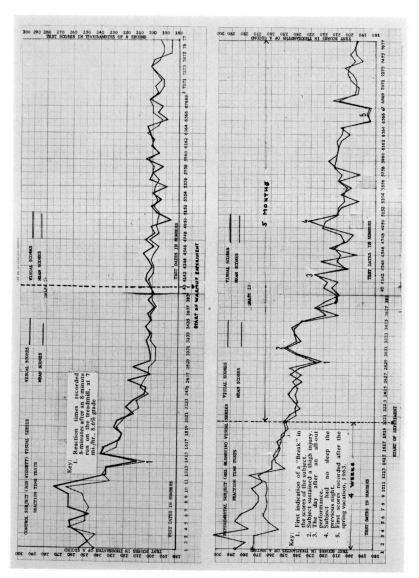

Figure 44. Control versus experimental subject, visual reaction time tests, 6 months (two matched sprinters).

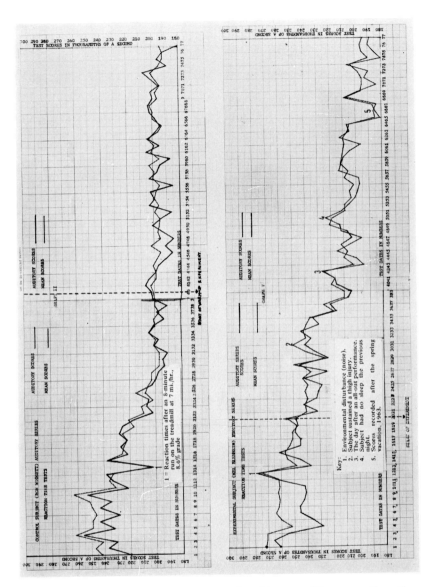

Figure 45. Control versus experimental subject, auditory reaction time tests, 6 months (two matched sprinters).

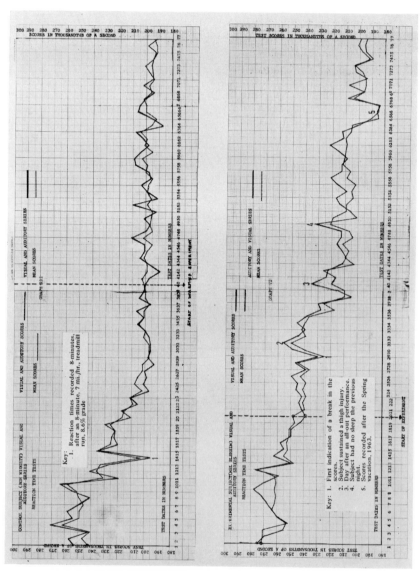

Figure 46-A. Control versus experimental subject, combined reaction time tests, 6 months (two matched sprinters).

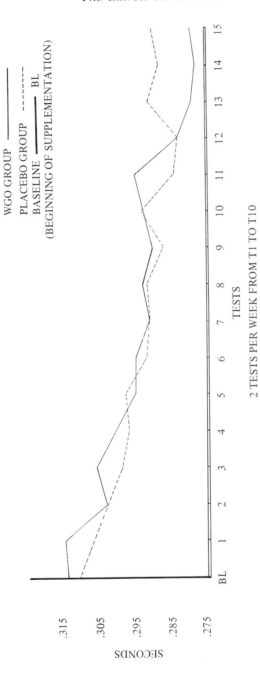

Figure 46-B. Total body average reaction time, group mean change, WGO versus placebo.

averaged to yield an "average total body reaction time." Nine adult subjects from the University of Illinois adult fitness program were given six weeks of preliminary testing for standardization and elimination of educational effect. The subjects were then matched into two groups on the basis of group means determined from an average of the last three reaction time testing sessions for each subject at the end of the preliminary testing period. The group means differed insignificantly by 0.003 seconds. One group was given ten six-minim capsules of WGO daily while the other group received ten six-minim capsules of placeboes daily. Neither the experimenter nor the subjects knew the contents of the capsules until the termination of the experiment. Fifteen serial reaction time testing sessions were held over a period of sixteen weeks, thirty tests per session.

Th results revealed that at no testing session did there emerge a significant difference between groups. Also, although the gains for both groups were large, no significant improvement was found in the within-group means. Figure 46-B shows the group mean differences. In the last three weeks, the twelfth through the fifteenth week, a favorable difference emerged giving an advantage to the WGO group over the placebo group. The analysis of individual changes showed significant improvements by three of the four subjects taking WGO; the fourth subject was very near to a significant improvement. Two of the five subjects taking placeboes failed to approach a significant improvement (Table CXVIII). The improvement of the remaining subjects taking placeboes were comparable to those of the WGO group. The results indicated a slight advantage for the subjects taking WGO.

No. 31, Milesis and Cureton Experiment

In this experiment (Exp. 31, 1960) thirty 10 to 13-year-old boys in the University of Illinois Sports-Fitness School were matched in three groups in a block design providing for systematic rotation. This was done to equalize learning and any possible fatigue in taking the fifteen preliminary trials and five trials on visual, auditory and combined signals, then averaging, using the Garrett-Cureton Total Body Reaction Timer apparatus as described. In double-blind feeding of placeboes, WGO and un-

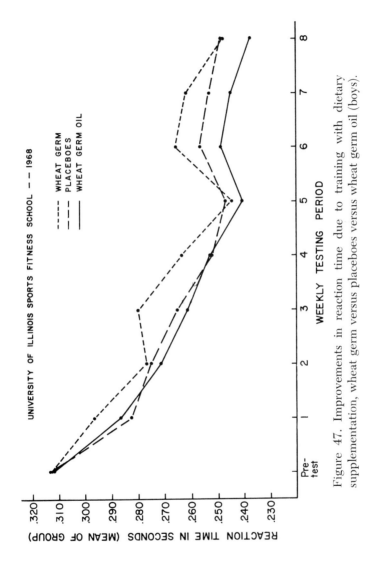

Figure 47. Improvements in reaction time due to training with dietary supplementation, wheat germ versus placeboes versus wheat germ oil (boys).

camouflaged wheat germ (1½ ounce) at the same time each day, in a rest period at 3:15 PM after they had been exercised, with one half pint of milk used to wash the capsules down. The testing was completed the first and last week of school and the dietary substances were given for six weeks in-between.

The t-test was used to test the significance of the differences between the groups. The data and results of the calculations are shown in Part Two of the study.

The conclusion was that the fifteen capsules four times per week of the six-minim size fed to the WGO experimental group reduced their average total body reaction time more than that which occurred in the controls ($t = <.15$). The wheat germ group failed to show this effect ($t = 0.19$). It was observed also (Fig. 47) that about four weeks were needed for the effect to show in a definite manner, with testing each week. The gains were 0.0648 for WGO, 0.0601 for the placebo group on devitaminized lard capsules, and 0.0601 for the wheat germ group. The slight favorable trend was for WGO compared to the placebo group.

CONCLUSIONS

1. Out of six experiments on the Total Body Reaction Times, WGO has shown a significant effect four times out of six and twice has shown trends favorable over the placebo substances used.

2. Octacosanol and wheat germ have also demonstrated a significant effect once out of two experiments in which these were used, the octacosanol also showing a favorable trend in one other experiment.

3. Swimming was shown in two experiments to have a detrimental effect upon the total body reaction times (as in the Forr and Marx experiments).

REFERENCES

1. Pierson, W. R. and Montoye, H. J.: Movement time, reaction time and age, *J. Geront.*, 13:418-421, Oct., 1958, and also, Henry, F. M.: the influence of the aging process on the ability to exercise, Professional Contributions of the *Amer. Acad. Phys. Ed.*, No. 2, 4-10, 1952.
2. Honet, J. C., Jebsen, R. H. and Tenckhoff, H. A.: Motor nerve con-

dition velocity in chronic and renal insufficiency, *Arch. Phys. Med.,* 47:647-652, Oct., 1966; also, Johnson, E. W. and Olsen, K. J.: Clinical value of motor nerve conduction velocity determinations, *J.A.M.A.,* 17:2030-2035, April 30, 1960.

3. Shock, Nathan W.: Kidney plasma flow related to age, in *Sci. Amer.,* 100-110, Jan., 1962.

4. Shute's: *The Summary* (of Vitamin E reports). London, Ontario, Canada, various issues.

5. Darlington, E. G. and Chassels, J. B.: Racing results in thoroughbred horses, *The Summary,* 8:1, 1956; and report of Lloyd Percival from Canada's Sports College, Toronto.

6. Brozek, Josef: Soviet studies on nutrition and higher nervous activity, *Ann. N. Y. Acad. Sci.,* 93:665-714,1962.

7. Armer, Eldon W.: An Experimental Study of the Effects of Training and Dietary Supplement (WGO) on Motor Fitness Tests of Adult Men, Urbana, M.S. thesis, Physical Education, University of Illinois, 1952, p. 59.

8. Forr, William A.: The Effects of Wheat Germ Oil (Vitamin E) on Physical Fitness, Urbana, Illinois, M.S. thesis in Physical Education, University of Illinois, 1950, p. 92.

9. Frank, Avis R.: The Relationship of Total Body Agility Reaction Time to the Agility Run Among College Women, Urbana, Illinois, M.S. thesis, Physical Education, University of Illinois, 1968, p. 77.

10. Grad, Carl: Reaction Time in Offensive Backfield Football Positions, Urbana, M.S. thesis, Physical Education, University of Illinois, 1949, p. 86.

11. Marx, E. I.: The Effect of a Dietary Supplement on Varsity Swimmers, Urbana, M.S. thesis, in Physical Education, University of Illinois, 1952, p. 48.

12. Von Ebers, D. A.: The Relationship Between Total Body Agility Reaction Time and Flexibility, Urbana, M.S. thesis, Physical Education, University of Illinois, 1950, p. 47.

13. Landry, F. J.: The Effects of the University of Illinois Sports-Fitness Summer Day School on the Motor Fitness of Young Boys, Urbana, M.S. in Physical Education, University of Illinois, 1955, p. 107.

14. Moore, George C.: A Factorial Study of Physical Fitness Test Variables, Urbana, Ph.D. thesis, Physical Education, University of Illinois, 1955, p. 133.

15. De May, Gilbert H.: The Relationship Between the Elasticity of the Calf Muscles and Total Body Reaction Time, Urbana, M.S. in Physical Education, University of Illinois, 1956, p. 70.

16. Griffith, C. R.: *Psychology and Athletics,* New York, Scribner's and Sons, 1938, p. 153.

17. Woodworth, R. S. and Schlosburg, H.: *Experimental Psychology,* New York, Holt and Co., 1954.

18. Garrett, H. E.: *Great Experiments in Psychology*, New York, Appleton-Century Co., 1930, p. 377.
19. Teichner, W. H.: Recent studies of the simple reaction time, *Psychol. Bull.*, 51:131, 1954.
20. Kleitman, N. and Jackson, D. P.: Body Temperature and Performance under Different Routines, *J. Appl. Physiol.*, 3:309-328, Dec., 1950.
21. Westerlund, J. and Tuttle, W. W.: The Relationship Between Running Events in Track and Reaction Time, *Res. Quart.*, 2:95-100, Oct., 1931.
22. Cureton, T. K.: *Physical Fitness of Champion Athletes*, Urbana, University of Illinois Press, 1955, pp. 94-102.
23. Beise, D. and Peasly, V.: The relation of reaction time, speed, agility of big muscle groups to certain sport skills, *Res. Quart.*, 8:133-142, March, 1937.
24. Henry, F. H.: Stimulus complexity, movement complexity, age and sex in relation to reaction latency and speed of movement, *Res. Quart.*, 32:353, Oct., 1955.
25. De May, G. H.: ref. 15.
26. Von Ebers, D.: The Relationship Between Total Body Agility Reaction Time and Flexibility, Urbana, M.S. thesis, Physical Education, University of Illinois, 1950, p. 40.
27. Moore, George C.: An Analytical Study of Physical Fitness Test Variables, Urbana, Ph.D. thesis, Physical Education, University of Illinois, 1955, p. 49.
28. Elbel, E. R.: A study of response time before and after strenuous exercise, *Res. Quart.*, 11:94, May, 1940.
29. Landry, J.: The Effects of the University of Illinois Sports-Fitness School on the Motor Fitness of Young Boys, Urbana, M.S. thesis, Physical Education, University of Illinois, 1955, p. 74.
30. Westerlund and Tuttle: Op. cit., ref. 21.
31. Thompson, C. A.: A Study of Various Reaction Times and Movement Times as Factors of Volleyball Playing Ability, Urbana, M.S. thesis, Physical Education, University of Illinois, 1962, p. 44.
32. Marx, E. I.: Op. cit. ref. 11.
33. Knowlton, G. A. and Himes, H. M.: The effect of Vitamin E deficient diet upon skeletal muscles, *Proc. Soc. Exp. Biol. Med.*, 38:246, 1938.
34. Weischler, I. S.: Recovery of amytrophic lateral sclerosis, *J.A.M.A.*, 114-950, 1940.
35. Marx, E. I.: Op. cit. ref. 11.
36. Forr: Op. cit. ref. 8.
37. Tillman, K. C.: The Effects of Dietary Supplements and Different Training Methods on Reaction Time and Agility, Urbana, M.S. in Physical Education, University of Illinois, 1958, p. 63.

Chapter VI

Effects of Wheat Germ Oil, Octacosanol and Wheat Germ on the Precordial T-Wave of the Electrocardiogram

MEANING OF THE T-WAVE

THE question, "What does the T-wave represent?" has never really been conclusively answered. The proponents of the repolarization theory[1, 2] contend that the positive T-wave deflection results from an imbalance of voltages that occurs when the stimulus current flows from the sinoauricular node from right to left across the heart and then reverses to flow back from left to right. On the other hand, the holders of the myokinetic theory[3, 4] argue that there is an exact mechanical counterpart to the large sum of action potentials (minute voltages) that innervate myocardial fibers, and that this mechanical counterpart is the result of stimuli causing the fibers to contract. Accordingly, they reason that the T-wave is the sum of a) electrical energies liberated by the mechanical action of the muscular fibers (action currents) and b) repolarization. Collen[5] emphasizes that the mechanical movement of the ventricles is necessary for the repolarization

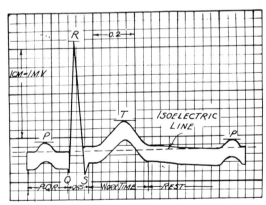

Figure 48. Precordial T-wave of the electrocardiogram, notation for mensuration.

185

4-CHANNEL OSCILLOGRAPH RECORDING

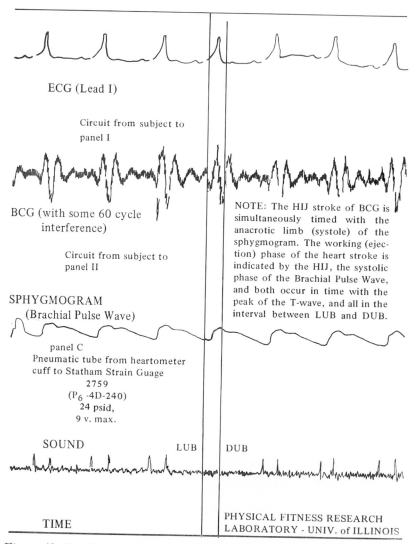

ECG (Lead I)

Circuit from subject to
panel I

BCG (with some 60 cycle
interference)

NOTE: The HIJ stroke of BCG is simultaneously timed with the anacrotic limb (systole) of the sphygmogram. The working (ejection) phase of the heart stroke is indicated by the HIJ, the systolic phase of the Brachial Pulse Wave, and both occur in time with the peak of the T-wave, and all in the interval between LUB and DUB.

Circuit from subject to
panel II

SPHYGMOGRAM
(Brachial Pulse Wave)

panel C
Pneumatic tube from heartometer
cuff to Statham Strain Guage
2759
(P_6 -4D-240)
24 psid,
9 v. max.

SOUND   LUB   DUB

TIME

PHYSICAL FITNESS RESEARCH
LABORATORY - UNIV. of ILLINOIS

Figure 49. Simultaneous recording of ECG, BCG, brachial pulse wave and sounds, single tape 4-channel oscillograph.

energy. It has long been known that myocardial dysfunction is related to thiamine deficiency, and this summary shows that it is also related to WGO deficiency (Eustis, A.: *New Orleans Med. Sci. J.,* 94:369, 1942) (Fig. 48).

Evidence supporting the myokinetic theory can be found in simultaneous recordings of the ECG, BCG, brachial or carotid sphygmogram and phonocardiogram, wherein it can be seen (Fig. 49) that the T-wave is synchronous with ventricular contraction as manifested in the BCG I-wave, the ejection period of the brachial or carotid pulse wave, and the mechanical systole (time interval between first and second heart sounds). Such evidence appears in simultaneous tracings recorded by several authors, du Toit,[6] Cundiff,[7] Sloninger,[8] Milesis[9] and Cureton.[10] The T-wave has also aligned well with the velocity and acceleration derivatives of the brachial pulse wave (Fig. 49).[11]

THE VALIDITY OF THE T-WAVE AS AN INDICATOR OF CARDIOVASCULAR FITNESS

Several studies have demonstrated the T-wave's relation to other important measures, its usefulness in differentiating levels of fitness, and the changes that occur in it in response to longitudinal training.

Massey[12] found a statistically significant curvilinear relationship between the T-wave in lead 4 and all-out treadmill run time. The ETA was 0.60.

Wolf[13] investigated whether or not the ECG could be used to differentiate levels of physical condition in *undiseased* subjects, with tracing taken before and after mild, fairly active, and vigorous exercise. The levels of fitness in the subjects he used ranged from cross-country runners to untrained college students classified as good, average, and poor fitness on the basis of an all-out treadmill run. He concluded the following:

1. The R. S. and T-wave amplitudes of training subjects increase in all leads following an all-out treadmill run at 7 mph/8.6 per cent grade.
2. Trained subjects show greater increases or greater decreases in amplitudes than the untrained subjects for the same amount of exercise. Following exercise, the P and S

waves increase and the R and T-waves decrease in the untrained subject. In contrast, in the trained subject the P-wave decreased while the R, S and T-waves increased after exercise.

3. Significant differences at the .05 level in the good and poor condition groups were found in changes from lying to sitting and lying to standing in the P, R and T-wave amplitudes.

In a series of ECG experiments, Cureton[14] has shown the effects of varying intensities of longitudinal endurance training (easy, moderate and hard) on the amplitude of the highest precordial T-wave. He reported that, in general, the very easy training programs of the sociorecreative type do not produce significant changes in the precordial T-wave, while the moderately intensive programs do produce some changes but they are not as great as programs progressively increased to severe intensity. The severely intensive programs, if continued for a long period of time without some kind of vacation or "training break" will sometimes increase the amplitude of the T-wave for a time, then the T-wave may diminish, perhaps due to accumulative fatigue. He also reports that, ". . . the high T-wave in the precordial waves is associated with endurance and high glycogen reserves." Other studies show too that high potassium reserves are a basic cause.

In a correlational study, Milesis[15] obtained a Pearson r of -0.466 (significant at the .02 level) between mile run time and resting ECG T-wave amplitude in middle-aged men.

Cureton[16] contended that a large T-wave probably meant a more forceful ventricular contraction, and that fatigue usually lowers the T-wave. In a subsequent report, Cureton[17] reviewed a large body of studies which demonstrated that the T-wave amplitude was distinctly higher in rested endurance athletes compared to normals.

Simonson and Keys[18] and Keys[19] have reported that *an acute or chronic nutritional deficiency will depress the T-wave amplitude.*

STUDIES PERTAINING TO THE EFFECTS OF WHEAT GERM DERIVATIVES ON THE PRECORDIAL T-WAVE OF THE ELECTROCARDIOGRAM

The first experiment to investigate the possible value of wheat germ oil to augment ventricular function was conducted by Forr.[20] Six groups of subjects were utilized, the first three consisting of college students being trained in a beginning swimming class and simultaneously receiving vitamin E (group A), WGO (group B) and corn oil placeboes (group C). The last three groups consisted of college fraternity men that served as inactive controls receiving corresponding dietary supplements. The dosage consisted of 144 three-minim capsules per week of the prescribed supplement. All supplementary feeding was conducted on a double-blind basis (cf. Exp. 1, Part Two). The swimming groups, like the fraternity groups, were matched on the basis of the sum of the standard scores in the following: a) Schneider Index, b) area under the curve in the brachial sphygmogram and c) Harvard 5-minute step test. After matching, all subjects were given a battery of physical fitness tests—initially T_1 (including the precordial T-wave of the ECG), at the eighth week, T_2, and at the twelfth week, T_3.

The findings with regard to the T-wave are presented in Figure 50. In the swimming class, the T-wave increased 23.8 per cent in the WGO group, 12.7 per cent in the corn oil placebo group, and 0 per cent in the vitamin E group. The advantage of the WGO group over the vitamin E group (2.30 mm versus 0.06 mm) was significant (T = 3.25, 0.5 level), using the ratio $\frac{D}{S.E._{\text{meas.}}}$, whereby the standard error of measurement was ± 0.724 mm. The placebo group advantage over the vitamin E group (1.20 mm versus 0.06 mm) proved insignificant (T = 1.58). Similar trends were found in the fraternity group. Such findings apply only to the group at hand.

An experiment by Maley[21] matched two groups of middle-aged men, one group receiving 20 six-minim capsules of WGO daily and the other group receiving 20 six-minim capsules of cotton-

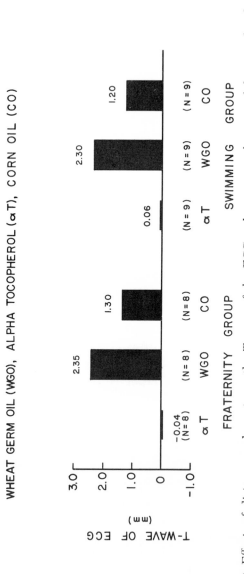

Figure 50. Effects of dietary supplements on the T-wave of the ECG: wheat germ oil versus alpha tocopherol versus refined corn oil.

seed oil placeboes daily, for an informal sports-exercise program. Tests were made on the subjects at T_1, four months later at T_2, and again six weeks later at T_3. The dietary supplements were fed only during the six-week period from T_2 to T_3. The findings were negative in terms of the ECG T-wave as well as all other tests. At T_2, the T-wave declined from 50.28 SS to 39.50 SS in the WGO group compared to a loss of from 46.67 SS to 44.67 SS for the placebo group; these and other T_1-T_2 changes were insignificant. From T_1 to T_3, both the WGO and placebo groups showed a statistically significant decline in the amplitude of the T-wave. Maley blamed these declines on the deleterious winter season and the lack of rigid control of the training, remarking that, "The training program was not hard enough to develop 'induced' nutritive deficiencies, hence, no changes are attributed to WGO or the placebo, and slight declines are due to the winter." This program was an informal one, without leadership.

The search to discover whether any benefits accrued from WGO supplementation continued with a study in 1953 by Susic[22] who investigated the effects of WGO supplementation on the T-wave of the ECG at ground level and at 10,000 feet simulated altitude. Six subjects served as experimental subjects in training, three subjects served as exercise-control subjects without WGO, and three final subjects comprised a "nonexercise" control group that took neither training nor WGO. ECG tests were administered initially (T_1), after a plateau had occurred following twelve weeks of hard training (T_2), and then again at T_3 after the experimental subjects had received WGO for six weeks in conjunction with their training (Figs. 51 and 52).

The six experimental subjects averaged 10.88 mm at T_1 and 12.00 mm at T_2, a gain of 1.12 mm due to a 12-week endurance training program. The change from T_2 to T_3 (endurance training plus a daily dietary supplement of WGO—10 six-minim capsules) was from 12.00 mm to 14.90 mm, a gain of 2.90 mm which was statistically significant ($T = 4.01$) at the .01 level (see Fig. 53). The S.E.$_{meas.}$ = ±0.723 (resting, at ground level; $\pm.924$ at 10,000 feet of simulated altitude).

The exercise control group averaged 8.5 mm at T_1 and 8.7 mm at T_2, then a loss of 1.9 m from T_2 to T_3 (8.7 mm to 6.8 mm).

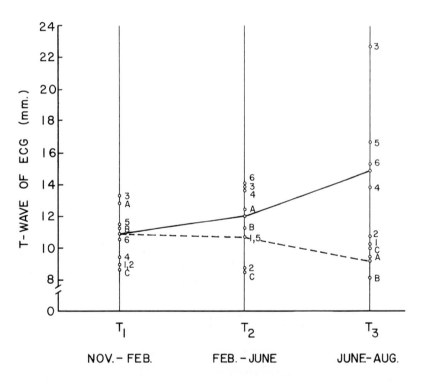

EXPERIMENTALS				CONTROLS			
SUBJ.	T_1	T_2	T_3	SUBJ.	T_1	T_2	T_3
1. HC	9.00	10.75	10.35	A. EM	12.80	12.50	9.5
2. GH	9.00	8.80	10.80	B. RR	11.25	11.35	8.2
3. WS	13.35	13.85	22.65	C. WVH	8.65	8.45	10.0
4. SS	9.50	13.75	13.85	MEAN	10.90	10.73	9.23
5. JT	11.50	10.75	16.70				
6. CW	10.60	14.10	15.25				
MEAN	10.88	12.00	14.90				

Figure 51. The effects of training with a dietary supplement on the T-wave of the ECG at ground level (WGO versus controls).

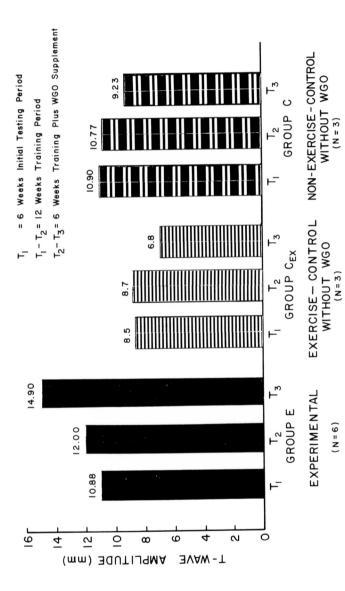

Figure 52. Changes in highest precordial T-wave of the ECG with and without WGO supplement.

The latter change was significant at the .05 level. The data were incorporated in a published report by Cureton[22] as the research was sponsored by the latter, aided by a research grant made to Cureton to pursue this research.[14]

Quite in contrast to the experimental group, the nonexercise control group (see Fig. 51) declined from 10.90 mm at T_1 to 10.77 mm at T_2. The period from T_2 to T_3 in this same group resulted in a further loss of 1.54 mm, from 10.77 mm to 9.23 mm. Both changes were statistically insignificant.

The results of testing the experimental subjects at 10,000 feet simulated altitude are shown in Figure 53. Here, the experimental subjects made a significant gain from T_1 to T_2 in connection with the training, but in the T_2 to T_3 analysis, when the influence of the WGO was to be critically tested, the experimental group lost (-1.24 mm), whereas, at ground level the corresponding gain apparently associated with WGO was impressive (a gain of 2.90 mm). This loss was partly attributed to some adverse influence (such as fatigue) which lowered one subject's score from 8.19 mm at T_2 to 3.5 mm at T_3, which is usually seen in comparing the pre- and post- all-out treadmill run. Oxygen intake, heartograph, stroke volume, and breath holding time tests all declined in this subject from T_2 to T_3, indicating that his T-wave decline was a real one and not due to the unreliability of the ECG.

The Cureton-Pohndorf[23] study of 1955 (given in detail, Exp. 13, Part Two) produced evidence that favored the exercise group on WGO, as the mean gain of this group in the precordial T-wave was from 9.84 mm (T_1) to 11.04 mm (T_2), an improvement of 8.3 standard scores (a significant change, $t = 3.13$). However, the exercise group on placeboes also made a significant gain ($t = 2.80$) of from 11.06 mm to 12.07 mm, an improvement of 5.9 SS. These two groups, A and B, were insignificantly different, hence the gains in each group must be credited primarily to the training. The changes within the control groups and between the control groups were not significant.

The experiment by Vohaska[24] (cf. Exp. 12) on two matched halves of a college wrestling team, resulted in small, insignificant

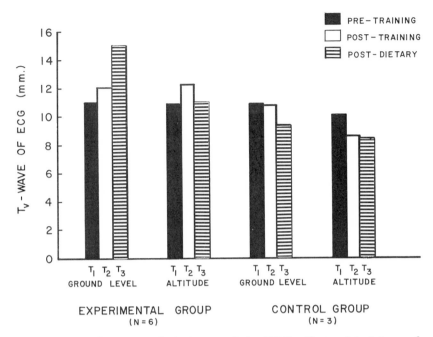

Figure 53. Highest precordial T-wave of the ECG, effects of training and dietary supplement (WGO) at ground level and at 10,000 feet simulated altitude (WGO versus controls).

changes from T_1 to T_2 in the R and T-wave amplitude for both the experimental group on WGO. The between-group analysis at T_2 showed that the two groups were insignificantly different. These negative findings were blamed partly on the late arrival of the supplements, allowing for only four weeks of supplementary feeding.

Bernauer and Cureton[24] divided a college track team into two matched groups on the basis of 440-yard run times. Twelve weeks of in-season training ensued during which one group received 10 six-minim capsules of WGO per day, while the other group received an equivalent dosage of devitaminized lard placeboes. The results showed that the T-wave was not appreciably altered following the twelve-week period of training in either the WGO or the control group. The within-group analyses favored the

WGO group with an improvement from T_1 to T_2 of 13.4 mm to 13.7 mm (a gain of 2.8 standard scores) over the control group which did not change (10.3 mm to 10.3 mm).*

The 1963 study by Cureton[26] was one of the better studies in this area from the standpoint of supervision of subjects, owing to the fact that the subjects were enrolled in a six-week course at the United States Navy Underwater Swimmer's School at Key West, Florida. The men were initially matched into an octacosanol group, a WGO group, and a placebo group on the basis of the average standard score on five muscular endurance tests. The supplementary feeding was then held daily for five weeks of the six-week training program with the men not knowing the contents of the capsules. Within-group changes in terms of standard score changes, favored octacosanol (+3.8 SS) over the placebo group (−0.5 SS) and the WGO group (−2.8 SS). None of the between-group differences in the T-wave were significant. Two limitations of this study may have hindered improvements in the T-wave. First, accumulative fatigue, insufficient sleep and inadequate time to make full cardiovascular adjustment probably handicapped the within-group improvements. Fatigue showed especially in the quiet cardiovascular tests. Second, the dietary supplements were fed for only five weeks, which may have been too brief to produce the intended nutritional effects. Most of the men developed considerable muscular soreness.

In Mayhew's Experiment[27] (No. 29) the 20-week training group on WGO gained from T_2 to T_3 in the ten weeks while on WGO 5 SS (0.99 mm), compared to a loss of (−1.0 SS; or −0.41 mm). With an S.E.$_{meas.}$ = ±0.44, the T-ratio for the difference of 1.40 mm is 1.40/0.44 or 3.19. This is posted as a favorable trend. Since the data are curvilinear, it was decided not to use the Fisher t test. It is shown in Figure 54 that in the ten weeks of preconditioning, the training group (N = 10) improved significantly as compared to the control group which did not exercise (N = 6), this in the test "quiet sitting T-wave" (subject sitting quietly on the ergometer bicycle). In Figure 55 it is further shown that in the second minute of the ergometer bicycle ride

---

* Cf. Exp. 18, Part Two.

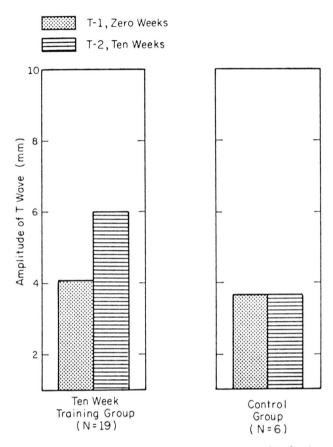

Figure 54. Effect of training on sitting T-wave amplitude (at rest).

time that again the ten-week training group (N = 19) significantly improved more than the control group (which did not
exercise). This part of the experiment aimed to bring the T-wave
up to a plateau in ten weeks, as had been done in previously
conducted experiments. In the last ten weeks the WGO training
group (N = 6) took ten capsules per day, 6-minim size, of Vio-
Bin WGO, while the placebo group took placeboes (N = 6) and
also continued in training parallel in the same workouts with the
WGO-training group (Fig. 56). A third group on no supplements
or placeboes (N = 7) also continued in training, just as the

others. Figure 56 shows the advantage for the WGO group as
compared to losses for the other two groups. These losses were
slight, the groups remaining practically at a plateau. Therefore,
this experiment supports Experiments 3, 4, 5, 6, 9 and 10, previously summarized. Table XXVI gives the reliability coefficients:
a) sitting rest T-wave, 0.802, b) end of second minute of recovery, 0.717; end of ten minutes of recovery, 0.896.

Only one study was found having a bearing on the same problem and this one was prompted by our previous work. It was
done to see if comparable results could be obtained by inde-

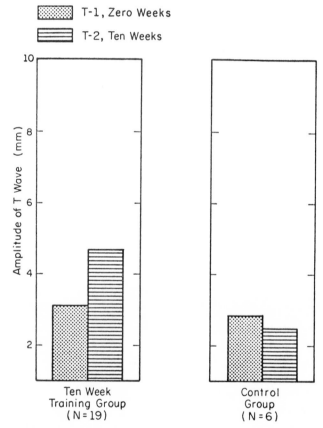

Figure 55. Effect of training on T-wave in second minute of ergometer ride
(25 kg-m/sec at 60 r.p.m.).

TABLE XXVI

RELIABILITY COEFFICIENTS*

Variable T Wave	Reliability Coefficients
Sitting rest	0.802
Last ten seconds of first minute of ride[†]	−0.748
Last ten seconds of second minute of ride[†]	0.717
Last ten seconds of first minute of recovery	0.995
Last ten seconds of second minute of recovery	0.991
Last ten seconds of third minute of recovery	0.005
Last ten seconds of fourth minute of recovery	0.974
Last ten seconds of fifth minute of recovery	0.729
Last ten seconds of sixth minute of recovery	0.867
Last ten seconds of seventh minute of recovery	−0.423
Last ten seconds of eighth minute of recovery	0.876
Last ten seconds of ninth minute of recovery	0.967
Last ten seconds of tenth minute of recovery	0.896

* N = 6, with one week between tests.
† Two-minute bicycle ergometer ride (25 kg-m/second at 60 rpm).

pendent investigators, at Stanford University by Poiletman and Miller.[28] Their subjects were highly trained athletes, divided into control and experimental subjects, and measured in twenty-four male cross-country athletes, 17-22 years of age, who were engaged in a heavy physical training program. After several weeks of preliminary workouts to determine a high level of fitness, the group was randomly divided into two groups of twelve, matched in the amplitude of the T-wave and measured on a Sanborn Model 500 instrument, using six precordial leads on the chest in the usual standardized positions. While training continued for another three weeks, one group of twelve men was given ten capsules of six-minim size daily. These workers eliminated the placebo capsules, saying "the use of placebo capsules was unwarranted since the ECG is a passive nonwillpower measure, and is unaffected by the presence or absence of a placebo." The measurements were basal, after fasting for twelve hours, and were taken under standardized laboratory conditions at the beginning and at the end of the experiment. The results are shown in Table XXVII.

The trend was found to be in the direction of a positive effect but was not significantly different by the $D/S.E._{diff.}$ procedure.

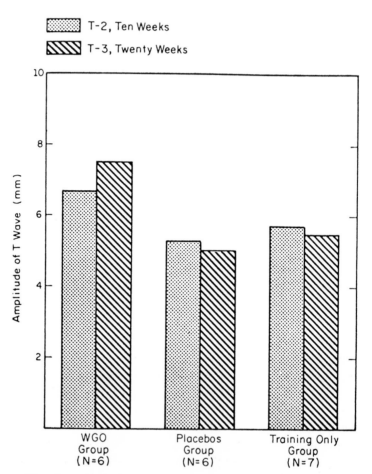

Figure 56. Effect of WGO on T-wave during sixth minute of recovery.

TABLE XXVII

WGO EFFECTS UPON THE PRECORDIAL T-WAVE OF THE
ELECTROCARDIOGRAM

(Poiletman and Miller, 1968)

Basic Data	Controls	After Three Weeks of WGO	Difference (mm)
N	12	12	
Mean Amplitude of Precordial T-Wave (mm)	11.9 to 12.4 S.E. = 0.6, 0.8	10.0 to 11.5 S.E. = 0.7, 1.0	0.99
		$T = \dfrac{D}{S.E._{meas.}}$	$T = 0.99/ 1.077 = 0.920$

It may be also mentioned that the capsules were not taken on an empty stomach under controlled conditions, when the body was still hot at the end of the workout, or with milk.

SUMMARY AND CONCLUSIONS FOR THE T-WAVE EXPERIMENTS

Seven studies produced five sets of results viewed as positive trends of advantage for the WGO experimental groups. The two experiments which did not show a favorable result were not run primarily for the T-wave effects and the data at T_1 were not matched carefully, so there is some doubt as to their worth (Maley, Exp. 11 and Vohaska, Exp. 12). In the Susic (Exp. 10) and Mayhew (Exp. 29) Experiments there was acceptable matching at T_1. In these the results favor WGO.

WGO affects the amplitude of the precordial T-wave positively, suggesting an improved nutritional state of the heart myocardium and a strengthening of the contraction action voltages.

Individual differences exist, as in all other measurements, and the data are curvilinear and not suitable for a t-test (Fisher) reliability checking. The S.E._{meas.} were determined and are used in the ratio $(T) = D/S.E._{meas.}$. The results cannot be generalized beyond the samples at hand. The coefficients of reliability are as follows: at rest—0.802; at the end of the second minute of exertion—0.717; and after ten minutes of recovery—0.896.

The naive nature of the precordial T-wave insures that the training changes and the WGO or octacosanol changes are not due to willpower.

The precordial T-waves are hard to change, especially after the subjects have been trained as athletes, as in Poiletman and Miller's study, and small changes of significance probably do relate to nutritional changes or fatigue. The advantage shown for the WGO-fed groups in Table XXVIII indicate that the nutritional state was improved, or that the subjects withstood the stress better (probably because of nutritional improvement).

Since high amplitude of the precordial T-waves has been shown to be related to relatively high plasma potassium levels by Braun (1955) and Winsor (1954), this might suggest a *nutritional* improvement brought about in the potassium levels of the plasma without any special potassium dosage except the one-half pint of milk used to wash down the capsules. Since both

TABLE XXVIII

CHANGES IN THE PRECORDIAL T-WAVE OF THE
ELECTROCARDIOGRAM DUE TO THE DIETARY SUPPLEMENTATION
WITH WGO, OCTACOSANOL AND WHEAT GERM (in SS)

Name of Study	Number of the Experiment	Relative Statistical Significance	Gains of WGO Experimental Group	Gains of the Octacosanol Group	Gains of the Group on Placeboes	Nonexercise Controls
Forr	1	**	8.0	(Syn. E)0.08	(CO) 1.25	
Maley	11	*	−12.7		1.0	
Susic	10	**	19.0		−11.0	
Cureton and Pohndorf	13	**	8.3		5.9	
Vohaska	12	*	−5.18		9.91	3.66
Bernauer and Cureton	18	**	3.8		−0.5	
Mayhew	29	**	5.0		−2.00	
			(0.99 mm)		(or −0.41 mm)	
		Average	3.746 SS		Average 0.623 SS	

Key to Statistical Significance:
*** Highly significant by *t* test (Fisher).
** Significant D/SE_meas. in favor of WGO.
* Negative or no experimental result.

experimental and control groups got the milk, there is no differential in this to explain the T-wave advantage on WGO.

REFERENCES

1. Einthoven, W.: The different forms of the human electrocardiogram and their significance, *Lancet,* 1:853, 1912.
2. Katz, L. N.: The significance of the T-wave in the electrogram and ECG, *Physiol. Rev.,* 8:447-500, Oct., 1928.
3. Groedel, Franz M. and Borchart, Paul R.: *Direct Electrocardiography of the Human Heart.* New York, Brooklyn Medical Press, 1948, p. 224.
4. Collen, George W.: *A New Concept Regarding the Genesis of T, Ta, U Waves and ST Segments, the Myokinetic Theory.* Los Angeles, The Enster Co., 1951, p. 101.
5. Ibid.
6. Du Toit, S. F.: Running and Weight Training Effects Upon the Cardiac Cycle, Urbana, Illinois, Ph.D. thesis, Physical Education, University of Illinois, 1966, p. 133.
7. Cundiff, D. E.: Training Changes in the Sympatho-Adrenal System Determined by Cardiac Cycle Hemodynamic, Oxygen Intake and Eosinopenia, Urbana, Illinois, Ph.D. thesis, Physical Education, University of Illinois, 1966, p. 188.
8. Sloninger, E. L.: The Relationship of Stress Indicators to Pre-Ejection Cardiac Intervals, Urbana, Illinois, Ph.D. thesis, Physical Education, University of Illinois, 1966, p. 214.
9. Milesis, C. A.: The Relationship of Vertical Deflections in the Brachial Pulse Wave, BCG and ECG to Endurance Performance, Urbana, Illinois: M.S. thesis, Physical Education, University of Illinois, 1965, p. 92.
10. Cureton, T. K. and Du Toit, S. F.: Effect of physical training on the latent period of electrical stimulation of the left ventricle of the human heart, *Proc. of the College Phys. Ed. Ass.,* Philadelphia, 69th Annual Meeting, 1965.
11. Banister, E. W., Cureton, T. K., Abbott, B. C. and Pollard, J. W.: A comparative study of the brachial pulse wave and its time derivatives among athletic, normal and pathological subjects, *J. Sports Med.,* 6:92-99, June, 1966.
12. Massey, B. H.: Prediction of All-out Treadmill Running from ECG Measurements, Urbana, Illinois, M.S. thesis, Physical Education, University of Illinois, 1947, p. 102.
13. Wolf, J. G.: The Effects of Posture and Muscular Exercise on the Electrocardiogram, Urbana, Illinois, Ph.D. thesis, Physical Education, University of Illinois, 1947; and *Res. Quart.,* 435-490, Dec., 1953.

14. Cureton, T. K.: Effects of longitudinal physical training on the amplitude of the highest precordial T-wave of the ECG, *Medicina Sportiva*, 12:259-281, July, 1958.

15. Milesis, C. A.: Op. cit., ref. 9.

16. Cureton, T. K.: Op. cit., ref 14.

17. Cureton, T. K.: In *Physical Fitness of Champion Athletes*. Urbana, University of Illinois Press, 1951, pp. 137-277.

18. Simonsen, E. and Keys, A.: The effect of age and body weight on the ECG of healthy men, *Circulation*, 6:749-761, Nov., 1952; and with Henschel, A. and Taylor, H. L.: Electrocardiographic changes in different nutritional states, *Fed. Proc.*, No. 1, March, 1945; and Simonsen, Henschel and Keys, The ECG of man in semi-starvation and subsequent rehabilitation, Amer. Heart J., 35:384-602, April, 1948.

19. Keys, A.: Some common conditions not due to primary heart disease that may be associated with changes in the ECG, *Ann. Intern. Med.*, 25:632-647, Oct., 1946.

20. Forr, Wm. A.: The Effect of Wheat Germ Oil (Vitamin E) on Physical Fitness, Urbana, Illinois, M.S. thesis, Physical Education, University of Illinois, 1950, p. 100.

21. Maley, A. F.: The Effects of Training and a Dietary Supplement on the Cardiovascular Fitness of Adult Men, Urbana, M.S. thesis, Physical Education, University of Illinois, 1952, p. 36.

22. Susic, Steve: The Effect of Training and a Dietary Supplement on the T-Wave of the ECG at Ground Level and at 10,000 Feet of Simulated Altitude, Urbana, Illinois, M.S. thesis, Physical Education, University of Illinois, 1953, p. 50.

23. Cureton, T. K. and Pohndorf, R. H.: Influence of wheat germ oil as a dietary supplement in a program of conditioning exercises with middle-aged subjects, *Res. Quart.*, 26:391-407, Dec., 1955.

24. Vohaska, Wm. J.: The Effects of Wheat Germ Oil on the Cardiovascular Fitness of Varsity Wrestlers, Urbana, Illinois, M.S. thesis, Physical Education, University of Illinois, 1954, p. 43.

25. Bernauer, E. M. and Cureton, T. K.: The Influence of Wheat Germ Oil as a Dietary Supplement in a Training Program of Varsity Track Athletes at the University of Illinois, Urbana, Staff Project, Physical Fitness Research Laboratory, 1958.

26. Cureton, T. K.: Improvements in physical fitness associated with a course of U. S. Navy Underwater Trainees, with and without dietary supplements, *Res. Quart.*, 34:440-453, Dec., 1963.

27. Mayhew, J. L.: The Effects of Training With and Without Wheat Germ Oil on the Pre-Cordial Lead of the T-Wave of the ECG and Other Selected Fitness Measures of Middle-Aged Men, M.S. thesis, Physical Education, University of Illinois, 1968, p. 128.

28. Poiletman, R. M. and Miller, H. A.: The Influence of Wheat Germ Oil on the Electrocardiographic T-Waves of Highly Trained Athletes, *J. Sports Med.*, 8:26-33, March, 1968.

29. Rose, K. D. and Dunn, F. L.: Physiology of running study by radio telemetry, and heart function in athletes by telemeter electrocardiography, and K. D. Rose, F. L. Dunn and D. Bargen: Serum electrolyte relationship to ECG changes in exercising athletes, *Nebraska State Med. J.*, 49:447, Sept., 1964.

Chapter VII

The Effects of Wheat Germ Oil and Octacosanol on the Systolic Amplitude and Area of the Brachial Pulse Wave (Sphygmograph) and Ballistocardiogram

MEANING OF THE BRACHIAL PULSE WAVE AND BALLISTOCARDIOGRAM

THE brachial pulse wave results from the contraction of the heart, which drives the blood upward through the aortic semilunar valves and into the aortic tree. The flow of blood resulting from the ejection (which follows the Ft = Mv impulse law) is basically impelled by a force (F) acting for a time (t) and equals the momentum of the ejected blood, i.e. mass of the blood times the velocity of the ejection. The pulse wave may be measured (Fig. 57) to reflect the velocity (the amplitude/time)

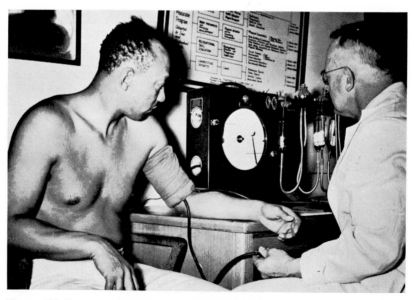

Figure 57. Testing a subject in the sitting position with the heartometer to record the brachial pulse wave.

or the rate of change of the anacrotic slope (acceleration). In the ballistocardiogram, the (F = Ma) law of accelerated motion is preferred, and here the F acts for a time (t) to produce the acceleration (a) of the mass of the body (M). Such an equation is only an approximation because of the friction of the person on the table. In this work a correction for this has been ignored, but a correlation was shown of 0.78 between the BCG wave (velocity) between the frictionless Ballisticor and the systolic amplitude of the heartograph wave as used in these experiments. The amplitude itself is proportional to velocity of the contracting force (or impulse from the force). It improves with training. Fig. 58.

It has been shown that the heartograph systolic amplitude is highly related to stroke volume, the rectilinear relationship being 0.91 in terms of correlation as determined on human subjects.[1] This relationship to stroke volume is represented in Figure 59. The Cameron Heartograph is depressed progressively as subjects are taken to 5000, 10,000 and 15,000 feet of simulated amplitude[2, 3] and is restored as the subjects are exposed to normal barometric pressure again. The oxygen to the heart muscle is involved. A shortage of oxygen to the heart muscle depresses the wave.

A factor analysis by Cureton and Sterling[4] demonstrated that the largest factor, taken out first by Thurstone factor analysis with rotation into orthogonal factor planes, resulted in the brachial pulse wave factor (ejection velocity) being the most dominant in the matrix of 104 cardiovascular variables, data on one hundred young men. It is not the same factor as maximum O_2 intake, as the pulse wave factor pertains particularly to the velocity of the ejected blood from the heart and the maximum O_2 intake is not so specific, being related to many factors but mainly to the ability of the muscle cells to utilize the oxygen, i.e. the lean body mass, or number of muscle cells in action in a given exercise.[5] While there is a moderate correlation between the maximum O_2 intake and systolic amplitude of the brachial pulse wave, the latter pertains more specifically to the heart. In an all-out endurance type of exercise the work is limited mainly by the ability of the heart stroke to maintain its vigor and largeness of stroke. Thus, Cureton[6, 7] demonstrated that trained ath-

AN IMPROVEMENT RECORD OF THE BRACHIAL PULSE WAVE (SITTING)

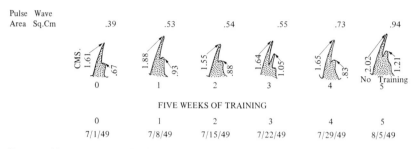

Figure 58. Exercising daily with hard endurance running and swimming, six weeks progression in brachial pulse waves.

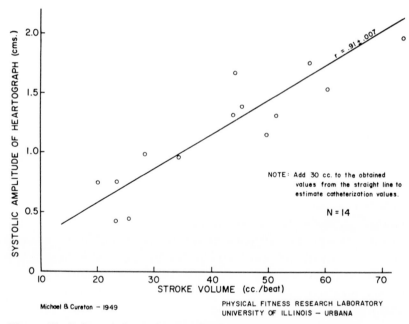

Figure 59. Relation of systolic amplitude of heartograph to stroke volume of the heart.

letes had larger strokes in training than out of training, and also
that top level endurance level athletes had larger and higher
relative velocity type strokes than nonathletic people, and that
moderately good predictions of endurance performance (mile
run, all-out treadmill run, 600-yard run times) could be obtained
from the velocity or area measures of the quantitated brachial
pulse wave at rest, and by measuring amplitude in the graph
taken while at work, or just after the work.[8]

That the pressure pulse wave is an important physiological
measure of circulatory dynamics and of heart function is attested
by many studies.[8, 9, 10, 11] Dontas[12] demonstrated a very close
agreement between the externally taken pulse waves and those
of the internal pressure pulse. Detection of early onset of arteriosclerosis is detectable by external pulse recording, and by
multi-channel recording to detect the pulse wave transmission
time.[13, 14, 15] The behavior of the arterial pulse waves after exercise compared to before exercise represents a valuable approach
to determining the ability of an individual to make a quick and
reasonably good adjustment to one minute of exercise, as an
oxygen deficit due to inadequate supply of blood to the heart in
view of the suddenly increased demand, whereas, an adequate
supply of blood may make possible an increased rather than a
decreased amplitude.[16] The condition of the coronary arteries
are involved. While it is not the purpose of this work, coronary
heart disease cases may be differentiated from normals by this
method, probably as well as by any method.[17, 18, 19] Stroke volume is a displacement measure, the amplitude of the brachial (or
carotid) pulse wave is a velocity measure, and the slope on the
forward wave face is highly related to acceleration of ejection
and to aging of the heart and attached arteries. It is of great
significance that during work the myocardium of the heart requires oxygen to keep right on pushing the blood from the heart
into the body. Any interference of this oxygen supply line will
cause the contractions to become relatively less (Cf. Fig. 62-B).
There is no difference really between just shutting off the oxygen
supply to the body, as by taking the subject to progressively
higher and higher levels of simulated altitude in a decompression
chamber, and interfering with the coronary arterial oxygen sup-

ply by any other manner. The immediate effect is the same—a diminished stroke of the heart. The amplitude, velocity and acceleration characteristics of the heart may, therefore, be traceable back to the oxygen supply to the heart myocardium through the coronary arteries.

Cundiff (Exp. 25, 1965-66) using a Brecht-Boucke capacitance transducer pick-up electrode under a cuff standardized for pressure at the diastolic level (set at 10 mm above DBP level to overcome loss of pressure in tube) found the following changes in resting systolic amplitude in matched groups of young boys, matched on the 600-yard run time: on WGO, systolic amplitude of BPW (2.93 to 3.08 cm, or 115 to 120 SS) compared to the placebo group on cottonseed oil (from 3.25 to 2.82 cm, or 130 to 110 SS); and on Kretchmer WGC (from 3.20 to 2.75 cm or 127 to 107 SS). The advantage here was +5.0 SS for WGO compared to −20.0 SS for the placebo group and −20.0 SS for the Kretchmer WGC group.

The study by Cureton, Ganslen, White, Susic (Exp. 10) demonstrated the effect of physical training on the brachial pulse wave (Fig. 60) showing the maintenance of a diastolic surge of the heartograph due to training compared to a sharp drop in amplitude in the untrained subjects (at ground level) and also the actual improvement of this measure of the physically trained group (at 10,000 feet of simulated altitude) compared to a loss by the control subjects, who were untrained. The data also show that the experimental group taking WGO, during the T_2 to T_3 stage, held up the diastolic surge while the comparable group in training showed a marked loss of amplitude, *at ground level.* Figure 60 also shows the maintenance of the *area under the wave* in terms of amplitude under the stress of altitude while taking WGO. These results indicate that WGO helps the subjects bear the stress.

Hupé studied matched groups of young boys from the University of Illinois Sports-Fitness School, 1958, and in the six-week training period obtained gains of 5.9 SS (WGO), 7.6 SS (OCTCNL), 14.0 SS (WGC). The average gain for these supplements was 9.17 SS for Systolic Amplitude of the BPW, compared to 8.4 SS on cottonseed oil placeboes. This was the only

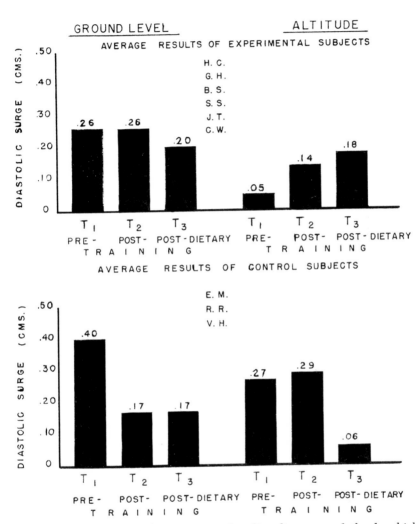

Figure 60. The effects of training on the diastolic surge of the brachial pulse wave (experimental subjects on WGO versus controls on placeboes, at ground level and at altitude).

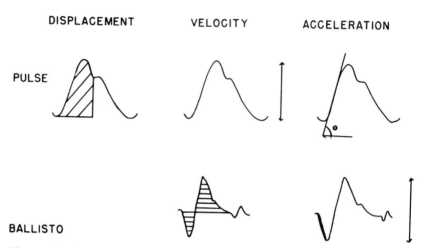

Figure 61. Aspects of cardiac functioning, displacement, velocity and acceleration (comparison of pulse waves with BCG waves), Starr.

time in the entire series of experiments that Kretchmer WGC turned up the best improvement. In the area of the HGF, the improvements were 14.2 (WGO), 6.0 (OCTCNL) and 7.0 (WGC) averaging 9.07 SS compared to 4.33 SS for the placebo group on cottonseed oil.

Tuma and Cureton (Exp. 17, 1959) compared three groups of United States Navy Underwater Demolition Trainees, at Little Creek, Va. (Marine Unit) from the beginning to the end of their training, these three groups being matched in three groups by a "composite muscular endurance index." The changes in the groups were as follows: OCTCNL group N = 5 (1.27 to 1.51 cm, 55 to 64 SS, gain of 9 SS); WGO group N = 6 (1.35 to 1.34 cm, or 57.0 to 57.0, gain of 0 SS); and the placebo group (cottonseed oil) N = 2 (0.89 to 0.65 cm, gain from 25.5 to 10.5 = −15.5 SS). Likewise, the area changes were 25.0 SS (on WGO); 15.0 SS (on OCTCNL) as compared to 2.0 SS gain on cottonseed oil placeboes. This experiment was reduced to the men listed because of a 70 per cent attrition due to injuries, failures and drop-outs. For the men still remaining at the end of the experiment the advantage was decidedly with those who were on either WGO or OCTCNL.

Bernauer and Cureton (Exp. 18, 1956) reported from an experiment in which a varsity track team was divided into two groups and compared for the twelve weeks of cross-country season, six men in each group, all distance runners. The gains for systolic amplitude of the BPW were for the WGO group (1.50 to 1.63 cm, or 76.8 to 92.7 SS) compared to the placebo group from 1.44 to 1.55 cm or 65.5 to 71.5 SS. The advantage was with the WGO group, 15.9 compared to 6 SS, a significant difference. Likewise, the gains in area of the BPW were as follows: WGO group (0.49 to 0.63 sq. cm or 55 to 70 SS) and for the placebo group from 0.46 to 0.55 sq. cm or 52.5 to 62 SS. The advantage was 15 to 9.5 SS, a significant difference.

THE BRACHIAL PULSE WAVE AS A BASIC CIRCULATORY MEASURE

The brachial pulse wave is considered to be a basic circulatory measure, highly correlated with the amount of circulation passing through the heart, aorta and coronary arteries. It has been used since about 1945 to show the circulatory effects of various exercise programs.[21, 22, 23] It is responsive to the effects of physical training and detraining in a wonderful way, and is more sensitive than oxygen intake measures. When the sympathoadrenal system is stirred up by exercise, the pulse wave is enlarged, especially its amplitude, as has been shown by injecting adrenalin into the venous system. In about five minutes there is an augmentation of the amplitude of the brachial pulse wave. By repetitious exertions the body carries a larger relative sympathoadrenal stimulus to the heart and the heart responds persistently with a larger stroke, a taller and sharper ejection angle of the systolic wave. It is also important to note that physical training results in a greater parasympathetic tone simultaneously, and the secondary (diastolic) portion of the wave is widened, so that the time of diastole to time of systole is a larger ratio, 3, 4, 5, 6, compared to the untrained pattern, 1:1, or a smaller ratio of *rest time* to *work time*. The Cameron Heartograph has long been used in exercise laboratories to trace the effects of exercise both instantaneously and in a persistently chronic way. It is not to be confused with an electrocardiogram (ECG) which is a voltage record, not capable of measuring the working capacity of the heart, or the responsiveness of the arterial system. The electrical propagation waves of the ECG are not used for dynamic force or velocity or acceleration but are used for propagation speeds and penetrability of the heart tissue, a scar, therefore, usually making a blemish on the record. The heartograph (HGF) measured instead the function and not the scar, or propagation speed of electricity flowing from the S-A node area, from auricles into ventricles, to the heart muscle and return.

In this section it is shown that WGO has affected the amplitude and area of the brachial pulse wave in a systematic way, and the generalization is that the effect is good, in the same direction of physical training, to augment the effect which would otherwise be obtained with the physical training alone, without WGO as a dietary supplement. It is shown that this added WGO effect is great enough to be of considerable consequence. This is considered an important finding.

TABLE XXIX

RELIABILITY OF THE EXPERIMENTS OF WGO, WGC AND OCTCNL
TO AFFECT THE BRACHIAL PULSE WAVE

Experiment	Statistical Significance < .10	Positive Trends but not < .10	No Experimental Result in Favor
1 (Forr)	WGO versus Synthetic E	WGO versus Corn Oil	
9 (Constantino) .		WGO versus Nothing	
12 (Vohaska)			WGO versus CSO
13 (Cureton and Pohndorf) ..	WGO		
15 (Hupé and Cureton) ...	Kretchmer WGC	WGO versus Lecithin Oil Octacnl versus Lecithin Oil	
17 (Tuma and Cureton) ...	Octacnl WGO		
18 (Bernauer and Cureton) ...	WGO		
25 (Cundiff)		WGO	Octcnl

The reliability of the eight separate experiments is tabulated in Table XXIX.

Lloyd-Thomas,[24] Tuttle[25] and others have shown that normal subjects show minimal changes or none at all in the S-T segments, the P-Q interval and the P-R segment after corrections are made for pulse rate. Young healthy competitors may show momentary ST-depression of more than 1 mm after swimming 100 yards at top speed.[26] Acceleration forward and backward may also make the ST-segment unstable without being attributable to heart disease. Almost as many middle-aged subjects develop heart disease with no abnormal ECG history as the reverse. In light of these facts, the carotid and brachial and popliteal arterial pulse waves are being used more and more to detect abnormal arterial circulatory conditions. By contrast, this work is *not* dealing with heart diseased subjects, and all have been medically examined as a prerequisite to taking part in the programs. We are most concerned with performance, and with circulation, and basic physiological condition of the heart and large arteries. The sphygmographic methods are commonly used for this purpose. The previous works show that reliability is as good and usually better for the brachial pulse wave compared to the ECG, but the electronic pick-up waves are not as reliable as the Cameron heartometer pulse waves.

SUMMARY AND CONCLUSIONS OF EIGHT PULSE WAVE EXPERIMENTS

Of eight different experiments, seven of these gave positive trends for WGO to affect the brachial pulse wave test. WGO was used eleven times and beat the placebo group nine times. The systolic amplitude experiment was used thirteen times and area of the brachial pulse wave experiment—six times. Unless otherwise mentioned, the criterion test is systolic amplitude. Octacosanol was used in four experiments and improved the group over the control group on all but one experiment with young boys who were overloaded and tired when they took the final brachial pulse wave test but fully recuperated three weeks later. The reliability of these experiments was as follows:

TABLE XXX

RESULTS OF STUDIES TO SHOW THE EFFECTS OF WGO ON THE BRACHIAL PULSE WAVE AMPLITUDE AND AREA (in SS)

Experiment Number	Experimenters	Experimental Supplement Group			Control Group			Net Difference SS
		T_1	T_2	Difference in SS	T_1	T_2	Difference in SS	
		Diff. in SS			Diff. in SS			
1	Forr and Cureton							
	Fraternity Sys. Amp.	47.2 to 52.8 (on WGO)		5.6	48.8 to 52.8		4.0 (E)	+1.6
					52.0 to 57.8		5.8 (CO)	– .2
	Swimming Sys. Amp.	47.8 to 49.4 (on WGO)		1.6	48.8 to 52.8		4.0 (E)	–2.4
					52.8 to 57.8		5.0 (CO)	–3.4
9	Constantine and Cureton Sys. Amp.	57.0 to 80 (on WGO)		23.0	57 to 60		3	+20.0
12	Vohaska and Cureton Sys. Amp.	49.6 to 54.6 (on WGO)		5.0	54.4 to 59.6		4.28	+0.72
13	Cureton and Pohndorf (Area) (S.A.)	41.0 to 62.0 (on WGO)		11.0	42.0 to 46.0		4.0	+7.0
		44.0 to 73.0 (on WGO)		29.0	50.5 to 53.0		2.5	+26.5
15	Hupé and Cureton	Sys. (on WGO)		5.9	(On CSO)		8.4	+0.77
		Amp. (on OCTCNL)		7.6				
		(on WGC)		14.0				
				Av. 9.17				
		Area (on WGO)		14.2	(On CSO)		–13.3	+22.37
		(on OCTCNL)		6.0				
		(on WGC)		7.0				
				Av. 9.07				

17	Tuma and Cureton	(S.A.)	55.0 to 64.0 (on OCTCNL)	9.0	25.5 to 10.5	−15.0	+24.0
			57.0 to 57.0 (on WGO)	0.0			+15.0
		(Area)	80 to 105 (on WGO)	25.0	40.0 to 42.0	+2.0	+23.0
			85 to 100 (on WGO)	15.0			+13.0
18	Bernauer and Cureton	(S.A.)	76.8 to 92.7 (on OCTCNL)	15.9	65.5 to 71.5	+6.0	+9.9
			115 to 120 SS (on WGO)	5.0	130 to 107	−20.0	−17.0
25	Cundiff and Cureton		127 to 107 SS (on WGC)	−20.0			
Improvements (Averages)				9.47 SS		−0.12 SS	9.59 SS

1. Three times the statistical significance was better than .05 level WGO as affecting the heartograph.
2. One time the statistical significance was better than .05 in affecting the IJ/t complex of the ballistocardiogram.
3. One time Kretchmer wheat germ cereal gave the best result.*
4. Nine out of eleven times the WGO affected the criterion test (HGF) favorably.
5. Nine out of eleven times the WGO experimental group bettered the placebo group; and three out of four times the octacosanol group won out.

It is concluded that the WGO and its derivative, octacosanol, have a positive effect on the brachial pulse wave, usually affecting most the Systolic Amplitude but also affecting the area under the wave in the quiet resting position.

The gains over the control group seem to be highly related to the total amount of work done. In Forr's study the men were only moderately active, three times per week and the *net* differences between the experimental and control groups were indefinite and statistically insignificant. With activity five days per week (Hupé), the net changes were larger, and they were largest with very heavy, daily work for sixteen weeks.

RESULTS OF STUDIES WHICH SHOW POSITIVE EFFECTS OF WGO AND OCTACOSANOL ON THE BRACHIAL PULSE WAVE

Forr (Exp. 1) in 1950 found little difference between the brachial pulse waves of his two groups after eight and twelve weeks of the program, with matched groups on WGO, synthetic vitamin E (alpha tocopherol acetate) and corn oil. The gains are shown in Table XXX to average 3.6 SS for the two groups on WGO, 0.40 SS for the two groups on synthetic vitamin E (equal amount to WGO) and −1.8 SS on corn oil. This is reported as a "trend" favorable but statistically insignificant for WGO. In these three groups, there were sixteen men taking WGO, sixteen men taking synthetic vitamin E and seventeen men taking corn oil.

---

* In this experiment, it was insisted that the wheat germ furnished by the Kretchmer Company be freshly milled, rather than bottles from the storage supplies.

Constantino (Exp. 9, 1952) found that three months of physical training increased both the systolic amplitude and the area of the brachial pulse wave significantly but the differential attributable to WGO was only slightly positive, as the group on WGO sustained the area (0.64 to 0.65 sq. cm), N = 6 men, whereas a control group not on a training or dietary supplement program lost from 0.66 to 0.51 sq. cm of area in the same time, a gain of 72 to 73 SS for the WGO group and a loss from 74 to 59 SS for the control group. Since the exercise group had plateaued off on three cardiovascular tests and also the bicycle ergometer ride, the advantage is probably with the WGO by a considerable amount. It is noticed that in the terminal stages of the program the WGO group lost in sytolic amplitude from 1.91 to 1.77 sq. cm (81 to 73 SS) compared to the control group losing from 2.01 to 1.76 cm (87 to 73 SS), the latter having a greater loss (Fig. 60).

Vohaska (Exp. 12, 1955) using college wrestlers found gains in area of the brachial pulse wave of 10.1 per cent for the WGO group (gain of 5 SS), 9.7 per cent for the matched group on cottonseed oil (gain of 4.28 SS) and a loss of 12.4 per cent for the control group (loss of 7.33 SS), all on the same exercise.

Cureton and Pohndorf (Exp. 13, 1955) obtained, in a six weeks long calisthenics plus swimming course with middle-aged men, a gain of 11.0 SS in area compared to 4.0 for the matched control group, and a gain of 29.0 SS in systolic amplitude compared to 2.5 SS for the control group. These gains in favor of the WGO group were significant by the $D/_{\text{S.E. meas.}}$ ratio.

EFFECTS OF A DIETARY SUPPLEMENT ON SELECTED BALLISTOCARDIOGRAPHIC INTERVALS AND AMPLITUDES IN YOUNG BOYS

The ballistocardiogram (BCG) measures "heart force" and is proportional to the velocity of ejection of the blood from the heart measured from I to J (Figs. 63 and 64).[*]

_____

[*] The BCG used in this work was the Arbeit direct shin-bar type (cf. S. R. Arbeit and N. Lindner): A new full-frequency range calibrated BCG, *Amer. Heart J.*, 45:52-59, Jan., 1953. The reliability of this device on human male subjects has been reported by Knowlton (I-J$_a$ = 0.94), Ph.D. thesis, Univ of Illinois, 1961.

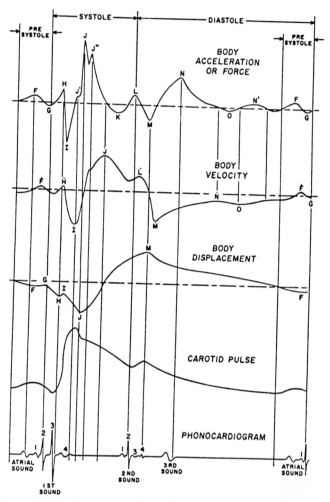

Figure 62-A. Direct body ballistocardiogram related to heart sounds in multi-channel tracing.

Dempsey (Exp. 22, 1963) studied the effects of training and a dietary supplement on seventy-six young boys. Fifty-six of the boys in the University of Illinois Sports Fitness School were equally divided into groups receiving wheat germ oil and lard placeboes. The other twenty boys were the control group which had neither the training nor the dietary supplement. The follow-

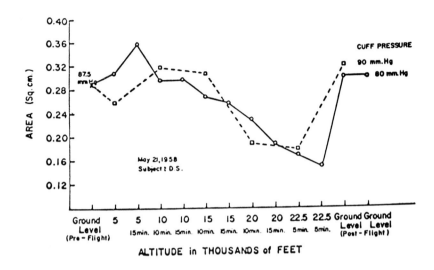

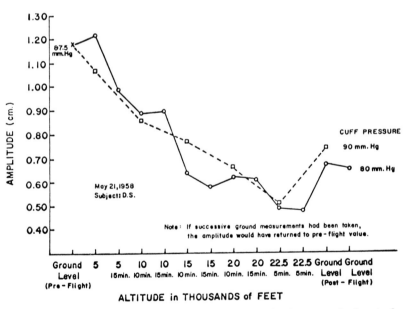

Figure 62-B. Failure of the ejection stroke of the heart with deprival of oxygen.

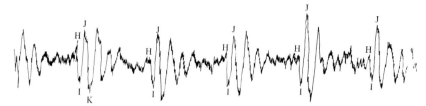

Figure 63. Type of BCG Record used with notation.

ing measures were determined from the velocity and acceleration settings of the ballistocardiogram (Fig. 62-A):† Amplitude of H, I, J, I-J and K waves; duration of H, I, J, K, I-J, I-K and I downstroke waves; angle of the I-wave downstroke and a ratio of velocity of body displacement (mm/sec.).* The BCG (V_a) is also highly related to the stroke volume (average per beat) designated V_s.

The wheat germ oil group made greater changes than either of the other groups in the following measures: Acceleration BCG amplitudes (BCG_a) J and I-J waves, duration of the J and K waves and angle of the I wave; velocity BCG, H wave amplitude, K wave duration, I downstroke duration and the ratio of velocity of body displacement; as well as heart rate, all-out treadmill run time and post-exercise pulse pressure. The training groups had larger changes than either of the other two groups in the acceleration BCG amplitudes of the H, I and K waves; duration of the H, I, I-K and I downstroke waves, and the ratio; velocity BCG amplitudes of the J, I-J, and K waves and duration of the H, J, and I-J waves and angle of the I wave. The control group had the greatest changes only in acceleration BCG I-J duration and velocity BCG I wave amplitude and I-K wave duration (see Table XXXI for raw scores). The stroke volume (V_s) is highly related to the I-J wave (Fig. 64).

The T wave of the ECG is skewed in relationship to performance. The Fisher t test is not a legitimate test to use in this re-

---

* From M. B. Rappaport: Displacement, velocity and acceleration ballistocardiograms as registered with an undamped bed of ultra-low natural frequency. *Amer. Heart J.* 52:643-652, Nov., 1956.

lationship, so the $D/$s.e.diff. was used. The trends are in favor of the WGO supplement. The large negative in Maley's Experiment (11) was due to averaging the standard scores for the R and T waves of the ECG, and this resulted in pulling the score down due to depressions in the R wave. In Experiment 12 by Vohaska, a composite CV index was used, on which there was an advantage for the WGO group but in Table XXVIII, a loss appears in the

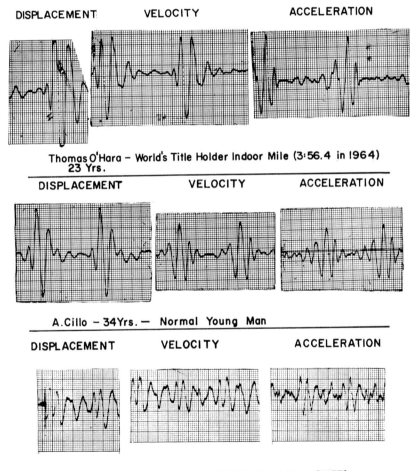

Figure 64. Strong, medium and weak ejection strokes of the heart from direct (Arbeit) ballistocardiograph.

TABLE XXXI

MEAN RAW SCORE CHANGES ASSOCIATED WITH THE TRAINING
PROGRAM AND WHEAT GERM OIL SUPPLEMENT

Variable (Unit of Measurement)	*Wheat Germ Oil Supplement and Training Program Group*			*Training Program Group*			*Control Group*		
	T_1	T_8	Change	T_1	T_8	Change	T_1	T_8	Change
Ballistocardiographic Measurements:									
Acceleration Wave:									
H-wave amplitude (mm)	5.79	7.17	1.38	6.21	7.70	1.49	6.54	6.14	−.40
I-wave amplitude (mm)	6.93	8.68	1.75	7.34	9.28	1.94	6.98	6.98	0
J-wave amplitude (mm)	14.79	18.05	3.26	15.94	18.58	2.64	16.34	15.21	−1.13
I plus J amplitude (mm)	21.69	26.73	5.06	23.08	27.92	4.84	23.33	23.32	−.01
K-wave amplitude (mm)	13.98	16.08	2.10	13.64	16.93	3.29	14.06	13.92	−.14
H-wave duration (mm)	2.40	2.39	−.01	2.23	2.39	.16	2.59	2.52	−.07
I-wave duration (mm)	1.40	1.35	−.05	1.26	1.33	.07	1.35	1.32	−.03
J-wave duration (mm)	2.41	2.48	.07	2.39	2.37	−.02	2.42	2.53	.11
I-J duration (mm)	1.73	1.78	.05	1.65	1.74	.09	1.78	1.88	.10
I downstroke (mm)	1.07	.69	−.38	.60	.63	.03	.73	.69	−.04
Angle I-wave (degrees)	76.61	82.65	6.04	81.54	81.52	.02	82.69	82.88	.19
M.R. ratio (mm/sec.)	5.73	6.84	1.11	6.37	7.75	1.20	6.33	5.82	−.51
Heart rate (beats/min.)	81.07	72.04	−9.03	77.71	73.75	−3.96	70.90	72.90	2.00
Velocity Wave:									
H-wave amplitude (mm)	5.86	7.20	1.34	6.56	7.74	1.18	6.44	5.95	−.49
I-wave amplitude (mm)	6.18	7.81	1.63	7.47	8.12	.65	8.07	11.15	3.08
J-wave amplitude (mm)	17.27	20.39	3.12	17.31	22.00	4.69	19.12	19.15	.03
I plus J amplitude (mm)	23.45	28.13	4.68	25.07	30.21	5.14	26.06	26.07	.01
K-wave amplitude (mm)	16.92	18.84	1.92	16.36	19.23	2.87	18.88	18.02	.86
H-wave duration (mm)	2.42	2.54	.12	2.46	2.87	.41	2.58	2.59	.01
I-wave duration (mm)	1.46	1.50	.04	1.47	1.48	.01	1.62	1.52	.10
J-wave duration (mm)	2.70	2.78	.08	2.62	2.78	.16	2.67	2.80	.13

K-wave duration (mm)	2.61	2.77	.16	2.74	2.77	.03	2.80	2.87	.07
I-J wave duration (mm)	2.08	2.15	.07	2.00	2.15	.15	2.13	2.19	.06
I-K wave duration (mm)	4.29	4.50	.21	4.36	4.49	.13	4.31	4.60	.29
I downstroke (mm)	.70	.73	.03	.67	.69	.02	.23	.13	–.10
Angle I-wave (degrees)	82.21	82.29	.08	78.74	83.75	5.01	82.58	79.06	–3.52
M.R. ratio (mm/sec.)	5.72	6.83	1.11	6.16	7.04	.88	6.29	6.02	–.27
All-out treadmill run (minutes)	1:43	2:43	1:00	1:39	2:34	:55	2:00	2:25	:25
Pulse pressure, post-treadmill run (mm/Hg)	63.68	69.75	6.07	66.25	69.64	3.39	72.60	64.46	–8.14
Composite (mm)	117.71	110.46	–7.25	104.14	96.54	–7.60	144.85	149.95	5.10
Gluteal adipose (mm)	24.68	20.25	–4.43	22.29	19.54	–2.75	22.35	24.20	1.85
Rear thigh adipose (mm)	24.86	22.14	–2.72	22.75	20.64	–2.11	23.85	22.05	–1.80
Height (inches)	54.16	54.71	.55	54.75	54.94	.19	55.29	55.68	.39
Weight (pounds)	75.51	78.22	2.71	70.97	71.18	.21	84.60	85.97	1.37
Heartograph:									
Pulse rate (lying) (beats/minute)	79.21	69.04	–10.17	80.75	74.93	–5.82	69.36	71.30	1.94
Systolic amplitude (lying) (mm)	5.85	7.43	1.58	5.90	8.35	2.45	7.32	6.67	–.65
Systolic amplitude (sitting) (mm)	5.61	7.90	2.29	5.38	7.50	2.12	5.66	5.75	.09
Change in systolic amplitude (mm) (sitting-standing)	2.05	1.22	–.83	1.56	1.14	–.42	1.57	1.88	.31

T_1 = Initial Test
T_s = Final Treatment Test

T wave and a gain in the placebo group. Here again the average of the R and T waves were used. It is seen now that it would have been better to have used only the T wave, because in some subjects as T increases, the R may decrease. While treating these two experiments as averages of R and T has hurt the case for WGO, the trend is favorable in spite of this, and generally supports the value of WGO.

MEASUREMENTS TO ESTIMATE STROKE VOLUME[*]

I-Wave	*H-Wave*	*J-Wave*
16.4	7.2	16.4
8.2	4.3	17.5
8.0	7.0	11.9
14.0	10.9	16.9
11.0	5.9	20.2

Av. 11.52 mm	Av. H = 7.06 mm	16.56 mm
− 2.82 corr.	× .40	4.51
I = 8.70 mm	2.82 mm corr.	J = 12.05 mm

$$V_s = 5 \sqrt{(3\ I + 2\ J)\ A\ c3/2}$$
$$V_s = 5 \sqrt{[(3 \times 8.70) + 2(12.05)]\ (14.6)\ (0.55)}$$
$$V_s = 100 \text{ cc per beat}$$

CONCLUSIONS

Within the scope of this study on young boys, the physical training increased the cardiac functions and intervals as measured by the amplitudes and durations of the waves of the ballistocardiogram, both velocity and acceleration deflections. Wheat germ oil appeared to have some effect; however, it was somewhat inconsistent. The effects of a dietary supplement on the measures from the ballistocardiogram in longer training programs with adults has not been studied; but the WGO group had a greater relative effect in lowering the pulse rate $(-9.03$ beats) compared to $(-3.96$ beats) the parallel training group not on WGO. The angle of the I_a-wave became more vertical and there was a five-second improvement advantage in the all out treadmill run and a larger increase in the post-run pulse pressure (6.07 compared to 3.39 mm. Hg.). The WGO group reduced the lying

---

[*] Committee on terminology, *Circulation*, 1:363-365, July, 1953; and Jokl, Arbeit, McCubbin, Grenier, Koskela and Jokl: BCGs of olympic athletes, *Am. J. Cardiol.*, 199-207, Feb., 1958.

pulse rate relatively more (-10.17 compared to -5.82) beats per minute; and there was a relatively larger improvement in the sitting and standing brachial pulse wave amplitudes and also in the IJ/t_v complex.

The concept that the heart muscle and also the muscular walls of the arteries can be nutrified is established in many studies. Myocardial dysfunction has been established as due to lack of thiamine. A. Eustis (*New Orleans M. S. J.*, 94:369, 1942), Keys (*Ann. Int. Med.*, 25:632-647, Oct., 1946), Henschel and Taylor (*Fed. Proc.* No. 1, Mar., 1945), and Simonsen, Henschel and Keys (*Amer. Heart J.*, 35:384-602, April, 1948), have shown that in semi-starvation there is a marked deterioration of the heart's T wave and contractility. Our own experiments both with the T wave and the Cameron and electronic pulse waves indicate *an apparent semi-starvation state exists for the fresh, natural, unboiled wheat germ oil, or the improvements shown in this section most probably could not have been obtained.* The BCG and HGF parts are in good agreement in that both show that WGO improved the heart myocardial action (and cardiovascular state) more than the placebo groups used. Other natural, fresh (uncooked) oils may also produce some of this same effect, as shown for corn oil but a lesser effect than for WGO.

REFERENCES

1. Michael, E. D.: Relationship of the Heartometer (Pulse Waves) and the Acetylene Method of Measuring Circulatory Fitness, Urbana, M.S. thesis, Physical Education, University of Illinois, 1949, p. 61.
2. Michael, E. D. and Cureton, T. K.: Effects of physical training on cardiac output at ground level and at 15,000 feet of simulated altitude, *Res. Quart.*, 24:446-452, Dec., 1953.
3. Cureton, T. K.: *Physical Fitness of Champion Athletes.* Rectilinear relationship of the systolic amplitude of the brachial pulse wave and the Grollman stroke volume of the heart. Urbana, University of Illinois Press, 1951; and p. 35 and p. 128 in Cureton's *Physiological Effects of Exercise Programs on Adults*, Springfield, Ill., Charles C Thomas, 1969.
4. Cureton, T. K. and Sterling, L. F.: Factor analyses of cardiovascular test variables, *J. Sport Med.*, 4:1-24, March, 1964.
5. Buskirk, E. and Taylor, H. L.: Maximal oxygen intake and its relation to body composition with special reference to chronic physical activity and obesity, *J. Appl. Physiol.*, 11:72, 1957; and Physiological

requirements for world-class performances in endurance running, *South African Med. J.*, 41:996-1002, Aug., 1969; and J. E. Coates, *et al.*: Factors relating to maximal oxygen intake in young adult male and female subjects, *Proc. Physiol. Soc.* (London), *J. Physiol.*, 189:70-80, Jan., 1967; and T. K. Cureton: The relative value of stress indicators, pp. 73-80 in *Biochemistry of Exercise*, Basel, New York, Karger, 1969.

6. Cureton, T. K.: The brachial pulse wave as a test of cardiovascular condition, pp. 228-254 in *Physical Fitness of Champion Athletes.* Op. cit., ref. 3.

7. Jokl, E. and Wells, J. B.: Exercise training and cardiac force, pp. 135-146, in Raab's, *Prevention of Ischemic Heart Disease*, Springfield, Ill., Charles C Thomas, 1966.

8. Editorial: What can be found in arterial pulse waves, *Am. Heart J.*, pp. 424-426, March, 1961.

9. Wiggers, C. J.: *Circulatory Dynamics*, New York, Grune and Stratton, 1952.

10. Hyman, C. and Winsor, T.: Application of the segmental plethysmography to the measurement of blood flow through the limbs of human beings, *Amer. J. Cardiol.*, 6:667, 1960.

11. Cureton, T. K.: Rating cardiovascular condition by the heartometer pulse wave tests, pp. 232-280 in Cureton's *Physical Fitness Appraisal and Guidance*, St. Louis, C. V. Mosby Co., 1947.

12. Dontas, A. S.: Arterial and pulse pressure contours in young human subjects, *Amer. Heart J.*, 61:676-683, May, 1961; and Comparison of simultaneously recorded intra-arterial and extra-arterial pressure pulse in man, *Amer. Heart J.*, 59:576, 1960 and 61:676-683, May, 1961.

13. Spencer, M. P. and Denison, A. B.: The aortic flow pulse as related to differential pressure, *Cir. Res.*, 4:476-484, July, 1956.

14. Robinson, Brian, I.: The Carotid Pulse, II. Relation of external recordings to carotid, aortic and brachial pulses, St. George's Hospital, London, *Brit. Heart J.*, 25:51-68, 1963.

15. Freis, E. D., *et al.*: Changes in the carotid pulse wave with age and hypertension, *Amer. Heart J.*, 71:757, June, 1966; and *Circulation*, 34:423, Sept., 1966.

16. Cureton, T. K.: Validity of testing cardiovascular fitness by the sphygmograph (external cuff, heartograph) method with the Cameron and related methods, pp. 118-191 in Cureton's *Physiological Effects of Exercise Programs on Adults*, op. cit., ref. 3.

17. Cooper, David, Hill, L. T., Jr., and Edwards, E. A.: Detection of early atherosclerosis by external pulse recording, *J.A.M.A.*, 199:449-454, Feb. 13, 1967.

18. Lax, H., *et al.*: Studies of arterial pulse wave, I. Normal pulse wave and its modification in presence of human arteriosclerosis, *J. Chron.*

Dis., 3:619-631, June, 1956; and B. L. Gilmore and Freis, E. D.:
Effect of amyl-nitrate on the height of the pulse wave incisura of
atherosclerotic patients, *Angiology*, 15:210-214, May, 1964; and
Woolam, G. L.: The pulse wave velocity as an early indicator of
atherosclerosis in diabetic subjects, *Circulation*, 25:533-539, March,
1962.

19. Starr, Isaac and Wood, F. G.: Twenty-year studies with the ballistocardiograph, *Circulation*, 23:714-732, May, 1961; and Rushmer,
R. A.: The initial impulse, a potential key to cardiac evaluation,
Circulation, 29:253-282, Feb., 1964; and Banister, E. W., Abbott,
B. C., Pollard, J. W.: A comparative study of the brachial pulse
wave and its time derivatives among athletic, normal and pathological subjects, *J. Sports Med.*, 6:92-99, June, 1966.

20. Starr, I. and Ogawa, S.: On the aging of the heart, *Amer. J. Med. Sci.*
549:No. 4, Oct., 1960; and 243:309, 1962.

21. Massey, B. H.: Changes in the Cameron Heartograph and Johnson
Oscillometer Pulse Wave Tracings with Progressive Loads of Work,
Urbana, Ph.D. thesis, Physical Education, University of Illinois,
1950, and pp. 134-147 in Cureton's Physiological Effects of Exer-
cise Programs on Adults, op. cit., ref. 3.

22. Cureton, T. K. and Massey, B. H.: Brachial peripheral pulse waves related to altitude tolerance and endurance, *Amer. J. Physiol.*,
159:566, Dec., 1949; and T. K. Cureton: What the heartometer
reveals that is of interest to physical education and physical fitness directors, *Phys. Ed. Today* (Manila), 7:10-14, March, 1960
and ibid., *Revue de l'Education Physique*, 1:No. 1, Sept., 1961,
pp. 796-1003; also T. K. Cureton: Review of Research to Determine Cardiovascular Condition, Proc. of the College P.E. Ass.,
1950-51.

23. Cureton, T. K.: Anatomical, physiological and psychological changes
induced in exercise programs, in *Exercise and Fitness*, pp. 152-182,
University of Illinois Colloquium Monograph, Chicago, The Athletic
Institute, 1960.

24. Lloyd-Thomas, H. G.: The effect of exercise on the electrocardiogram
in healthy subjects, *Brit. Heart J.*, 23:260-270, May, 1961.

25. Tuttle, W. W. and Korns, H. M.: Electrocardiographic observations on
athletes before and after a season of physical training, *Amer. Heart
J.*, 21:104-7, Jan., 1941.

26. FIMA Medical Research Committee: *Medical Research on Swimming,*
pp. 74-73, by E. A. Hunt, Electrocardiographic study of 20 champion swimmers before and after a 100-yard sprint swimming competition, pp. 70-73, 1969; also Forbes Carlile: T-wave changes in
strenuous exercise, Aus. Sports in *Carlile on Swimming*, pp. 99-122;
Medical Ass., Apr. 15, 1959. London: Pelham Books, Ltd., 1959;
and in *Phys. Ed. J.* (Melbourne), No. 17, 10-20, Nov.-Dec., 1959.

Chapter VIII

The Effects of Wheat Germ Oil, Octacosanol and Wheat Germ on the Schneider Index, Progressive Pulse Ratio and Harvard Five-Minute Step Test in Exercised Groups Over Control Exercised Groups on Placeboes

NINE studies are presented which investigated the effect of WGO, wheat germ or octacosanol, taken in conjunction with physical training, on the Schneider index,[1] progressive pulse ratio,[2] and five-minute step test.[3] Table XXXII presents the results of these studies in terms of standard score improvements within groups, including the swimming and fraternity classes of Forr's study and ground level and altitude conditions. Of the eight experiments involving the Schneider index as the criterion, six resulted in an advantage for the dietary supplements. Of the two experiments involving the progressive pulse ratio, all three favored the WGO supplements. Of the one study involving the five-minute step test, the octacosanol group bettered the placebo group on the terminal pulse rate −13.60 versus −10.0 (placebo group) and 0.20 beats (diff. stat. insignificant) (WGO group) in Experiment 21.

These studies have demonstrated the following:

1. The dietary supplements (WGO and octacosanol) favorably influenced the condition of the autonomic nervous system in the subjects described herein to such a degree that improvements in the Schneider index occurred in six out of eight experiments.
2. Wheat germ oil had slight positive influence on the cardiovascular efficiency of performing increasing intensities of submaximal exercise, as evidenced by improvements in all three of the progressive pulse ratio studies made by groups taking wheat germ oil as opposed to placeboes.
3. Vagal tone, as inferred from resting pulse rate, was not generally improvable by means of WGO supplementation.

The gains were made in favor of WGO when the pulse rates were taken during standard increments of work and indicated an economy reflected in relatively slower pulse rates.

THE TESTS OF CARDIOVASCULAR FUNCTION

Quiet Resting Pulse Rate

Although it is highly desirable to develop and maintain high sympathoadrenergic capacity in order to cope with physical stress through strong reactions of the "fight or flight" mechanism, it is also important to possess high vagal (cholinergic or parasympathetic) capacity, so that in the absence of stress one is able to rest, relax, sleep, digest food well, and free himself from nervous tension and anxiety. Cureton[4] summarized that endurance training augments both aspects of the autonomic nervous system, after noting that training increased the inotropic (vertical) deflections of the brachial sphygmograms as well as decreased the vagal-dominated pulse rate. Du Toit[5] reached the same conclusion. Traditionally, only the parasympathetic tone was affected.

It is generally considered that a shift of autonomic tone towards sympatheticotonia, when this is produced *not by stressful exercise training* but by chronic nervous tension, is conducive to necrotic and fibrous myocardial degeneration. Raab[6] and Weissler[7] point to the protective value of exercise in restoring adequate cholinergic activity to the myocardium; corroboration of this concept is found in studies by Raab,[8] Franks and Cureton.[9] Subsequently, in follow-up work studies on wheat germ and its derivatives (WGO and OCTCNL) were undertaken to determine if training plus dietary supplements improved vagal function more so than training alone. Measurement of vagal function was accomplished through tests of resting pulse rate, the Schneider index and progressive pulse ratio, and the Harvard five-minute step test.

It is widely accepted that a slower resting pulse rate in response to endurance training is indicative of improved vagal tone. It has been generally accepted that vagal stimulation results in bradycardia. Although the resting pulse rate may be considerably accelerated by apprehension during the time it is being counted, it nonetheless represents a valuable test of vagal tone.° The convenience of the resting pulse rate test adds to its usefulness.

Progressive Pulse Ratio

The progressive pulse ratio test, as standardized by Cureton,[10] is one of the few submaximal tests that is able to differentiate levels of fitness while requiring almost no equipment. It is explained that,

> If the subjects are able to exercise, there is no doubting the superiority of the interpretation which can be made of the progressive pulse ratio tests (12, 18, 24, 30, 36 steps per minute) compared to a single or two point pulse ratio test. The quiet, resting "sitting pulse rate" is carefully determined. Then the subject steps for exactly one minute up and down on a 17-inch stool at the rate of twelve steps per minute. Beginning ten seconds afterwards, the heart rate is counted with a stethoscope for two minutes. This count is divided by the "sitting pulse rate." After the pulse rate has leveled off, the next rate of stepping is used. Each succeeding rate is carried out with enough rest between trials to permit the pulse rate to come back to its lowest rate. These several pulse ratios are plotted against the rates of stepping on standardized graph paper. . . . There is an excellent relationship between the ratings by the brachial pulse wave and the progressive pulse ratio test; also, the average of the five pulse ratios is highly related to gross oxygen intake in the 10 mi/hr, 8.6 per cent grade treadmill run

Well-trained subjects have relatively low pulse ratios at all rates of stepping and the plotted points fall in a straight line closely approximating the horizontal. A sharp upward break in the slope of the line indicates the limit of aerobic tolerance and the onset of O_2 debt.[†]

° While this may be usually so, there are many exceptions as in the case of a very large heart, lack of vitamin B_1 in the diet, unusually large blood volume and in cases of psychological depression. These diverse causes of slow resting pulse rate make this measure more uncertain than the working pulse rates.

† The proof of this has been obtained from research work in which the O_2 intake and O_2 debt for many subjects on each rate of stepping throughout the entire series (cf. pp. 90-117 in Cureton's *The Physiological Effects of Exercise Programs on Adults*, 1969).

Schneider Index

The Schneider index is a composite score based on the ratings of changes in pulse rate and blood pressure in response to postural change (lying to standing) and very mild exercise (five steps on a chair in fifteen seconds). Good cardiovascular function is indicated by higher scores, with a maximum attainable score of twenty-two points. Cureton[11] gives a typical description of the meaning and interpretation based on the following categories:

    12-22 Functionally fit autonomic nervous system.
    9-11 Average range.
    0-8 Functionally unfit.
    −1 to 10 Chronically fatigued.

The Schneider index is an approximate measure of the state of training of the autonomic nervous system, the blood, the heart and the respiratory mechanism. It is able to differentiate only gross categories of cardiovascular condition, and will not adequately measure power, strength, motor skill, or the energy capacity of the central nervous system. It correlates moderately with endurance performances requiring circulatory-respiratory efficiency. Adverse environmental influences such as overwork, lack of sleep, worry, fatigue, chronic nervous tension and fear will lower the score whereas good sleep, moderate eating on a well-balanced diet and moderate endurance exercise on a regular basis will raise the score.

RESULTS OF STUDIES PERTAINING TO THE EFFECTS OF WHEAT GERM DERIVATIVES AND RESTING PULSE RATE, PROGRESSIVE PULSE RATIO AND SCHNEIDER INDEX

Forr[12] used two classes, an active swimming class and an inactive fraternity class to test the effects of differential supplementation on certain physical fitness tests, one of which was the Schneider index. Each class was divided into three groups for purposes of feeding the supplements according to the following scheme: group A received alpha tocopheral acetate (synthetic vitamin E), group B received WGO and group C received corn oil placeboes.

The results for the Schneider test are shown in Figure 12. An analysis of the difference in mean changes between groups in each class, treating the T_1 to T_3 change in each subject as an individual measure, then applying the *t* test, revealed no significant differences between the groups in each class.

Most of the within-group changes were losses rather than gains. In the swimming class, the mean T_1 to T_3 changes in Schneider index raw scores (standard scores in parentheses) were as follows: group A (alpha tocopherol) lost one point (−2.0 SS); group B (WGO) lost .77 of a point (−1.4 SS); and group C (placeboes) lost 2.4 points (−6.2 SS). The reason for these losses was not fully disclosed. At first, it may only be said that in the swimming class the WGO group declined the least (and in the swimming groups TBRT was slowed).

Corresponding changes in the fraternity group (inactive) were as follows: Group A (alpha tocopherol) lost three points (−11.5 SS); group B (WGO) lost 2.25 points (−7.9 SS); and group C (placeboes), the only group that improved, gained 1.1 points (+6.1 SS).

Toohey[13] used the progressive pulse ratio criteria of a) the average angle of inclination and b) the average pulse ratio to determine the effects on six experimental subjects of six weeks of training plus wheat germ oil supplementation, after the subjects had already reached a plateau of performance resulting from prior training without WGO. A control group was used which did not partake in either training or dietary supplementation during the entire course of the experiment. The six experimental subjects and the four control subjects were each given at least two tests at ground level and altitude at each of three testing sessions (pre-training, T_1; post-training, T_2; and post-training plus WGO, T_3). His findings are as follows:

A. *Experimental group:*

    1. Training alone (T_1 to T_2) produced a significant ($t = 2.45$) improvement of 10 SS in the average pulse ratio at ground level of from 2.32 to 2.19; at altitude, the average pulse ratio improved 14.9 SS from 2.42 to 2.22 (significant). Training alone gave similar results for the average angle of inclination. It improved signifi-

cantly from 20.50 degrees to 15.83 degrees at ground level, and from 22.25 degrees to 17.00 degrees at altitude.

2. The training-plus-WGO program (T_2 to T_3) resulted in an insignificant improvement (2.19 to 2.16, a gain of 2.1 SS) in the average pulse ratio at ground level; at altitude, another insignificant gain of from 2.22 to 2.17 (a gain of 3.5 SS) was observed. The average gain in angle of inclination gave similar gains of from 15.88 degrees to 13.08 degrees at ground level and from 16.70 degrees to 13.20 degrees at altitude, both insignificant.

3. Significant gains were reported for the entire experimental period involving nine weeks of training followed by six weeks of training plus WGO. In this analysis (the T_1 to T_3 interval) the average pulse ratio gained significantly ($t = 3.40$, .02 level) from 2.32 to 2.16 at ground level; this was also a significant gain.

4. At an altitude there were the following changes. ($t = 3.87$, .02 level) in the average pulse ratio at an altitude of from 2.41 to 2.17 (a 17.8 SS). For the average angle of inclination, there was a significant gain ($t = 3.76$, .02 level) of from 20.5 degrees to 13.08 degrees at ground level, and an insignificant gain of from 22.25 degrees to 16.30 degrees at altitude.

5. The T_1 to T_2 changes in the control group at ground level and at altitude were both insignificant; the average pulse ratio regressed from 2.30 to 2.32 (a 1.4 SS loss) at ground level and from 2.34 to 2.35 at altitude (a loss of .7 SS).

It must be remembered that although the gains resulting from training plus WGO (T_2 to T_3) were not significant, they are nonetheless important because the group had already reached a plateau of physical fitness beyond which it is difficult to improve. Any slight positive trends of improvement from T_2 to T_3, therefore, should not be minimized.

White[14] studied the effect of physical training and WGO on the Schneider index at ground level and at 10,000 feet simulated altitude. His six experimental subjects were tested at three stages: T_1 (pre-training); T_2 (post-training) and T_3 (post-dietary). From

T_1 to T_2 these subjects underwent a ten-week physical training program until a plateau in the Schneider index had been reached; from T_2 to T_3 they were given WGO while they continued their training for an additional six weeks. Four control subjects, who did not train nor supplement their diet, were tested at T_1 and T_3. The standard error of measurement for the S.I. was $\pm$ .40 points at ground level and $\pm$ .52 points at 10,000 feet simulated altitude.

Figure 65 illustrates the mean change in the experimental group from T_1 to T_2 and from T_2 to T_3. At ground level, the experimental group lost 2.5 SS during the T_1 to T_2 stage (16.8 points to 16.3 points), but made a statistically significant improvement (based on standard errors of measurement) of 11 SS in going from 16.3 points at T_2 to 18.5 points at T_3. The T_2 to T_3 improvement presumably reflects the influence of WGO. At altitude, the experimental group averaged 15.0 points at T_1, 16.3 at T_2 (a gain of 6.5 SS) and 17.7 points at T_3 (a gain of 7 SS over T_2). The control group mean Schneider test for T_1 and T_3 were

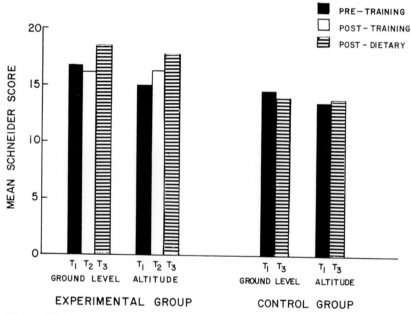

Figure 65-A. Mean Schneider index scores, effects of training on WGO versus placeboes at ground level and at 10,000 feet simulated altitude.

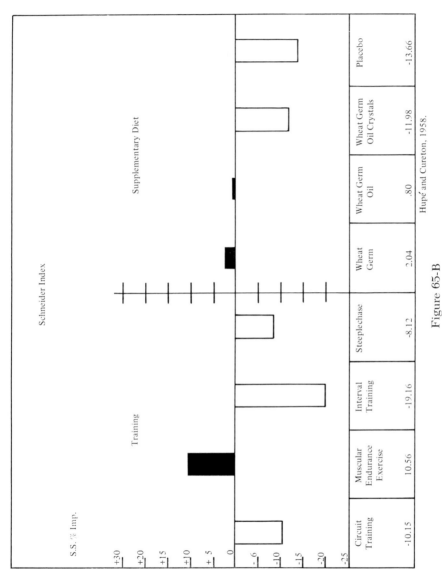

Figure 65-B

Hupé and Cureton, 1958.

nearly equal at both ground level and altitude. The ground level scores were 14.5 points at T_1 and 14.0 at T_3; the altitude scores were 13.5 at T_1 and 13.7 at T_3.

Maley's study (Exp. 11, 1952) matched nine experimental subjects with nine control subjects on the basis of age and composite standard scores on five cardiovascular tests (T_1). These tests were repeated after both groups had undergone four months of physical training consisting of calisthenics and games (T_2). The final tests (T_3) were given after both groups had partaken in a six-week program of continued training plus a dietary supplement; the experimental group received WGO and the control group received placeboes.

The five cardiovascular tests included heartograph (from which pulse rate was derived), ECG R and T waves, Schneider index, progressive pulse ratio and five-minute step test. Evidently Maley[15] neglected to administer the Schneider test and the progressive pulse ratio test at T_2, for these results are missing in his data presentations and raw data sheets. This is unfortunate because the T_2 to T_3 changes in these particular tests critically determine the interpretation of how the dietary supplements affect these measures of cardiovascular fitness. As it stands, only a T_1 to T_3 analysis can be made for the Schneider index and progressive pulse ratio.

The T_1 to T_3 changes, then, are as follows:

1. For the experimental group, the Schneider index gained from 55.56 standard scores to 56.11 SS, while the progressive pulse ratio gained from 41.56 SS to 44.00 SS.
2. For the control group, the Schneider index regressed from 58.89 SS to 58.33 SS, while the progressive pulse ratio regressed from 46.89 SS to 41.83 SS.
3. Differences at T_3 in the Schneider index and progressive pulse ratio between the two groups were insignificant. See Figure 65-A and B for graphical presentation of the T_1 to T_3 changes.

The pulse rate changes in standard scores from T_1 to T_2 to T_3 are as follows:

1. In the experimental group, the pulse rate fluctuated only slightly, gaining from a T_1 value of 66.22 SS to 66.66 SS at T_2, then regressing to 65.66 SS at T_3.
2. In the control group very slight gains were made as the pulse rate went from 64.22 SS at T_1 to 65.00 SS at T_2, and to 66.66 SS at T_3.
3. Between-group differences in pulse rate were insignificant at all three testing periods.

Maley[15] ascribes the decline in the experimental group's pulse rate standard scores to the lack of progression in the training program. He believes that the training was too easy and informal to provoke and maintain cardiovascular improvements in the face of the deleterious winter season. This belief is somewhat corroborated by similar negative results in the other cardiovascular tests he used, namely, the R and T waves of the ECG and the five-minute step test. Quite likely, any training effect which this mild program induced was negated by neuromuscular economy and circulatory-respiratory adaptation which ensued as a result of the program lacking progression.

Vohaska[16] split a college wrestling team into two matched halves, one taking WGO and the other taking placeboes, to determine if WGO would improve the Schneider index from T_1 to T_2 more so than placeboes. The feeding was administered for four weeks during the competitive wrestling season. A control group partaking in neither training nor dietary supplementation was also used.

The between-group analyses at T_2 revealed no significant differences in the Schneider index between the three groups.

Within-group changes from T_1 to T_2 were insignificant in all three groups. The training-plus-WGO group gained only slightly from 66.45 SS at T_1 to 67.91 SS at T_2; the training-plus-placeboes group made a better improvement, going from 64.36 SS at T_1 to 69.18 SS at T_2; the control group, ironically enough, improved the most, going from 60.44 SS at T_1 to 65.67 SS at T_2.

The short feeding period and the accumulative fatigue of the competitive wrestling season may have been partially responsible for the negative results. It is known that fatigue, overwork, and chronic nervous anxiety will cause reductions in the Schneider index.[17] These adverse nervous influences are not uncommon among athletes and teams that undergo regular competition.

The study by Cureton and Pohndorf,[18] involving four matched groups of middle-aged men, lends considerable support for the beneficial effects of WGO to improve the Schneider index. The group which exercised and took WGO for five weeks improved from 12.75 to 15.0 in the Schneider index. This gain of 2.25 points was equivalent to 17.65 per cent (9.7 SS), and was significant at the .05 level ($t = 2.33$). No other group made a significant change. The matched group which exercised and took placeboes changed from 13.87 to 14.12, a mean gain of 0.25 points (1.25 SS); the inactive group on WGO changed from 14.4 to 13.6, a loss of 0.8 points (−4 SS); and the inactive group on placeboes improved from 9.8 to 10.1, a gain of 0.3 points (1.5 SS).

Bernauer's[19] experiment, whereby two halves of college track team were matched on the basis of 440-yard run times, showed only a slight advantage in the Schneider index for the WGO group over the placebo group. The WGO group improved from 13.7 points at T_1 to 14.0 points at T_2 (a gain of 1.1 SS), whereas, the placebo group declined from 16.2 points at T_1 to 15.5 points at T_2 (a loss of 4.1 SS). The difference between groups at T_2, reflecting the net effect of WGO, was not significant.

The resting heart rate changes in Bernauer's data were only trifling and insignificant, favoring slightly the placebo group over the WGO group. The placebo group improved from 57.2 beats/minute to 55.7 beats/minute, an insignificant ($t = 1.38$) gain of 2.0 standard scores. The WGO group declined from 70.0 beats/minute to 70.6 beats/minute, an insignificant ($t = 0.02$) loss of 0.8 SS.

Hupé[20] found some declines in the Schneider index for the placebo and octacosanol groups of his experiment (Fig. 66), with only small gains made by the wheat germ and WGO groups. He attributed the declines to accumulated fatigue that may have remained throughout the T_2 testing period. In any case, the WGC group gained 2.04 standard scores, the WGO group gained 0.80 SS, the OCTCNL group declined 11.98 SS, and the placebo group declined 13.66 SS.

In Cureton's study[21] on the United States Navy underwater trainees, three groups of men were matched initially and fed dietary supplements as follows: Group A received octacosanol, group B placeboes, and group C received WGO. Although most of the variables in this study favored WGO and/or octacosanol, the Schneider index results clearly favor the placeboes. Within-group changes, expressed in standard scores, were as follows: Group A (octacosanol) gained 4.9 SS, group B (placeboes) gained 15.0 SS ($t = 2.32$, significant at the .05 level), and group C

TABLE XXXII

RESULTS OF SCHNEIDER INDEX, PROGRESSIVE PULSE RATIO, PULSE RATE AND 5-MINUTE STEP TEST (HARVARD) AS AFFECTED BY WHEAT GERM OIL

(in Standard Scores, SS)

Experiment No.	Experimenters	Experimental Group Training Plus WGO	Experimental Group Training Plus Octacosanol	Placebo Group in Training	No Training and No WGO
1 (Schneider)	Forr and Cureton	− 1.4 (swim) − 7.9 (Frat)		−2.4; − 2.0 +6.1; −11.5	
4 (PP Ratio)	Toohey and Cureton	3.5			− .7 −1.4
5 (Schneider)	White and Cureton	2.1 (ground level) 11.0 (ground level) 7.0 (altitude)		− 2.5	1.0
11 (Schneider) (PP Ratio)	Maley and Cureton	.55 2.44		− .56 − 5.06	
12 Schneider	Vohaska and Cureton	1.46		4.82	5.23
13 Schneider	Cureton and Pohndorf	9.70		1.25	
15 Schneider	Hupé and Cureton	0.80	−12.0	−13.7	
18 Schneider	Bernauer and Cureton	1.10		− 4.10	
21 Schneider 5-minute ST	Cureton, *et al.* (Navy)	− 2.30 (Schneider) − 1.5 (5-minute ST)	4.9 17.0	15.0 10.7	
22 Pulse Rate	Dempsey and Cureton	15.0		5.0	
Comparative Improvements (Average)		2.41	3.97	−0.63	

TABLE XXXIII

RELIABILITY OF THE SCHNEIDER INDEX, PROGRESSIVE PULSE
RATIO, PULSE RATE AND HARVARD STEP TEST EXPERIMENTS
AS AFFECTED BY WHEAT GERM OIL, OCTACOSANOL AND
WHEAT GERM (in Standard Scores)

Experiment No.	Experimenters	Statistical Significance $p < .10$	Positive Trend but Not Statistically Significant	No Experimental Result in Favor of Supplement
1 (Schneider)	Forr and Cureton			WGO
4 (P P Ratio)	Toohey and Cureton		WGO WGO	
5 (Schneider)	White and Cureton	WGO WGO		
11 (Schneider) (P P Ratio) (5-min. ST)	Maley and Cureton		WGO WGO WGO	
12 (Schneider)	Vohaska and Cureton			WGO
13 (Schneider)	Cureton and Pohndorf	WGO		
15 (Schneider)	Hupé and Cureton	WGO		
18 (Schneider)	Bernauer and Cureton	WGO		
21 (Schneider) (5-min. ST)	Cureton et al. (Navy)	OCTCNL		WGC and OCTCNL
22 (Pulse rate lying)	Dempsey and Cureton	WGO		

(WGO) gained 2.3 SS. The *t* value for the improvement within the octacosanol group fell .01 point shy of being significant at the .05 level (a *t* of 1.79 was obtained, whereas, a *t* of 1.80 is required for .05 significance). The .10 level of significance was obtained.

None of the differences between groups at T_2 was significant at the .05 level, but the difference in favor of the placebo group over the WGO group was significant at the .05 level ($t = 2.03$).

The reasons for the greater Schneider index improvement made by the placebo group in this study are not known exactly. It was rather surprising that any of the groups improved in the Schneider index, in view of the short (six weeks) intense nature of the training and insufficient sleep, both of which may have prevented full cardiovascular adjustment. Such conditions usually lower, rather than improve, the Schneider index.

Table XXXII shows the overall average of the experimental group to be an improvement of +2.41 SS for the WGO group in training, +3.97 SS for the octacosanol group in training and −0.63 SS for the control group in training on placeboes.

Table XXXIII shows that in six experiments there were statistically significant results seven times; favorable trends five times in two more experiments and in three experiments there were no statistically significant results in favor of the dietary supplements.

CONCLUSIONS

There is a moderate advantage of 3.04 SS for WGO and 4.60 SS for octacosanol over the placeboes, which is interpreted as advantageous economy for the groups on the dietary supplements compared to the control group taking the same exercise program.

Octacosanol had a decided advantage over the WGO group and also over the controls on the same exercise program.

Wheat germ oil and octacosanol, one of its ingredients, appears to stabilize the nervous system, which is reflected by lowered pulse rates, shown consistently in such tests as the pulse rates at the end of work (as in the 5-minute step test), the Schneider index and the progressive pulse ratio test (working pulse rates).

The effects are more consistent on the working pulse rates (or pulse rate immediately after work) than on the quiet pulse rates, although some lesser effect was observed here too. The lower pulse rates indicate better resistance to the stress.

REFERENCES

1. Cureton, T. K., Huffman, W. J., Welser, L., Kireilis and Latham, D. E.: Analytical and normative studies of the Schneider test, pp. 195-222 in *Endurance of Young Men*, Washington, D. C., National Research Council, Society for Research in Child Development, Vol. X, Serial No. 40, Monograph No. 1, 1945; and also Schneider, E. C.: A cardiovascular rating as a measure of fatigue and efficiency, *J.A.M.A.*, 74:1507-10, May 29, 1920; and editorial: The measure of physical fitness, *J.A.M.A.*, 74:110, July 10, 1920.
2. Cureton, T. K.: Progressive pulse ratio test as an indicator of oxygen

shortage (or exercise tolerance) and predictor of oxygen availability for progressively harder work increments, pp. 90-117, in *The Physiological Effects of Exercise Programs on Adults,* Springfield, Thomas, 1969.

3. Cureton, T. K.: Experimental and statistical analysis of the step test, pp. 187-194 in *Endurance of Young Men,* op. cit. (ref. 1); and Johnson, R. E., *et al.:* A test of physical fitness for strenuous exertion, *Rev. Canad. Biol.,* 1:491-503, June, 1942; and Brouha, L.: The step test: A simple method of measuring physical fitness for muscular work in young men, *Res. Quart.,* 14:31-35, March, 1943.

4. Cureton, T. K.: The nature of cardiovascular fitness in normal humans, *J. Ass. Phys. Ment. Rehab.,* 11:186-196, Nov.-Dec., 1957, No. 1 (and continued, Nos. 2, 3, 4).

5. Cureton, T. K. and Du Toit, S. F.: Effect of progressive training on the latent period of electrical stimulation of the left ventricle of the human heart, *Proc. Coll. P.E. Ass.,* Philadelphia (69th Annual Meeting), 1965; and S. F. Du Toit, ibid., Ph.D. thesis, Physical Education, University of Illinois, 1966.

6. Raab, W.: Training, physical inactivity and the cardiac dynamic cycle, *J. Sports Med.,* 6:38-47, 1966.

7. Weissler, A. M.: Relationships between the left ventricular ejection time, stroke volume and heart rate in normal individuals and patients with cardiovascular disease, *Amer. Heart J.,* 62:367-76, 1961.

8. Raab, W., *et al.:* Adrenergic and cholinergic influences on the dynamic cycle of the normal human heart, *Cardiologia,* 33:351-64, 1958; and Raab, W. and Krzywanek, H. J.: Cardiovascular sympathetic tone and stress response related to personality patterns and exercise habits, *Amer. J. Cardiol.,* 16:42-53, 1965.

9. Franks, B. D. and Cureton, T. K.: Orthogonal factors of cardiac intervals and their response to stress, *Res. Quart.,* 39:524-532, Oct., 1968.

10. Ibid., Effects of training on time components of the left ventricle, *J. Sports Med.,* 9:80-88, June, 1969.

11. Cureton, T. K.: *Physical Fitness Workbook.* Urbana, Stipes Pub. Co., pp. 115-119, 1944.

12. Forr, Wm. A.: The Effects of Wheat Germ Oil on Physical Fitness, Urbana, M.S. thesis, 1950, p. 88.

13. Toohey, J. V.: Variations of the Progressive Pulse Ratio with Altitude, Training and Wheat Germ Oil, Urbana, M.S. thesis, Physical Education, University of Illinois, 1951, p. 103.

14. White, C. H.: The Effect of Physical Training and Dietary Supplement on the Six Item Schneider Index at Ground Level and at a Simulated Altitude of 10,000 Feet, Urbana, M.S. thesis, Physical Education, University of Illinois, 1951, p. 96.

15. Maley, A. F.: The Effects of Training and a Dietary Supplement on the Cardiovascular Fitness of Adult Men, Urbana, M.S. thesis, Physical Education, University of Illinois, 1952, p. 36.

16. Vohaska, W. J.: The Effects of Wheat Germ Oil on the Cardiovascular Fitness of Varsity Wrestlers, Urbana, M.S. thesis, Physical Education, University of Illinois, 1954, p. 43.

17. McFarland, R. A. and Huddleson, J. H.: Neurocirculatory reactions in the psychoneuroses studied by the Schneider method, *Amer. J. Psychiat.*, 93:567-99, Nov., 1936.

18. Cureton, T. K. and Pohndorf, R. H.: Influence of wheat germ oil as a dietary supplement in a program of conditioning exercises with middle-aged subjects, *Res. Quart.*, 26:391-407, Dec., 1955.

19. Beranuer, E. M. and Cureton, T. K.: The Influence of Wheat Germ Oil as a Dietary Supplement in a Training Program of Varsity Track Athletes at the University of Illinois, Physical Fitness Research Laboratory, Staff Project, 1958.

20. Hupé, A. S.: The Effects of Training and Supplementary Diet on the Cardiovascular Condition of Young Boys, Urbana, M.S. thesis, Physical Education, University of Illinois, 1958, p. 74.

21. Cureton, T. K., Improvements in physical fitness associated with a course of U. S. Navy Underwater Trainees, with and without dietary supplements (WGO and OCTACOSANOL), *Res. Quart.*, 34:440-453, Dec., 1963.

Chapter IX

Effect of Wheat Germ Oil and Wheat Germ on the Pre-Ejection Intervals of the Heart

INTRODUCTION

INTEREST has been sustained for many years in the latent time period (TP) from the instant of the Q point of the ECG to the first instant of blood leaving the heart (beginning up-stroke of the pulse wave).[1] By putting the ECG, the brachial or carotid pulse wave and the heart sounds on the same tape simultaneously, this latent period (TP—tension period) may be measured (Fig. 66). This procedure has been known as Blumberger's method.[2] It has been used in the first of two studies to be presented to see if wheat germ oil, or wheat germ or octacosanol would affect this interval. When the interval is too short, the tension is high internally in the left ventricle and is related to relatively higher stroke volume.[3] When it is lengthened relatively, a lower stroke volume results, and a more relaxed state prevails for tension within the left ventricle of the heart. Raab[4] has reported that long, moderate exercise routines (cycling, dancing) cause a lengthening of the TP if persistently followed. He also experimented with repetitious phone calls to heart disease patients in the hospital and found a shortening. Various studies have shown that stress shortens the TP interval. Raab also warned that disturbing noises, resulting in irritation, may be a factor in precipitating heart attack.

By using the sound waves, ECG and carotid pulse wave (or brachial pulse wave), the TP interval may be split into the EML (electromechanical) and ICP (isovolumic) intervals. Franks and Cureton[5] discovered that these two intervals were negatively correlated, and hence should be used separately. Nevertheless, if the stress is great enough, both intervals shorten. The faster the contraction of the left ventricle, the shorter is the TP or ICP interval, which may be highly desirable for a young athlete, yet of doubtful value in an "out of condition" adult. It was found that

246

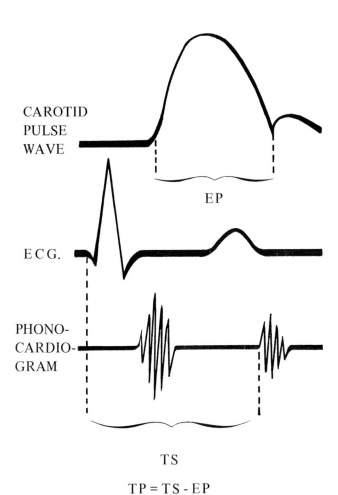

TP = TS - EP

Figure 66. The tension (TP) pre-ejection interval of the left ventricle (Blumberger's method).

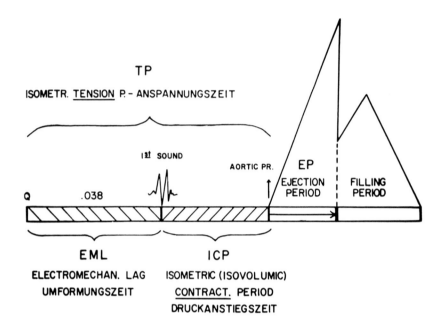

TP = Tension Period
EML = Electromechanical Lag
ICP = Isovolumic Period
EP = Ejection Period
EP + Filling Period = Mechanical Systole
Pulse Wave Area = Work Done by Heart

Figure 67. The heart cycle and the pre-ejection interval of the left ventricle (Cureton, Franks, Wiley).

a fast, powerful ejection of blood from the heart and a relatively long recovery time for filling, are highly desirable characteristics of the "trained state."[6]

RESULTS OF THE EFFECTS OF DIETARY SUPPLEMENTS ON SELECTED CARDIAC INTERVALS IN THREE GROUPS OF YOUNG BOYS

Cundiff[10] reported the effects of dietary supplements on young boys while enrolled in the University of Illinois Summer Sports Fitness School. Three groups, matched on a 600-yard run, in-

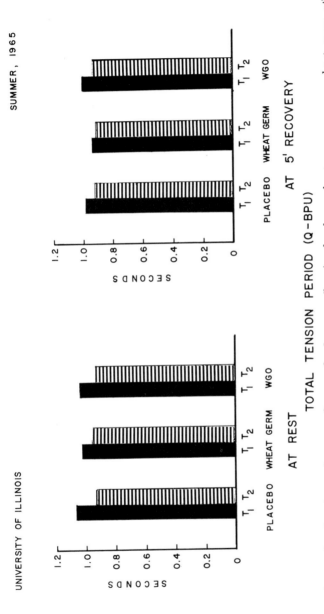

Figure 68. Results of eight weeks sports fitness school course (boys), placebos, wheat germ, versus wheat germ oil on TP interval (at rest and at five-minutes of recovery).

cluded placebo (N = 16), wheat germ (N = 19) and wheat germ oil (N = 18). The cardiac intervals (Fig. 69) were from the beginning of stimulation to the beginning of the brachial pulse wave (picked up with a Brecht-Boucke capacitance transducer under a sphygmomanometer pressure cuff set at 10 mm above diastolic blood pressure), as measured from Q (ECG) to the beginning of the rapid ascent of the brachial pulse wave; beginning of stimulation to an estimated beginning of ejection, as measured from Q to the peak of G_a (BCG, acceleration setting); pulse wave transmission time, as measured from G_a to the beginning of the brachial pulse wave; and the total cycle time, measured by R-R′ (ECG) (Fig. 69).

The sports-fitness training decreased the pulse wave transmission time (Fig. 70) and Q to BPU (Fig. 68) at rest and post-exercise (2′ step test, 16 inch bench, 30 steps per minute) in all groups, but there was little difference among the groups. There were almost no changes in the Q to G_a intervals (Fig. 69). The total cycle time increased at rest and post-exercise for all the groups (see Table XXXIV for group means).

A number of preliminary studies were made in the department of Physical Fitness Research Laboratory to perfect the system and to determine the reliability of the several intervals.[7] At rest the reliability of all of the intervals was good, but in work they were not very good. Wiley[8, 9] devised a way to immobilize the hips and greatly improved the reliability of the intervals taken during ergometer bicycle work in the supine position, but too late for this study, which data were taken sitting. It was found by Cundiff[10] that the reliability of the ICP interval was not very good with young boys, so the decision was made to use the TP interval, which was not much better (0.21 to 0.30), and the PWTT interval reliability was 0.47, and the cycle 0.53. These are too low to guarantee a satisfactory level of reliability (PWTT = pulse wave transmission time).

It was found in the Cundiff-Cureton study with young boys in the Sports-Fitness School that the program built up, week to week, an increasing "transient" sympatheticotonia, with faster pulse rates and depressed pulse wave amplitudes, and relatively shorter TP intervals, showing the transient stress to which the

TABLE XXXIV

RESULTS OF EIGHT WEEKS SPORTS FITNESS COURSE
UNIVERSITY OF ILLINOIS—SUMMER, 1965

Measurement	Placebo T_1 T_2	WG T_1 T_2	WGO T_1 T_2	Comments
(1) At rest — Total tension period, Q to BPU, (brachial up-stroke) seconds	1.06 0.93 D = 0.130 t = 4.11	1.02 0.95 D = 0.070 t = 2.22	1.04 0.94 D = 0.101 t = 3.02	N = 16 (Pl); 19 (WG); 18, 17 (WGO) WG and WGO groups stood stress best with relatively less shortening. All significant at 5% level.
(2) At 5' recovery (after 2' step test, 17 inch bench) — Total tension period, Q to BPU, seconds	0.980 0.927 D = 0.053 t = 3.02	0.944 0.906 D = 0.038 t = 1.26	0.998 0.928 D = 0.070 t = 3.42	All groups were shorter. Changes between groups were insignificant.
(3) At 5' recovery — Inotropic effect Vertical amplitude of the acceleration pulse wave of the brachial artery millimeters	2.90 2.73 D = 0.170 t = 3.09(–)	2.93 2.41 D = 0.519 t = 2.09(–)	2.64 2.89 D = 0.250 t = 0.95(+)	WGO is only one with gain in amplitude, showing favorable adjustment to exercise in terms of circulation. Placebo and WG groups show fatigue.
(4) At rest — Pulse wave transmission time (PTT) secs. Peak of G in acceleration Wave of BCG to beginning of up-stroke from brachial pulse wave	0.247 0.182 D = 0.065 t = 2.61	0.242 0.154 D = 0.087 t = 2.23	0.274 0.174 D = 0.100 t = 2.93	WGO group had more shortening of PTT, indicating tenser brachial artery, stood stress better. All groups shortened.

boys were exposed, due mainly to the "between sides" competition increasing in tempo and spirit as the end of the eight-week period of the summer session waned. This resulted in a type of temporary fatigue, carried around the clock, and which affected the tests. It was eliminated by two or three weeks abstinence from such competitions. The excitement attending the competitions or in making points for their side in individual competitions,

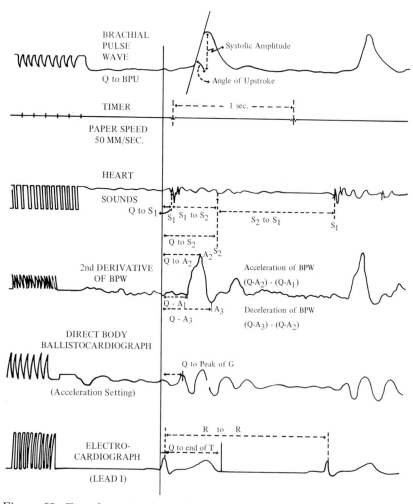

Figure 69. Five-channel polygraph variables, typical multichannel record describing intervals measured.

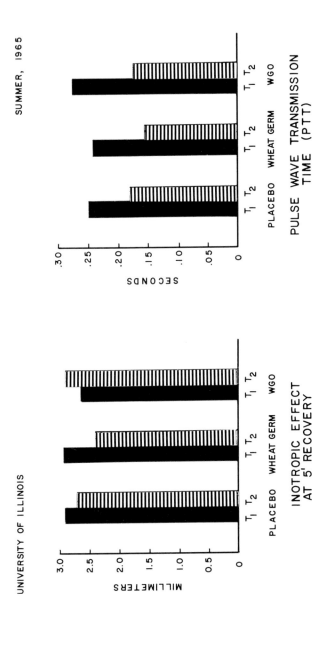

Figure 70. Results of eight weeks sports fitness course (boys) comparing placebo, wheat germ and WGO groups on electronic pulse waves and pulse wave transmission time.

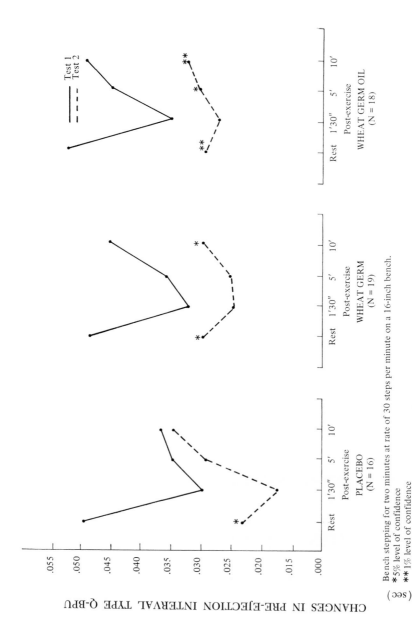

Bench stepping for two minutes at rate of 30 steps per minute on a 16-inch bench.
* 5% level of confidence
** 1% level of confidence

Figure 71. Changes in Q to brachial pulse wave upstroke as result of training and comparison of placebo, wheat germ and wheat germ oil effects (boys).

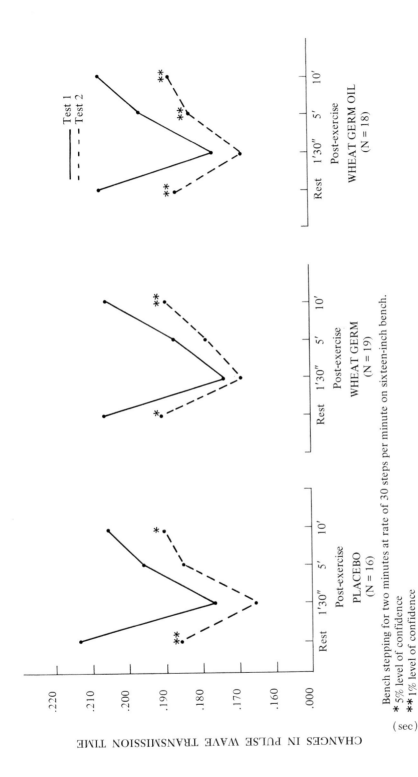

Bench stepping for two minutes at rate of 30 steps per minute on sixteen-inch bench.
* 5% level of confidence
** 1% level of confidence

(sec) Figure 72. Changes in pulse transmission time as result of training and comparison of placebo, wheat germ and wheat germ oil effects (boys).

TABLE XXXV

GROUP STANDARD SCORE CHANGES IN THE 600-YARD RUN TIME
RESULTING FROM EIGHT WEEKS OF TRAINING ON WHEAT
GERM, IN THREE MATCHED GROUPS

Group	Test	Mean (sec.)	Standard Score (SS)	SS Change
Placebo	1	151	61	
	2	131	75	+14
Wheat germ	1	149	62	
	2	132	70	+ 8
Wheat germ	1	154	58	
oil (N = 18)	2	130	76	+18

In actual time, Table XXXV shows the advantage to be with the WGO group.

contributed to the sympatheticotonia and resulting fatigue. When
the pulse rates were faster, the TP and ICP intervals were generally relatively shorter. The measurements taken are diagrammed
in Figure 69. The results of the Cundiff study show that, while
the differences are small (0.070, 0.053, 0.038, for WGO, Placebo
and WG cereal groups in that order), in the post-exercise, 2-
minute step test, 16 inch bench, between the three groups, the
least amount of shortening was with the wheat germ cereal
group; and at rest before exercise the differences were again
least for WGC—0.070, 0.101 and 0.130 seconds for WGC, WGO
and placebo groups, respectively (Table XXXIV). The interpretation is that the dietary supplement groups resisted the fatigue
the best (cf. Figs. 71 and 72), but the difference is marginal and
not larger than the S.E.$_{meas.}$ even though it came up statistically
significant by the t-test.

As a result of Cundiff's experiment, the resting latent interval
Q to the brachial upstroke changed significantly because of the
training but the placebo, wheat germ and wheat germ oil groups
were not significantly different from each other with respect to
these improvements, the *t* values being 4.11 (placebo group),
2.22 (WGC group) and 3.02 (WGO group). All were significant
< .05 level. The actual differences due to training were 0.130
second (placeboes), 0.101 second (WGO) and 0.070 second
(WGC). Since all groups *shortened* because of the training, it

is noticeable that the WGC group shortened the least, then next the WGO group and the most was the placebo group. It appears that the WGC group resisted the shortening the most (Table CII). For WGC versus WGO (t = .300, insignificant); and for WGO versus placeboes, t = 5.87, significant < .01; whereas, WGC versus placeboes, t = .02, insignificant.

After five minutes of recovery the same Q to BPU interval was shortened least during training by the same WGC group (0.038 second) compared to 0.053 for the placebo group and 0.070 second for the WGO group.

Two groups were depressed in terms of the inotropic (vertical) displacement in the brachial electronically picked-up wave but in this the placebo group was depressed 0.170 mm, the WGC group 0.519 mm.; whereas, the WGO group increased 0.250

TABLE XXXVI

CHANGES IN VARIOUS MEASURES OF THE HEART CYCLE
WHILE IN TRAINING ON WGO

(Means, Standard Deviations and Mean Changes of Groups Used for
Determining the Effects of Wheat Germ Oil)
(On WGO, N = 7 and on Placeboes N = 7)

Group	T_2 Mean	T_2 S.D.	T_3 Mean	T_3 S.D.	Change in Mean from T_2 to T_3
Rest (Supine)					
Cycle time (sec)					
On WGO	1.009	0.123	1.057	0.125	0.048
On placeboes	1.062	0.189	1.096	0.223	0.034
Diastole (sec)					
On WGO	0.598	0.109	0.639	0.119	0.041
On placeboes	0.654	0.165	0.683	0.197	0.029
Electromechanical lag (sec)					
On WGO	0.054	0.005	0.055	0.005	0.001
On placeboes	0.055	0.007	0.055	0.008	None
Isovolumetric contraction period (sec)					
On WGO	0.053	0.002	0.056	0.002	0.003
On placeboes	0.050	0.003	0.052	0.003	0.002
Ejection period (sec)					
On WGO	0.304	0.013	0.308	0.010	0.004
On placeboes	0.302	0.025	0.306	0.023	0.004
Percent diastole in cycle time					
On WGO	58.9	3.8	60.0	4.1	1.1
On placeboes	60.9	4.7	61.4	5.0	0.5

TABLE XXXVII

SIGNIFICANT DIFFERENCES OBTAINED WITHIN TRAINING GROUPS
OVER TEN WEEKS, COMPARABLE GROUPS ON WGO, PLACEBOES
AND ON NO SUPPLEMENTATION AT ALL*

(N = 7 on WGO; N = 7 on placeboes; N = 8 on nothing)

Variable	Significance Level		Significant Differences in Adjusted Group Means[†]		
	T-2	*T-3**	*TW*	*TP*	*TO[‡]*
Electromechanical Lag		(Significant)		(Not Significant)	
Rest (sitting)	—	0.05	0.055	0.054	0.053
Last ten seconds of ride	—	0.05	0.043	0.041	0.041
Thirty seconds post-exercise	—	0.10	0.048	0.046	0.046
Five minutes post-exercise	—	0.05	0.056	0.053	0.053
Isovolumetric Contraction Period					
Rest (supine)	—	0.10	0.055	0.054	0.053
Thirty seconds post-exercise	—	0.01	0.042	0.039	0.040

* The testing periods were at ten (T-2) and 20 (T-3) weeks of the training period. Group on nothing (N = 8) was dropped from Table XXXVII.

[†] Determined by Duncan's multiple range. All means underlined by the same line are *not* significantly different (0.10 level). Means not underlined by the same line are significantly different.

[‡] TW = training with wheat germ oil group (N = 7); TP = training with placeboes group (N = 7); TO = training only group (N = 8).

mm. The reliability of these measures by test and retest was poor.[10]

The pulse wave transmission time (PWTT) was shortened the most in the WGO group (0.100 second), the WGC group next (0.087 second) and the placebo group least (0.065 second). Thus it would seem that the arterial tone increased most in the two groups on the experimental nutritive supplements (Table CII), as these shortened somewhat more than the control group on placeboes.

PRE-EJECTION INTERVALS OF THE HEART CYCLE
(TP and ICP)

Wiley[8, 9] conducted a similar experiment (Exp. 30 in Part Two) on middle-aged men in 1968 at the Physical Fitness Research Laboratory, University of Illinois, Urbana. Simultaneous tracings were made of the carotid pulse wave, ECG and phonocardiogram on thirty-two sedentary, male adults, of whom twenty-two participated in a longitudinal physical training program for twenty weeks with testing at 0, 10 and 20 weeks (known as T_1, T_2 and T_3). Analysis of variance showed the group means to be insignificantly different at the start. Two of the groups were thusly matched and trained 50 mins. per day on Cureton's continuous, rhythmic, low-middle gear program, allowing some gradual progression in intensity of the work and in total kilocalories expended (from *Physical Fitness and Dynamic Health*, New York, Dial, 1965). Then, in the T_2 and T_3 stage of the training, one of these groups took WGO (10×6 capsules, 5 days per week at the end of the workout). The WGO group lengthened the ICP and TP intervals slightly more than the placebo group, also on the same physical training led by the same instructor. While the training effect was much greater than the effect of the WGO, the result was slightly favorable to WGO in the direction of lengthening the "stress indicator" intervals, which shorten under stress (Table XXXV). Perhaps, the WGO group was able to bear the stress of training slightly better.

The experimental group in Wiley's experiment (Exp. 30, 1968), seven male middle-aged subjects lengthened the ICP interval 0.003 second while on WGO, whereas, the control group taking placeboes lengthened the ICP interval 0.002 second, and the difference between these two groups, 0.001 second was significant $< .10$ level (Table XXXV). Likewise, the cycle time lengthened in this same period of ten weeks, T_2 to T_3 0.048 for the WGO group and 0.034 second for the placebo group; and similarly, the *diastole time* was lengthened during this period of physical training, T_2 to T_3 over ten weeks, 0.041 for the WGO group and 0.029 for the placebo group. This difference is very slight in ICP interval but, otherwise, the differences are large enough to be of some consequence.

There was a greater reduction of diastolic blood pressure at rest and in recovery over the whole twenty-week period of physical training for the groups in training compared to the reductions at ten weeks of physical training. This is to show that the length of training in weeks is important to get real differences (Fig. 73). If there are no differences, nothing can be shown to

be statistically significant. Likewise, the Brachial Pulse Wave had
higher amplitude at 20 weeks compared to 10 weeks of training.

The significance of the difference between the WGO and the
placebo groups, seven men in each group, is shown in Table
XXXVII for the T_2 to T_3 period of ten weeks. There is a slight
advantage for the WGO group over the placebo group.

A parallel study was made by Mayhew,[11] who collaborated
with Wiley, the former followed the precordial T-wave of the

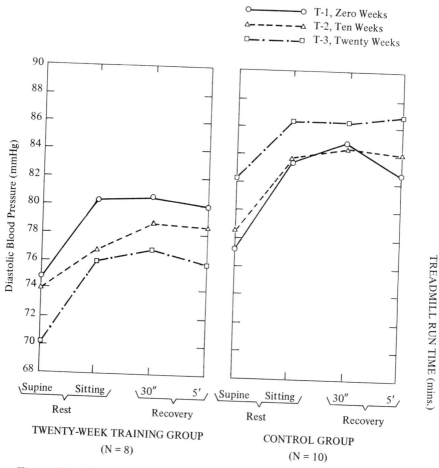

Figure 73. Effects of twenty weeks of training on diastolic blood pressure
(men).

ECG on twenty-five of the adults in Wiley's study. The men were matched by mile run times at the start of the experiment and then divided into three groups. Two groups trained for ten weeks without dietary supplementation, then one of these groups took WGO for ten weeks more, and the other group took placeboes for the same ten weeks. The third group was tested at 0, 10 and 20 weeks but took no supplements or physical training, serving just as controls. Both groups in Cureton's *"continuous rhythmic progressive training program"* improved significantly more than the controls, as would be expected, and both groups lengthened the TP and ICP intervals also more than the controls. But the T-wave was depressed in both exercised groups, the WGO group showing relatively less depression, consistent with standing the stress better.

CONCLUSIONS

The wheat germ cereal group shortened the Q to the BPU interval relatively the least in the Cundiff-Cureton experiment, indicating that the stress was withstood relatively better by the WGC group; and this was also true for the WGO group over the placebo group (Fig. 72). In the latter, t = 5.87 significant < .01.

Also, in the Cundiff-Cureton experiment (Exp. 25) the WGO group improved relatively more over the WGC group and the placebo groups in the vertical amplitude of the brachial pulse wave test (acceleration, in the electronically picked-up waves) compared to the placebo and the WGC groups, both of which lost in amplitude at five minutes of recovery after the two minute standardized bicycle ergometer bicycle ride.

The WGO group Experiment 25 also developed relatively more arterial tone and pulse wave transmission speed than the control group or the WGC group.

The WGO group in Wiley and Cureton's experiment (Exp. 30) lengthened the ICP interval slightly more than the group on placeboes in the last ten weeks of physical training, and more than the control group. The difference at rest was only .001, yet computed significant < .10 by the Fisher *t* test. Similar favorable differences were shown for the WGO group over the placebo group in the last ten seconds of the five-minute ergometer bicycle ride in *cycle time,* and this similar advantage held also at five minutes of recovery time.

In the Wiley-Cureton experiment (Exp. 30) it is noted that the diastolic blood pressure at rest and in recovery reduced markedly at twenty weeks of physical training, compared to 10 and 0 weeks. This may have been due to the effect of the WGO on the subjects in the last ten weeks. Likewise, the amplitude of the brachial pulse wave was higher at twenty weeks, than at 10 or 0 weeks of training, again probably reflecting the advantage for the WGO supplement.

REFERENCES

1. Blumberger, K.: Die Wirkungen des peripherischen Kreislaufs auf die zeitliche Dynamic des Herzens beim Menschen, *Vhdlgn. d. dtsche. Ges. f. Kreislaufforschg.,* 22:79, 1956.

2. Blumberger, *et al.*: In Luisada's *Cardiology and Encyclopedia of the Cardiovascular System.* New York, McGraw-Hill, 1959, pp. 372-7.

3. Weissler, A. M., *et al.*: Relationships between left ventricular ejection time, stroke volume and heart rate in normal individuals and patients with cardiovascular disease, *Am. Heart J.,* 62:367-76, 1961.

4. Raab, W., *et al.*: Cardiac adrenergic preponderance due to lack of physical exercise and its pathological implications, *Amer. J. Cardiol.* 5:300-20, 1960; and (Ed.) *ibid., Prevention of Ischemic Heart Disease,* Springfield, Ill., Charles C Thomas, 1966.

5. Franks, B. D. and Cureton, T. K.: Effects of training on the time components of the left ventricle, *J. Sports Med.,* 9:80-88, June, 1969, and ibid., Orthogonal factors in cardiac intervals and their response to stress, *Res. Quart.,* 39:524-532, Oct., 1968; and Orthogonal factors and norms for time components of the left ventricle, *Med. Sci. Sports,* 1:171-176, Sept., 1969.

6. Rushmer, R. F., *et al.*: Mechanisms of cardiac control in exercise, *Circ. Res.* 7:602-627, July, 1959; and Cureton, T. K.: Sympathetic versus vagus influence upon the contractile vigor of the heart, *Res. Quart.,* 32:553-557, Dec., 1961, Glick, G. and Braunwald: Relative roles of the sympathetic and parasympathetic nervous systems in reflex control of heart rate, *Circ. Res.,* 16:363-375, 1965.

7. Cureton, T. K., Pollard, J. W., Cundiff, D. E., Du Toit, S., Liverman, R. D., Babister, E. and Sloninger, E. L.: Studies of the Isovolumic Interval of the Heart at Rest, After Exercise and After Longitudinal Physical Training (Including Reliability Data), paper before Amer. College of Sports Med., Dallas, Texas, Mar. 16, 1965.

8. Wiley, J. F.: Effects of Training With and Without Wheat Germ Oil on Cardiac Intervals and Other Fitness Measures of Middle-Aged

Men, Urbana, Ph.D. thesis, Physical Education, University of Illinois, 1968, p. 199; also, Effects of body position and exercise on left ventricular intervals, *Med. Sci. Sports*, 2:132-136, Fall, 1970.

9. Wiley, J. F.: A method for positioning the subject to increase reliability of the pre-ejection intervals in work, *Res. Quart.*, Oct., 1971.

10. Cundiff, Linda: Reliability of the Cardiac Intervals, p. 29 in Effects of Training and Dietary Supplements on Selected Cardiac Intervals of Young Boys, Urbana, M.S. thesis, Physical Education, University of Illinois, 1966, p. 59.

11. Mayhew, J. L.: The Effects of Training With and Without Wheat Germ Oil on the Precordial T-Wave and other Selected Fitness Measures of Middle-Aged Men, Urbana, M.S. thesis, Physical Education, University of Illinois, 1968, p. 128.

Chapter X

Experiments on Basal Metabolism Rate, Effects of Physical Training with and without WGO and Wheat Germ Supplements

STUDIES ON MIDDLE-AGED MEN

D URING 1953 and 1954 as part of the summer school program,* at the University of Illinois, experiments were run
to determine the possible effects of wheat germ oil and wheat
germ compared to cottonseed oil placeboes used with a matched
group design—to observe the possible effects on basal metabolic
rate (BMR). The BMR test had been studied both in the University of Illinois Physical Fitness Research Laboratory and at
other laboratories[1, 2, 3] and it was known that this test is not as reliable as many other tests, even when standardized conditions
(STPD) are observed. The tests were given principally on the
McKesson Metabolator but with occasional comparisons made
with the Douglas Bag procedure.[4] Normally, after a thirty-minute
rest period on a bed, in post-absorptive state, and relative inactive
state for twenty-four hours, the six-minute graph of O_2 used in
the quiet state was taken. This was repeated several times, and
the lowest of those obtained was used on any one day to indicate
the most acceptable test. Preliminary work on the reliability of
the BMR test of this type gave:

Bender N = 74 σ = 4.49% (on adults) $\sigma_{meas.}$ = 0.526%
  s (9 cases retested) = 13.427% $\sigma_{meas.}$ (8 cases re-tested) = ±1.70%

---

* The summer school at the University of Illinois lasted eight weeks from the
middle of June to the middle of August. The first week was used for testing
(T_1) and the second week to seventh week the main program was run, and the
eighth week was used for T_2 testing. The *difference* between T_1 and T_2 was the
training difference considered, which was tested for significance by the ratio of
the Diff. to the S. E. $_{meas.}$ The resulting T (ratio) was then evaluated by the
normal probability tables, the assumption being that the chance errors distributed
normally from such chance errors about the mean. An alternative mehod was to
compute the mean difference and the $\sigma_{diff.}$ from the actual scores for the denominator of the ratio.

264

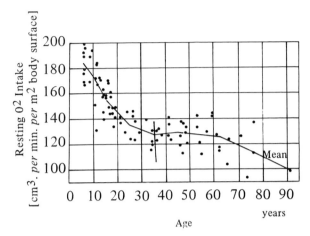

Figure 74. The resting O₂ intake of fasting subjects in relation to age (Shock).

The stability of this test on young boys was worse, and as many as five trials were necessary to get reliability between the two lowest trials to agree as well as r = 0.80. Van Huss[3] and Cureton[5] made extended studies of the factors which affect the BMR test at the University of Illinois.

It is also noted that the basal metabolic rate deteriorates very sharply from ten years of age to thirty-six, this slope corresponding somewhat to the data reported by Dr. Hardin B. Jones (Fig. 74).

Cureton-Pohndorf Experiment

Findings

The results of the 1953 and 1954 experiments are shown in Table X. In general there were statistically insignificant differences attributable to the WGO but some positive effects due to the exercise training program itself. The gross results (1953) are as follows:

Changes in BMR

Group A	Eight middle-aged men in six weeks of physical training with supplement of cottonseed oil placeboes (ten 6-minim capsules per day, five days per week)	10.6 SS
Group B	Five middle-aged men in six weeks of physical training with WGO supplement (ten 6-minim capsules per day, five days per week)	2.0 SS
Group C	Four middle-aged men on the same WGO supplement but relatively inactive as controls	3.25 SS

Group D   Two professional (younger) middle-aged men in
a control group, relatively inactive as controls
on placeboes   –5.0 SS
                                                                 (loss)

CALCULATIONS FOR STATISTICAL SIGNIFICANCE

Group A *Exercise with Wheat Germ Oil*	*Versus*	*Group B* *Exercise with Placeboes*
D_{AB} = 8.87		11 degrees of freedom:
t_{AB} = 1.43 .10 level		.05 level = 2.201
favor placeboes		.01 level = 3.106

Group C *Inactive (Wheat Germ Oil)*	*Versus*	*Group D* *Inactive (Placeboes)*
D_{CD} = 8.10		4 degrees of freedom:
t_{CD} = .862 .5 level		.05 level = 2.776
favor WGO		.01 level = 4.604

Summation of Results on BMR

Group A (exercised group on WGO) raised the BMR 1.75 per cent compared to group B (exercised group on placeboes) raising the BMR + 10.62 per cent. Group C (inactive controls on WGO) raised the BMR 3.25 per cent and Group D (professional control group on placeboes) lowered the BMR −4.82 per cent. The WGO effect with exercise seems to be depressive to the BMR compared to the exercised group on placeboes (significant at the .10 level) 8.87 per cent; this effect is reversed with the normal, inactive, middle-aged group C raising the BMR 8.10 per cent compared to the inactive professional group D, on placeboes, which dropped in BMR after going out of training. The exercised group B on placeboes had the greatest actual difference with group C on placeboes, a difference of 15.44 per cent (significant at the .05 level) the difference being due presumably to the exercise effect. Also the "economy effect" of the WGO shows strongly in comparing group A (exercised on WGO) but the difference is statistically insignificant, 1.53 per cent (t = 0.202).

Repeat Experiment in 1954

In 1954 the experiment was repeated with the following results:

Ten middle-aged men in six weeks of training, taking WGO
(same dosage as above)   (+ .11 SS)

Ten middle-aged men in six weeks of training, taking wheat germ   (−3.25 SS)

Nine middle-aged men in six weeks of training on cottonseed oil placeboes (same dosage as above)   (+9.89 SS)

Five professional middle-aged men, who went inactive as controls, taking placeboes   (−15.0 SS)

Summation of Results (1954)

Whereas, the exercised WGO and WGC groups made statistically insignificant *changes* of −0.11 SS (on WGO) and −3.25 SS (on wheat germ), the exercised group on placeboes improved 9.89 SS (t = 1.77) a value nearly significant with a definite trend for the BMR to be higher. This last group of men had eight out of the nine who raised the BMR. The most outstanding set of differences are, however, group II-B, which went out of training just for the time of the experiment and lost in BMR rate, averaging a drop from +2.34 per cent (56 SS) to −12.74 per cent (−15.0 SS). This last group must be compared on a different basis as most had been quite active before entering the experiment. The results indicate that the men on WGO and WGC maintained a lower BMR in the face of the work, compared to their normal control group, which showed the greatest change in BMR. We interpret the trend to mean that the men who maintained the BMR closest to normal made good adaptations to the work, whereas the control group on cottonseed oil placeboes did not adapt as well. A marked rise in BMR above normal is interpreted as indicating metabolic inefficiency.

It also seems that, as a trend, the physical activity itself had an effect of raising the BMR (stirring up the sympathoadrenergic system for a longer time or to a greater relative extent). The opposite effect is seen when a group of relatively active men went out of training just to be controls for a period, whereupon their BMR dropped from +2.34 per cent (56 SS) to −12.74 per cent (41 SS), a drop of −15.08 per cent (−15 SS). These opposite trends seem to check each other and confirm the effect of the exercise as a sympathoadrenergic stimulator.

It is inferred that the WGO has a stabilizing effect upon the BMR, probably due to the well-known vitamin E effect which typically lowers the BMR[6] or provides more adequate nutrition for strenuous work. But this may be due to WGO.

The reported effect in the literature is confirmed again and again that vitamin E is useful to improve the conservation of oxygen, and also to prevent its premature oxidation before reaching the body cells involved in basal metabolism. There are no experiments to show that such a small amount of vitamin E would actually increase the working performance itself. But it is clear from various experiments herein described that WGO and OCTCNL do aid the working performance and improve the cardiovascular efficiency.

THE ADAPTATION PHENOMENON

In certain training experiments where changes are being determined due to the effects of the exercise itself, an increase in the BMR may usually mean a carry-over effect from stirring up the sympathoadrenergic activity, and a rise in the BMR means that the subjects show relatively more stress effect and are only partially recovered, day to day. The metabolic upheaval from working out may last around the clock with some poorly trained subjects. It has been shown to last over a week from very exorbitant workouts.[10, 11] The effect of the WGO is consistent with faster recovery.

An example of adaptation versus lack of adaptation is shown with the data taken by an experiment completed in 1968 by Samson[12] on eighteen subjects. The subjects were trained for twenty weeks in Cureton's low gear, middle gear and high gear progression, following Cureton's book, *Physical Fitness and Dynamic Health* (1966, The Dial Press, New York), with tests of BMR at 0, 10 and 20 weeks. From 0 to 10 weeks, the three groups of six men each trained together and followed their leader (Samson). Tests were also taken on six nonexercising controls. At the end of the ten weeks, the changes were insignificant for the BMR in both the groups (exercising and nonexercising) indicating that the program was a gradual one and did not induce severe metabolic upheavals, although the training group changed +1.84 per cent in BMR. The inactive control group changed 0.76 per cent, but after the T_2 tests given at the end of the first ten weeks, the three groups of six men each were trained another ten weeks, somewhat harder as specified in the program. The group on WGO

TABLE XXXVIII

BMR ADAPTATION REFLECTED IN ATHLETES AFTER TRAINING
COMPARED TO OTHER GROUPS (Missiuro) (in cc/min)

Group	N	Values for group at beginning of training	Changes due to the program of training
Beginners (Untrained)	24	261 ± 6.84 $\sigma = 33.51$	420 ± 0.92 $\sigma = 4.49$
Men with two years of training in the physical education school ...	20	236 ± 9.81 $\sigma = 44.11$	37.5 ± 1.40 $\sigma = 6.25$
Olympic athletes at end of training season	13	196 ± 12.44 $\sigma = 44.84$	30.9 ± 1.83 $\sigma = 6.60$

(group A) made a significant change in BMR but it was the *least* change, compared to group B taking placeboes (moderate increase) and the third, group C, taking nothing at all. These results are shown in Tables XXXVII and XXXVIII. The data indicate that the group on WGO adapted quite fully to the exercise, whereas the other two groups adapted less well. This means that for group A on WGO the work became relatively easier, using less O_2 in the resting state, with recovery not fully made, even after twenty-four hours.

Data reported by Missiuro (Institute of Physical Culture, Warsaw, Poland) show that veteran athletes have acquired, over years of training, good adaptation to the work of athletics, and show the lowest BMR.[13]

Table XXXVIII illustrates that seasoned Olympic athletes change the least, due to a season of training. It is recognized that mental excitement will raise the metabolic rate, as on the morning of a football game. It will lower on other days when there is no game.[18]

Impressive supporting data have been published by a group of Russian experimenters (T. A. Allik, A. V. Korobkov, E. A. Matvyeva and I. M. Epshtein in the volume edited by S. Firsov and E. Jokl, *Medical Research on Swimming* sponsored by FINA, 1968), to quote:[14]

At the end of the training season under study, practice loads were further increased over several months. Oxygen (basal) consumption did not rise proportionately but decreased. Within the ensuing months oxygen consumption reached levels of between +5 and –10 per cent of the Harris-Benedict standards, while performances continued to improve. Levels of oxygen consumption at rest dropped to –30 per cent, with some individuals even to –50 per cent of the Harris-Benedict standards, without deterioration of the athletes' well-being and performance. In order to attain this physiological state, special training methods are required. If an athlete performs with 80 to 85 per cent of his maximal capacity, his oxygen consumption at rest decreases the next morning, but if he performs at maximal capacity, his oxygen consumption at rest shows an increase the next morning. In overtrained athletes the basal oxygen value becomes stabilized at a higher than normal level.

The training experiment by Ganslen[15] also demonstrated the "adaptation phenomenon." Six graduate students were tested at T_1 in a series of trials and averaged 0.219 L/minute in resting O_2 intake. After twelve weeks of progressive training on the track, in which they ran repetitious 600-yard runs with gradually increasing speed, the T_2 value of resting metabolism (sitting) was 0.265 L/minute. The subjects continued to train at the same type of work for another six weeks and also day by day, five days per week, took WGO (10 × 6 minim capsules). At T_3 the BMR had dropped to 0.235 L/minute. This did represent adaptation but it could not be determined with certainty that the reduction between T_2 and T_3 had been brought about by the WGO. In the light of data which have accumulated since, however, it is reasonably certain that this reduction was facilitated by WGO. Between T_2 and T_3 there were marked improvements in the all-out bicycle ride time and in various other fitness performance measures. The all-out maximal O_2 intake progressed from 2.166 at T_1 to 2.571 at T_2 to 2.681 L/minute at T_3. In spite of this, the BMR declined, indicating an adaptation along with higher fitness performance (cf. Fig. 75 and Fig. 79 in Part Two).

Knowlton and Weber[16] reported the results of training a young college-age, female athlete, the track training continuing over a 17-month period. There was phenomenal increase of her working capacity from 17,972 foot pounds of work to 27,625 at the end of the fifth testing period (half way through) up to 64,400 foot

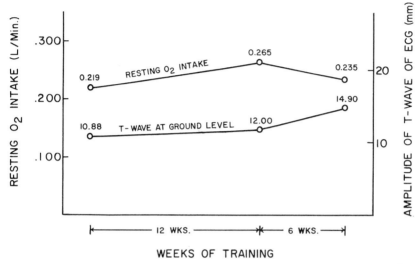

Figure 75. Relationship of highest precordial T-wave to the resting O_2 intake.

pounds of work at the end of the period. There was also during this time a marked increase in the contractile energy of her left ventricle, as measured by ultra-low frequency BCG technique. Basal oxygen consumption increased from 242 cc/minute (19.14%) to 256 (24.82%); at T_5, adaptation apparently occurred in the second half of the program, as at T_{10} when her working capacity was the highest, the basal O_2 was down to 209 cc/minute (4.01%).

CORRELATIVE STUDIES, EFFECT OF EXERCISE ON BASAL METABOLIC RATE

Whether basal metabolic rate will change or not depends upon the state of the subject at the beginning of the experiment. Bender[17] reviewed the literature of this problem, and also ferreted out the cause of some of the errors of other investigators. Zuntz and Schumberg,[18] Lusk-Graham and DuBois,[19] de Almedia[19] and Cureton[5] all reported increases in the BMR due to physical training, whereas, Schneider, Clarke and Ring[20] reported slight losses, and several others reported no change. Review of these works shows certain lack of controls. For instance, exercise of a very strenuous nature may affect the BMR for several days immediately afterwards; athletes on a heavy diet of carbohydrates are not similar to those who restrict the carbohydrates, as the storage CHO in the tissues is a factor, even if no food has been eaten for twelve hours. Anxiety is more manifest in some subjects than in others and it is a factor even though there are excellent temperature controls. It is also shown that when subjects have adapted to a program of exercise, they may then relax and the BMR is lower than when they were just starting; and subjects in a relatively hard, progressively harder and harder, program such as engaged in by many people in training are not always free of their tensions and fatigue, and their influence may go around the clock, and show in BMR tests—*the more violent the program and the newer the subject is to it, the higher will be the BMR, and the lower the RQs.* While several studies such as those by Benedict[21] show that athletes with mesomorphic body build usually have more lean body mass and a somewhat higher metabolism, many thin people of ectomorphic body build also have a relatively high percentage of lean body tissue, very active thyroid glands, and have relatively high metabolism. If subjects in training eat more carbohydrate food than normal and exercise, they will generally show an increase in BMR, but if they starve themselves it may be the opposite.

Leilich[22] found in a sample of seventy-three college men tested three times each, with the lower figure taken, that the twenty relatively sedentary men averaged −4.0 per cent (DuBois-DuBois Tables), twenty in moderate physical training from physical education classes averaged +2.8 per cent and twenty varsity athletes averaged +3.0 per cent, and highly trained, top-level athletes in track work averaged +3.5 per cent.

Bender[23] measured five experimental subjects and four controls repeatedly, a minimum of eight times at first, after which he trained them one hour per day in repeat walk and run work on a track for eight weeks, five days per week. The lowest value was accepted in each series as closest to "true" BMR, with the laboratory ambient temperature 78-80 F for all tests throughout the experiment. Measurements were made between 6:00 AM and 8:00 AM, the subjects being free of any food intake for the previous twelve hours and rested in the horizontal position for thirty-five minutes before each test, using the Sanborn Metabulator. Oral temperatures were taken before and after the test, and the subjects were measured for height, weight and surface area obtained from a nomogram. They were also then tested for maximum dynamometer strength, pinch-up fat folds in six places, and were also tested in a pool for bouyancy and specific gravity. One control subject had a lowered BMR and three others did not change significantly as controls. Of the five experimental subjects who took the exercise training program, the results showed the following: in cubic centimeter per minute changes +3.5 (insignificant), −1.5 (insignificant), 7.9 (significant 5 per cent level), 14.8 (significant 1 per cent level) and −11.0 (significant 5 per cent level). *It was concluded that subjects in good condition to begin with did not change significantly but those in poor condition to begin with increased their BMR by participating in the exercise program.* Bender attributed the increase to their increased *lean body mass.*

Cureton, Wolf and Harrison[24] trained fifteen middle-aged men in a fitness-swimming course, at the noon hour five days per week for six weeks. The work was almost nonstop and about as hard as the men could take. The average BMR shifted from an average of −21.9 per cent to −14.2 per cent, a rise of +7.7 per cent, presumably due to the exercise program.

In another experiment Cureton[25] reported training a forty-six-year old man (R. L.) in a mixed running and swimming experiment, in which after three months the man exercised an hour, twice per day. His improvements were very conspicuous; the BMR changed from −18.8 per cent to −11.04 per cent, an increase of 7.76 per cent in the five-month period of training. Quite likely this man worked hard enough to bring about an appreciable metabolic upheaval which went around the clock day-by-day, as he lost appreciable weight. Heusner's[26] progressive training in swimming showed a fluctuating change at first, within 4-8 per cent for five months of moderate work, then in the two months of actual competition increased to 14-15 per cent, and remained as high as 13 per cent for a month afterward and then, as soon as the hard training was stopped, decreased to +7 per cent in the next two months.

Du Toit[27] found that a progressive walking-jogging interval-type program, fifty minutes per day, four times per week, changed eight middle-aged men from an average of 245 cc/minute of basal oxygen intake to 286 cc/minute (increase of 16.75 per cent) for twelve weeks of training, whereas, a comparable group of men in a weight lifting program decreased from 311 to 264 cc/minute (−15.12 per cent). Apparently the walk-jog type of interval training program had more total work to it and stirred up the sympathoadrenergic system relatively more.

Pallandi[28] trained thirty middle-aged men in a walk-jog interval type program supplemented by various exercises for other parts of the body, following Cureton's continuous rhythmical exercise system (from *Physical Fitness and Dynamic Health*, 1966) in four weeks of low gear work, then in six weeks of middle gear work, three days per week. The control subjects did not change significantly but the experimental subjects made the following types of changes (by averages):

    Pulse pressure .... 35 changed to 49 mm Hg
    Systolic blood pressure . 126 changed to 130 mm Hg
    Diastolic blood pressure . 91 changed to 81 mm Hg
    Pulse rate .... 71.6 changed to 61.9 beats/minute
    Stroke volume .... 64 changed to 79 cc/beat

The figures by the Gale formula computed −8.8 per cent before training and −6.9 per cent after training, a relative increase of +1.9 per cent in the Gale estimated metabolic rate.

Whether a person will lose fat or not in an exercise program is seemingly very dependent upon whether the metabolic rate will increase, and the total calories used raises enough; this is estimated to be at least to the 300 to 500 kcal level per day.

Results

The results of the experimental training on BMR are shown in Table XXXIX.

Table XL shows that between T_2 and T_3 there were some statistically significant changes.

It may be observed in Table XL that the smallest change in BMR was in group A (on WGO), and the next greatest change was in group B (on lard placeboes), and the *greatest* change

TABLE XXXIX

BMR EFFECTS OF TRAINING (in %) (Sampson, Exp. 28, 1968)

	T_1 Mean	σ	T_2 Mean	σ	T_1 to T_2 D	Significance of Change°
Training group .... N = 18	3.77	15.97	5.61	13.54	1.84	N.S. $D/\sigma_{diff.} = 0.572$
Control group .... N = 8	0.75	11.13	1.50	11.06	.76	N.S. $D/\sigma_{diff.} = 0.108$

was in group C which took nothing. It appears, therefore, that the effect of the WGO was to maintain an economical BMR in the face of the progressive training, thus holding the homeostasis to the best of the three groups. This may be attributed perhaps to the effect of vitamin E in the WGO, and possibly also to the octacosanol fraction in the WGO, as shown in the Farrell-Gier animal experiment. The lard placeboes were least effective in holding the BMR down relatively close to the level tested at T_2, hence, group C was least economical of oxygen.

By the usual t test the differences between the three groups A, B and C did not meet the .05 level of significance. This might be expected because of the small size of the samples of six men in each group, and they were *not* random samples. Therefore, it is appropriate to look at the experiment as a single experiment, and

TABLE XL

EFFECTS OF TRAINING AND WHEAT GERM OIL (in %)

(second ten weeks)

	T_2 Mean	σ	T_3 Mean	σ	T_2 to T_3 D	Significance of Change
On WGO group A .. N = 6	14.83	5.53	17.33	13.85	2.50	$D/\sigma_{diff.} = 2.91$ significant
On placeboes group B .. N = 6	.33	11.65	5.00	5.02	4.67	$D/\sigma_{diff.} = 0.637$ insignificant
On nothing group C .. N = 6	1.67	17.40	18.17	16.10	16.50	$D/\sigma_{diff.} = 1.208$ insignificant

not generalize its reliability by the *t* test. This step, to determine whether the groups A, B and C were different from each other calls for computing the S.E.$_{meas.}$ for each of the three groups from the r_{11} data, which were determined in the experiment by retesting the subjects for reliability at the beginning of the experiment to determine the magnitude of the chance errors of *measurement*. Then this would permit this one experiment to be evaluated, without resorting to inference statistics to estimate how many times out of one hundred samples, of the size used, would give results as good as obtained, and/or how many times such results could be obtained theoretically by chance. Marked curvilinearity invalidates the *t* test.

The T-ratio (D/S.E.$_{diff.}$) between the WGO training group and the placebo group was 1.612 (near significance) < .20 level; and the T-ratio between the WGO group and the group taking nothing was 10.43. This indicates that the WGO had an effect on BMR but the placebo also had some effect, hence was not a "true" placebo. The lard placeboes had as much vitamin E in them as the WGO.[7, 8]

All three groups were improved by the training program, as might be expected in endurance and various other measures. The "oxygen economizing effect" has also been noted in several other experiments, compared to the groups taking nothing, which very usually increase in the BMR, indicating that they were slower to make an adaptation to the work compared to the groups on WGO, vitamin E or cottonseed oil or lard placeboes which contain vitamin E. The octacosanol effect may be much like the vitamin E effect in preventing oxygen wastage. That this "economy effect" is correlative with physical fitness may also be noted in the advantage of the WGO over the placebo group (T = 3.0/0.114 = 26.35), indicating that the force of the heart stroke was strengthened (referring to the I$_{accel.}$ wave). Dempsey[9] also found that WGO increased the I + J/time in young boys.

CONCLUSIONS

While no irrefutable conclusion can be made from the data at hand, it is of great interest that both sets of experiments shown in this section show similar trends for the effects of WGO or BMR, namely that the WGO has an economizing effect in relationship to the use of oxygen. In various training experiments it has been shown that BMR usually goes up in the first few weeks but by ten weeks has stabilized and declined somewhat, as adaptation to the training effort has been gradually achieved. The interpretation is, therefore, that the use of WGO was helpful and made possible a more economical use of oxygen relatively, and facilitated adaptation to the work. It is impressive in the second experiment by Samson (1968) that the changes at ten weeks were statistically insignificant within each group but after ten more weeks an adaptation had occurred which favored the WGO group. This trend is in accord with experiments by Allik, Korobokov, Matvyeva and I. M. Epshtein reported in *Medical Research on Swimming* (1968) and also with independent experiments summarized by Cureton.[25]

By the $D/\sigma_{diff.}$ ratio, T, the group A in the second ten weeks changed 2.50 per cent (T = 2.91, significant); the group B on placeboes changed 4.67 per cent (T = 0.637, insignificant); and the group C on nothing changed 16.50 (T = 1.208, insignificant). The results in this single experiment show that WGO was effective in holding the BMR nearest to normal value with less change due to the training program. The T-ratio ($D/S.E._{diff.}$) between the groups in the second ten weeks of training while taking WGO and the placebo group B was 1.612 (near significance < .20); and between group A on WGO and group C on nothing was 10.43 (significant < .01). This also suggests that both the WGO and the placeboes had an effect in holding the BMR relatively stable and closer to the normal level than if they had taken nothing.

REFERENCES

1. Benedict, F. G.: *Vital Energetics.* Washington, D. C., Carnegie Institute of Washington, 1938, p. 215.
2. Benedict, F. G. and Carpenter, T. M.: *Metabolism and Energy Transformations.* Washington, D. C., Carnegie Institute, 1918, p. 236.
3. Van Huss, Wayne: Factors Related to Basal Metabolism, Urbana, M.S. thesis, Physical Education, University of Illinois, 1949, p. 99.
4. Unpublished data, Physical Fitness Institute, University of Illinois.
5. Cureton, T. K.: The lying basal metabolism test of physical fitness, pp. 286-313 in *Physical Fitness of Champion Athletes.* Urbana, University of Illinois Press, 1951, p. 458.

6. Tappel, A. L.: Where old age begins, *Nutrition Today,* pp. 2-7, Dec., 1967.

7. Garrett, H. E.: *Statistics in Psychology and Education,* New York, Longmans, Green and Co., 1933, pp. 8-133.

8. Peters, C. C. and Van Voorhis, W. R.: The reliability of differences, pp. 60-170, in *Statistical Procedures and Their Mathematical Bases.* New York, McGraw-Hill Book Co., Inc., 1940.

9. Dempsey, Cedric W.: A Ballistocardiographic Investigation of Cardiac Responses of Boys to Physical Training and Wheat Germ Oil, Urbana, Ph.D. thesis, Physical Education, University of Illinois, 1963, p. 196.

10. Bender, Jay A.: The Effects of Exercise on Basal Metabolism, Urbana, Ph.D. thesis, Physical Education, University of Illinois, 1951, p. 124.

11. Cureton, T. K.: *op. cit.,* ref. 5.

12. Samson, Jacques J-H-J.: Effects of Training with and without Wheat Germ Oil on Basic Metabolism and Selected Cardiovascular Measures of Middle-Aged Men, Urbana, M.S. thesis, Physical Education, University of Illinois, 1968, p. 124.

13. Missiuro, W.: Influence de l'Entrainment Physique sur les Exchanges Respiratoires, *Przeglad Fizjologji,* Ruchu, 5:1, 1933.

14. Allik, T. A., Korobokov, A. V., Matvyeva, E. A. and Epshtein, I. M.: *Medical Research on Swimming.*

15. Ganslen, R. V.: The Influence of Training upon the Aerobic and Anaerobic Metabolic Variables, Urbana, Ph.D. thesis, Physical Education, University of Illinois, 1953, p. 98.

16. Knowlton, R. G. and Weber, Herbert: A case study of training responses in a female endurance runner, *J. Sports Med.,* 8:228-235, Dec., 1968.

17. Bender, Jay A.: ref. 10, *op. cit.*

18. Benedict, F. G. and Smith, H. M.: The metabolism of athletes as compared with non-athletes of similar height and build, *J. Biochem.,* 20:243-252, 1915.

19. Leilich, Roy E.: The Comparison of Various Physical Education Groups on Basal Metabolism, Urbana, M.S. thesis, Physical Education, University of Illinois, 1948, p. 60.

20. Bender, J. A.: ref. 10, *op. cit.*

21. Cureton, T. K., Wolf, J. G., Harrison, Aix B.: Improvements in middle-aged men swimming for endurance 6 weeks, 5 days per week, pp. 72-74 in Cureton, *The Physiological Effects of Exercise Programs on Adults.* Springfield, Illinois, Charles C Thomas, 1969.

22. *Ibid.,* p. 78.

23. *Ibid.,* pp. 80-82.

24. *Ibid.,* p. 47.

25. *Ibid.,* p. 39.

Chapter XI

The Effect of Wheat Germ Oil on the Flicker Fusion Frequency (Krasno-Ivy) Test

CENTRAL FLICKER FREQUENCY

VISUAL fatigue or what may be called "asthenopia" (from the two Greek words for "weakness" and "eye") can produce such discomforting symptoms as: pain in the eyes or immediately around the eyes, headaches, tearing, blinking, drowsiness, vertigo and spasmodic twitchings. Close work, overwork, flare and poor illumination usually aggravate these symptoms. Rohracher and Schwartz[1] recognized that visual fatigue frequently parallels nervous fatigue. Patients with organic or functional nervous disorders such as hysteria and neurasthenia were commonly afflicted with asthenopia. Such people can improve the condition of their eyes by adhering to general hygienic measures, including proper exercise, rest and adequate nutrition. These measures are aimed at restoring the normal function of the voluntary and autonomic nervous systems, since it is the dysfunction of these systems which caused the visual fatigue in the first place. Simonson and Brozek,[2] Misiak[3] and Landis[4] have provided extensive documentation of the *flicker fusion frequency test.*

Extensive studies have been conducted on the effect of experimental conditions on visual fatigue, using Critical Flicker Frequency (c.f.f.) as the criterion. Steinhaus and Kelso[5] found that cold hip baths significantly improved the c.f.f. scores in forty-seven males aged 17 to 45. It seems likely that the improvement resulted from the shunting of blood from the skin capillary beds to the central circulation, thereby creating more circulation to the eye. The stimulation to the central nervous system offered by the cold bath must also be considered as a possible reason for the improvement. At our own laboratory, Cheever[6] studied the effects of training and untraining on the c.f.f. of three subjects at ground level and at 15,000 feet simulated altitude. The c.f.f. of all three subjects steadily improved with training, in a twelve-week program, five days per week, as tested on the Krasno-Ivy Flicker Fusion Frequency Meter but subjects deteriorated at a higher altitude, a fact also noted by Birren.[7] From the beginning of training until its conclusion, the three subjects declined after eight weeks of untraining. Also, generally higher c.f.f. scores were made at ground level as opposed to altitude, although during training c.f.f. improved under both conditions at approximately the same rate. Simonson and Brozek, Ryan and Bitterman[2] found that one of the best tests to show visual fatigue during or after prolonged visual work was the c.f.f. Attempts to show visual fatigue trends with other visual function tests have proved disappointing due to the insensitivity of the tests.

After observing that the improvement in c.f.f. parallels the shift towards sympatheticotonia in adult men undergoing a regular exercise program, the interpretation is that the c.f.f. improvement is indicative of improved sympathetic nervous functioning with a concomitant lessening of blood ptosis, and is in the same directional shift as physiological "warm-up."

Even routine everyday living frequently entails the use of reaction time. The driver of an automobile must react quickly in applying the brakes to avoid striking a pedestrian, while the pedestrian must react quickly in order to remove himself from the car's path. It is higher in threshold with greater sympatheticotonia.

Finally, fast reaction-seeing time is a virtual prerequisite to the hunter or fisherman. Hunting quail, pheasants and many other game birds will only prove frustrating to those with slow reaction times; and setting the hook too late on a striking fish can be equally disappointing.

Velocity of nerve conduction declines with age[8, 9] and with unfitness. The c.f.f. is affected by circulatory unfitness.[10] The significance of the Krasno-Ivy, for which research the American Medical Association awarded these researchers its gold medal, is that the c.f.f. is affected by the number of functioning capillaries in the retina of the eye, and that this condition is paralleled by similar activity in the heart. These authors measured the response of heart patients to a standardized dose of nitroglycerine to test their responsiveness.

ADMINISTRATION OF THE CFF TEST

In administering the critical flicker frequency test (c.f.f.) extreme caution must be exercised to insure standardized testing conditions, especially with respect to atmospheric conditions, emotional attitude of the technician (and the subject, if possible), time allotted for dark adaptation of the eyes, distance of subjects' eyes from photometer and time of day.[3] The test measures the subject's ability to detect visually the flickering of a small light that is flickered at progressively increasing or decreasing frequencies. In progressing from high to low frequency, the testor records the frequency at which the subject is first able to see the flicker. In progressing from low to high frequency, the testor records the frequency at which the subject can no longer see the flicker, but instead sees the fusion of the flicker into a continuous light. Then the procedure is reversed.

The total body reaction time apparatus consists of a) a control box with switches to initiate the stimulus (light, buzzer or both), b) a reaction platform off which the subject jumps to break the electrical circuit and c) a Standard Electric Time Clock, Model SW-1, D-C clutch, which records the reaction time in thousandths of a second. The reaction time recorded with this apparatus is thus the time elapsed between the presentation of the stimulus and the breaking of the platform's electrical circuit. Recent evidence comparing the reaction times obtained from two different methods of jumping off the platform suggests the need to standardize the jumping method. Rapidly flexing the lower legs while the rest of the body was pulled down slightly by gravity and the leg-flexing muscles elicited significantly faster reaction times than an upward translatory hop.

If the concept of reaction time is restricted to nerve conduction velocity, it may be more appropriate to refer to the test described above as "response time," since movement is involved in jumping off the platform. At least fifteen "warm-up" preliminary trials are considered necessary before the five tests of auditory, visual and combined reactions are given "to count."

DIRECTIONS FOR USE OF FLICKER PHOTOMETER

1. The subject should not smoke (two hours), drink alcohol (four hours), or take vasodilator drugs (twenty-four hours) prior to test.
2. Subject rests in dark room at least ten minutes.
3. If glasses are normally worn, they should be used during test.
4. Record machine used (A or B), name, date, age, weight, height and activity for the previous twenty-four hours.
5. Turn on machine.
6. Subject seated one yard from machine with eyes approximately horizontal to the small window in the front of the machine.
7. Make sure that there are no distractions in the room—it is important for the subject to concentrate solely on the window.
8. Hand the stop button to the subject and instruct him to push it as soon as he sees the first flicker.
9. Set the dial at the back at 1600 and turn it on (a trial run to let the subject see the flicker and press the button to stop it).
10. Give three trials (setting the dial at 3100, 2900 and 3000, respectively, unless his threshold is above one of these).
11. Record each trial, total and average scores.
12. If the trials are extremely variable (more than 150-200 difference on any two trials), have the subject rest for a few minutes and repeat.

STUDIES PERTAINING TO THE EFFECTS OF WHEAT GERM DERIVATIVES ON CRITICAL FLICKER FREQUENCY AND TOTAL BODY REACTION TIME

In our laboratory Bernauer experimented with six young male subjects, and found very individualized reactions in the c.f.f. test over a period of twelve weeks of physical training (Figs. 76, 77

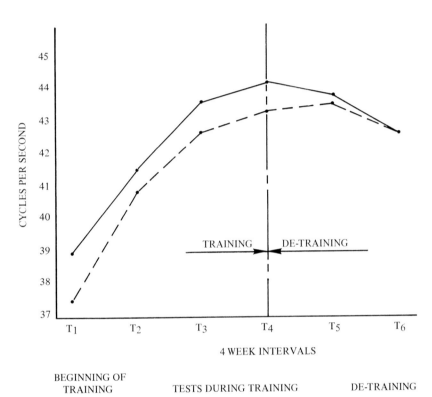

Figure 76. Changes in critical flicker fusion of the mean of the three subjects at ground level and at altitude.

and 78A). Fatigue reduced the frequency threshold, as in the 5-minute step test. Five of six subjects gave markedly reduced frequencies after this test, comparing pre-training to post-training (after twelve weeks). The physical training lowered the frequency in four and raised it in two while taking the test in the rested state. But in a single period the harder work stirred up the sympatheticotonic state relatively more than a quiet sitting position or a mild treadmill exercise (Fig. 78A).

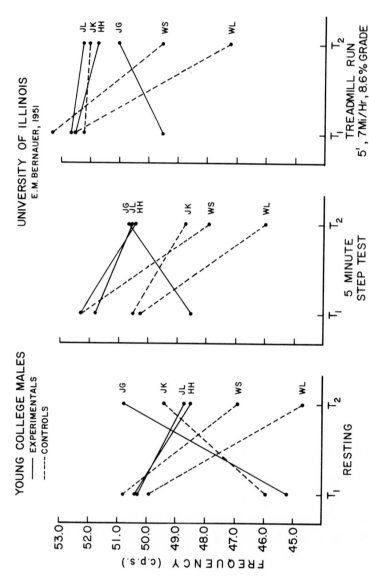

Figure 77. Critical flicker fusion frequency before and after training (resting, five-min. step test effect and treadmill run effect).

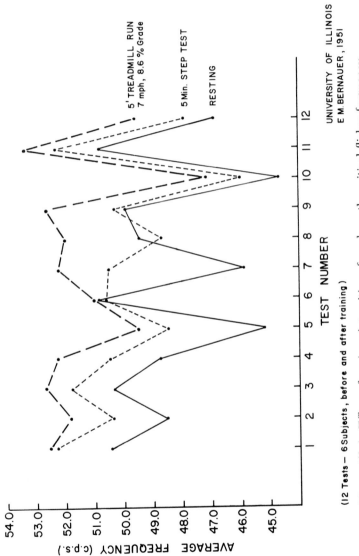

Figure 78-A. Effect of various intensities of work on the critical flicker frequency.

THE FRANKS-CURETON STUDY

Although the c.f.f. has been used as a criterion of visual fatigue in a wealth of studies, only one study exists in which wheat germ or wheat germ oil comprised the experimental variable. This study was conducted at the University of Illinois Physical Fitness Research Laboratory during the summer of 1967 by Cureton and Franks (Exp. 27). Sixty-three boys from the University of Illinois Summer Sports-Fitness School were placed into three matched groups on the basis of 600-yard run times. Group A (N = 20) received 10 of the 6 minims of WGO, compared to the placebo group C (N = 20) receiving the same amounts of devitaminized lard and group B taking wheat germ cereal (N = 20). The goups which took the dietary supplements of WGO and WGC were more adapted at rest, following eight weeks of strenuous physical training in a hot summer, finishing with lower pulse rates and flicker fusion frequency than the placebo control group.

The three groups were satisfactorily matched in the principal variable, i.e. the flicker fusion frequency, twenty subjects in each group initially. Analysis of covariance was used to determine the matching and the significance of the differences in the improvements. There were insignificant differences between the groups in age, height and weight.

The placebo and wheat germ oil groups improved most in the eighteen-item motor test (6.58 and 5.95 points, respectively, compared to 3.15 points for the wheat germ group). The covariance F was insignificant between all three groups, this was due to the relatively large errors in administration.

The softball throw gave an advantage to the wheat germ cereal group by 4.26 feet over the placebo group (significant at the .01 level); and a similar advantage of 2.0 feet to the wheat germ oil group over the placebo group (F = 1.22, significant at the .30 level). The distance was greatest in the wheat germ cereal group (124.57′) compared to the placebo group (108.05′); and the wheat germ oil group improved 69.89′ (F = 1.45, significant at the .20 level).

The broad jump improved the most in the wheat germ oil

group (2.06″) compared to the wheat germ cereal group (1.73″) and the placebo group (1.16″) (F = 0.23). Since several other experiments have shown trends of advantage for wheat germ oil in total body reaction time and in strength/weight, this might be a favorable trend for the sample in hand which took WGO.

Pull-ups improved insignificantly in all groups, averaging 0.34, 0.42 and 0.45 of one chin for the placebo, wheat germ cereal and wheat germ oil (F = 0.23). All results are statistically insignificant.

The 50-yard dash improved insignificantly in all groups, 0.13 second in the placebo group, 0.16 second in the wheat germ cereal group, and 0.13 second in the wheat germ oil group (F = 0.30).

In the 600-yard run group the largest improvement was in the placebo group (13.58 seconds) compared to the wheat germ oil group (11.11 seconds) and then lastly, the wheat germ cereal group (9.89 seconds). All differences were statistically insignificant between groups (F = 0.21). The placeboes were devitaminized lard, 15 × 3 minim capsules per day.

The criterion test flicker fusion frequency changed the most in the placebo group (113.45 f/second), next in the wheat germ cereal group (33.35 f/second) and lastly, in the wheat germ oil group (1.50 f/second) (F = 3.23). The between-groups F was 3.23, significant at the .05 level.

The fact that the training experiment, which included about three hours of activity work per day, including one period of conditioning gymnastics and one period of running endurance, improved the 600-yard run time *in all groups* is of some significance. The differences are large in terms of converting the times to distance in feet. The advantage with the placebo group was statistically insignificant.

If the program left the boys with a higher relative sympathoadrenergic condition, at least this persisting through the period of the final tests, T_2, we might expect to find somewhat faster pulse rates and higher c.f.f. and brachial pulse waves. This has typically been the case and such stimulation has been shown to last for a week or more in some boys. However, after two or three weeks, almost every boy was shown to have relaxed to slower pulse rates. It is admitted that the intensity of the program in the last week or two built up some cumulative fatigue. The supplemented groups with wheat germ and WGO were more relaxed (held hemostasis better at rest) than the placebo group.

Pull-ups have also been shown to give similar insignificant results in all other similar short-term training groups, as in our experiment on young men in the Underwater Scuba (swimming) Group at the United States Naval Base, Key West.

CONCLUSIONS

The c.f.f. test reflects circulatory fitness and increased sympatheticotonia. In the face of stress over 10-12 weeks it increases with increased sympatheticotonia if the work is hard and full adaptation not reached, after which it would level off or reverse by decreasing. The stress at 10,000 feet of simulated altitude caused a fairly constant decrease in c.f.f. (Fig. 76). The decrease was attributed to relatively poor circulation without full adaptation.

The addition of WGO to the diet of one of the three matched groups of young boys resulted in the WGO group remaining more stable, less excitable, or showing relatively less fatigue at the end of the eight weeks of physical training and sports, this program finishing normally with boys showing some appreciable fatigue for a week or two. It is temporary and disappears in about two weeks, as retests have shown.

The interpretation is that the WGO helped the boys withstand the stress, so the c.f.f. test changed relatively less in the group which took WGO.

REFERENCES

1. Rohracher, L. and Schwartz: Retinal sensitivity to fatigue, *Zeitsschrift für Sinnesphysiolie*, 66:164, 1935; *ibid.*, 67:227, 1938.
2. Simonsen, E. and Brozek: The influence of age on the fusion frequency of flicker, *J. Exp. Psychol.*, 29:252-255, 1941; also *ibid.*, *J. Consult. Psychol.*, 9:87-90, March-April, 1945; Work vision and illumination, *Illumination Engineering*, 47:355-349, June, 1952; *ibid.*, A work test for quantitative study of visual performance and fatigue, *J. Appl.*, *Psychol.*, 31:519, Oct., 1947.
3. Misiak, H.: The flicker-fusion test and its applications, *Trans. N. Y. Acad. Sci.*, Series II, 29:616-622, March, 1967.

4. Landis, C.: Determinants of the critical flicker-fusion threshold, *Physiol. Rev.*, 34:259-286, 1954.

5. Steinhaus, A. H. and Kelso, A.: Improvement of visual and other functions by cold hip baths, *War Medicine*, 4:610-17, 1943.

6. Cheever, E. G.: The Effect of Training Upon Critical Flicker Frequency at Ground Level and at 15,000 Feet of Simulated Altitude, Urbana, M.S. thesis, Physical Education, University of Illinois, 1952, p. 42.

7. Birren, J. E., *et. al.*: Effects of anoxia on performance at several simulated altitudes, *J. Exp. Psychol.*, 36:35-49, 1946.

8. Simonsen and Brozek: *op cit.*, ref. 2; and C. Landis, *op cit.*, ref. 4.

9. Wagoner, H. P. and Keith, N. M.: Diffuse arteriolar disease with hypertension and the associated retinal lesions, *Medicine*, 18:317-430, Sept., 1939.

10. Ganslen, R. V.: Variation in the Electrical Sensitivity of the Optic Nerve as an Index of Fatigue, paper presented to the American College of Sports Medicine, New York City, June 8, 1957.

Chapter XII

Summary of Part One

THIS review of thirty-one group studies and eleven individual studies conducted at the University of Illinois from 1950 to 1969, with support from a few other studies made in other places, show that the VioBin wheat germ oil (WGO) and a substance derived from it, octacosanol, produce significant physiological changes in experimental subjects compared to control subjects on placeboes. With adults, the dosage has been ten capsules of the 6-minim size per day, and with children, twenty capsules of the 3-minim size, or a somewhat smaller number by one-third.

The gains for the WGO over the placebo substances (cotton-seed oil, refined corn oil with an equivalent amount of vitamin E to equate to that in WGO, lecithin oil, refined corn oil and de-vitaminized lard with an equivalent amount of vitamin E to match the WGO) are fairly remarkable because some of the placebo substances also have some biological effects. It was difficult to find a placebo substance of the same calorific value as WGO which was absolutely without biological value to humans. Each experiment states exactly what type of placebo was used.

The principal research method used, and that considered the best, was the use of *matched groups* in parallel experimentation on the same physical training program (for exercise) for the same number of minutes and under the same instructor. Both groups worked together in the same type of physical work (Experiments 1, 7, 8, 11, 12, 13, 14, 15, 16, 17, 18, 19, 20, 21, 22, 23, 24, 25, 26, 27, 28, 29, 30, 31). Of these, seven experiments were on young men, ten were on young boys 7-13 years of age, and seven were on adult men 26-60 years of age.

The second research method used was *single group*, training to a plateau in twelve or more weeks, then adding the dietary supplement capsules daily at the end of the workouts, to show their effect over and above the effect of the physical training (Experiments 2, 3, 4, 5, 6, 9, 10, all on young men).

The third research method used was that of *individual longitudinal experimentation* with variations introduced in different years to show contrasting effects with wheat germ oil (WGO), or with octacosanol (OCTCNL), or with wheat germ cereal (WGC) (Experiments 32, 33, 34, 35, 36, 37, 38, 39, 40, 41, 42; all on adult middle-aged men).

While the usual variations (sickness, various body types, different levels of physical fitness, slight indispositions, etc.) were encountered by using human subjects, all three research methods show impressive results, for the WGO and OCTCNL supplements to have favorable effects in the same direction for improvement as the physical training effects themselves, but over and above these physical training effects, the dietary substances mentioned have induced additional improvement. Wheat germ cereal (WGC) has also some traceable effects too but only once outdid the WGO and OCTCNL, this when absolutely fresh material was demanded.

Possibly the most uncontrollable variation was that of extraneous activities of the subjects in the form of additional exercise other than that taken in the experiments; and some smoking and using alcohol and others not; and some with indisposition on certain days due to fatigue from the previous day's work or competition (events for time or number). The latter was a definite interference in the case of the boys.

Endurance was affected in the same direction of improvement in eleven out of thirteen experiments, ten times reaching the level of statistical significance accepted (i.e. Fisher $t < .10$ level, or the mean difference $2 \times$ S.E.$_{meas.}$ from test and retest deviations). Only once was there no difference and this was with Brown's experiment involving wheat germ. The average advantage was 12.51 standard scores (SS) compared to 6.77 SS for the placebo substances averaged (Table XIII). Wheat germ oil (VioBin) and octacosanol appear to have about equal effects, and synthetic vitamin E has virtually no effect in the small amounts fed. Wheat germ cereal averaged 5.71 SS, sedentary subjects on WGO 2.6 SS, sedentary subjects on placeboes 1.0 SS, and sedentary subjects on nothing 4.22 SS.

Oxygen intake in all-out treadmill runs gave indeterminate results, as some subjects were affected and some were not, about one-fourth of the boys used in this work did not improve in this test at all. From an analysis of the errors involved, and the large probable effect of heredity and lean body mass over the oxygen intake capacity test, it was concluded that this test was unsatisfactory as a measure of the marginal effect of the dietary substances. The aerobic oxygen intake improvements were smaller in these experiments than any other type of test, except "chinning" the "bar." Obviously, with almost no change due to the training, this small difference also nullified the statistical significance calculation. The difficulties associated with this test are discussed in full (Chapter IV). Net oxygen debt was ruled out of consideration because of the large variable errors involved, although the experiments of Prokop and also Farrell-Gier showed some advantages for WGO with the test, the advantage being significantly in favor of OCTCNL in animal work (Farrell-Gier) and WGO with humans (Prokop) but only in recovery.

Six experiments using the total body reaction time test (Cureton-Garrett) resulted in favorable advantages to speed the reactions five times out of the six experiments, four times with WGO, OCTCNL once and in one part of one experiment WGC affected the visual reaction time. Statistical significance was claimed in five of the six experiments for WGO (Table XXV). Swimming was shown to slow the TBRT test compared to required non-swimming physical education (Exp. 1, Forr and Cureton). Four to five weeks were required for the feeding to develop large enough changes to permit statistical significance to be satisfactorily achieved. It is believed that one experiment failed because of too short a time for feeding the WGO (Exp. 12).

Seven experiments were made with the "highest" T-wave of the precordial lead of the electrocardiogram. The average gain in favor of the dietary experimental materials was 3.746 SS compared to 0.623 SS for the placebo substances. Five times statistical significance was obtained $< .10$ and twice the trend of advantage over the placeboes favored the WGO. Octacosanol was not used.

The brachial pulse wave test (heartograph or sphygmograph) was used in eight experiments (Experiments 1, 9, 12, 13, 15, 17,

18, 25) and six times WGO was credited with positive effects of improvement, OCTCNL twice and WGC once. The area or amplitude of the brachial pulse wave is reflective of stroke volume and also of "velocity of ejection" when measured for this characteristic. These measurements are reflective of the innervation and also the nutritive state of the heart muscle. One OCTCNL experiment turned up negative because of excessive fatigue nullifying the gains in a group of boys which the dietary supplement could not overcome; this may have occurred also in Vohaska's (Exp. 12) experiment, although the time that the WGO was fed was only four weeks, judged to be a minimum time to get significant effects. The average of all experiments gave a gain of 9.47 SS for the WGO, OCTCNL and WGC supplemented groups, compared to (−0.12 SS) for the placebo substances (Table XXIX). Satisfactory statistical significance is claimed in four of eight of these experiments and four additional times there were favorable trends for WGO; and once no result (Vohaska, Exp. 12) and once no result for OCTCNL (Table XXX).

Ten experiments were conducted which used pulse rates (Schneider index, progressive pulse ratio and Harvard five-minute step test). A moderate advantage was shown for the dietary supplemented groups: 2.41 SS for WGO, 3.97 for OCTCNL, and −0.063 SS for the placebo substances (Table XXXII). Satisfactory statistical significance was shown six times for WGO and once for OCTCNL (Table XXXIII). In three experiments the results were not in favor of the supplements. The lowering of the pulse rates indicate relatively better tolerance of the stresses imposed.

The pre-ejection intervals of the left ventricle were used in two experiments. Wheat germ cereal (WGC) used with boys shortened the ICP interval the least in a program which induced definite temporary fatigue (which caused all comparative groups to shorten, rather than lengthen); and the WGC group also shortened relatively less than the placebo group. The generalization is made that the WGC substance permitted the boys taking them to stand the stress better. Wiley's experiment (Exp. 30) resulted in a similar trend, a slight lengthening of the ICP interval to the group taking WGO, compared to the placebo group.

In Wiley's experiment there was a slight tendency, 0.001 second for the ICP interval to lengthen more in the same type of work than the control group on the placebo substance. However, in this experiment there were also some advantages shown in the WGO group compared to the control group on the amplitude of the brachial pulse wave and diastolic blood pressure.

The experiments by Ganslen (Exp. 6), Cureton and Pohndorf (Exp. 13) and Sampson (Exp. 28) show that WGO exerts a stabilizing effect on the basal metabolic rate in the face of stress, in that the WGO groups increased the BMR less than the control groups on placeboes. The OCTCNL group was also slightly better in this regard than the placebo group.

The flicker fusion frequency test is deleteriously affected by altitude as shown in the experimental decompression chamber experiment, but WGO acts to resist such a deleterious change as the result of physical training stress or altitude stress. One experiment (Franks-Cureton, Exp. 27) gave results similar to those given for basal metabolism.

Because of skewed distributions the Fisher t test was not always applicable. The small samples used in these experiments were not always normal; the nonparametric procedures were used for statistical reliability, but usually the method of testing the consistency of the testing for the groups at hand was used, i.e. the $S.E._{meas.}$ was determined and evaluated in a similar manner to the t test but against the normal probability tables.

The correlative experiments on WGO and octacosanol using animal protocol, reviewed by Professor W. Richard Dukelow (*Acta Endocrinol.* Suppl., 121, Wheat germ oil and reproduction, a review, Vol. 56, Copenhagen: *Periodocia*, 1967) shows sixty-nine related references dealing with his topic. While this work on human subjects was not on reproduction, as such, it is believed that the influence shown for the effect of WGO on reproduction reflects better physical health in the WGO-fed animals. The experiment by Farrell and Gier at Kansas State University shows similar supporting evidence. The part of this animal work that is analogous to the human fitness experiments just summarized is the work of Farrell-Gier, which shows that very fatigued rats, from swimming to all-out exhaustion in a water vat, used less oxygen in recovery while being fed octacosanol than while being fed placebo materials. Mr. Levin has also reviewed this evidence (Foreword).

Mr. Ezra Levin has long been involved in animal studies, and he has presented evidence that octacosanol influenced the growth of combs on young roosters when properly mixed with phosphorylizing materials such as lecithin or calcium phosphate in solution. The same conditions apply to the use of WGO; it is used better in the muscles when taken with 2 per cent milk on an empty stomach.

All studies, both animal and human, have resulted in a new United States Patent, No. 3031376. It is a fact that WGO and octacosanol make biological changes. These changes in humans are slow, taking 4-5 weeks for gains to accrue sufficiently to make a real statistically significant difference. Octacosanol ($CH_3 \cdot (CH_2) 26 \cdot CH_2OH$) is not vitamin E and is most likely the critical factor affecting our physical fitness tests than vitamin E.

Physical training itself is a powerful biological process, which makes physiological changes much greater than the WGO or octacosanol but when used in conjunction with the feeding of these substances catalyzes the formulation of glycogen in the muscles. The exercise causes an efflux of enzymes to come from within the cells into the interstitial spaces between the cells and then into the blood, where "digestion" is assisted to facilitate the utilization of the WGO supplements. Several times (Experiments 6 and 13) it was shown that with WGO taken after exercise on a daily basis, the effects were relatively greater than WGO taken by sedentary subjects.

The under-nutrition of heart muscle is probably quite general in the United States, where such a large amount of atherosclerosis and coronary disease and hypertension exist. No doubt this is related to the fact that only 4 per cent of American people take enough exercise to make any difference in these diseases (Gallop Poll Report). Keyes *et al.*, have shown the deleterious effect of such semistarvation on the T-waves of the electrocardiogram. We certainly could not have shown such changes favorable to WGO and OCTCNL if there were not such a basic deficiency present in the United States for the fresh, unheated or unfried, natural

TABLE XLI

SUMMARY TABLE FOR ELEVEN INDIVIDUAL CASES, SHOWING
EFFECTS OF WGC WHEAT GERM OIL VERSUS OTHER
CONTROL SUBSTANCES OR NOTHING

Subject	Tests Showing Definite Effect from WGO versus Control	No Response from WGO > Control	Explanation of Loss from WGO versus Control
T. K. C. Exp. 32	Precordial T-wave and performance		Nothing
S. L. T. Exp. 33	Precordial T-wave, heartograph, Schneider index and performance		Once, not fed long enough Placeboes No program
D. H. Exp. 34	Treadmill performance and T-wave changes		WGC No program
H. S. Exp. 35	WGO (twice) on T-wave WGC (twice) on T-wave		No program
C. B. Exp. 36	WGO (twice) Schneider index Placeboes Schneider index		WGC No program
R. D. Exp. 37	WGO on heartograph and T-wave WGC on heartograph and T-wave WGC on T-wave	WGC on heartograph	WGO Placebo No program
F. K. Exp. 38	WGO (three times) on heartograph	Placebo	No program
D. S. Exp. 39	WGO on T-wave WGC	WGC	No program
E. R. Exp. 40	WGO (three) on TM run WGC on TM run Placebo (slight)		No program
M. S. Exp. 41	WGO on T-wave (twice)		WGO (once) No program
J. R. Exp. 42	WGO on mile time (ten times)		

oil. The use of these supplements has already been widespread among athletic coaches, who have watched the published reports with interest.

There seems to be truth in the preliminary assumption that the VioBin WGO, fresh, uncooked and chemically extracted at a low temperature, furnishes a type of nutrition more effective (due to octacosanol) than previously considered a possibility. But also, Lars Carlson of Stockholm, Grafe and Van Belle seem to accept the role of such polyunsaturated fats, in this light. Grafe states that such fresh, natural oils (if uncooked) have a turnover rate of forty times that of glycogen. Linoleic acid itself is a very fine nutrient for the heart muscle and muscular walls of the blood vessels. It is present in WGO to about 52.5 per cent. It converts to arachadonic acid and then to glycogen in the body. B. Connor Johnson's experiments with pregnant mothers of guinea pigs, transmitting a "survival factor" to the newborn progeny, saving their lives in the first three weeks because of the mothers' feeding on WGO before they were born, and the young shown to have more glycogen in the tissues resulting from such feeding of the mothers, is suggestive of the power of this nutrient.

The trends of the Russian studies (Brozek's monograph, Soviet studies on nutrition and higher nervous activity, *Ann. N. Y. Acad. Sci.*, 93:665-716, 1963 indicate that the nervous system is affected by such "pin-pointed" added supplementary feeding of extra vitamins (B_1 and C) and wheat germ oil. The Russian work shows results in terms of improved conditioned reflexes, not greater "oxygen transport," and Brozek comments on this in his monograph, "Americans have probably overemphasized oxygen transport compared to nervous reflexes." Our results, in general, agree with this view.

The highly individualized responses of humans to training and to the WGO and OCTCNL supplements is certainly to be expected, this is in line with Dr. Roger Williams' extensive treatments of "biological individuality."

Cholesterol Pathology in Rabbits Reduced by Wheat Germ Oil

H. T. Gier and G. B. Marion

THE experiments involved nine groups of rabbits fed for sixty days on various diets involving VioBin wheat germ oil, octacosanol and cottonseed oil. Experiments show the effect of wheat germ oil in depressing the increase of blood cholesterol. Statements from the text* are quoted: "The differences in blood cholesterol level of the C group were significantly lower (P<.01) than the cholesterol level of any other group. This suggests that wheat germ oil permits a much greater stabilization of blood cholesterol and metabolism, elimination, or storage of excess cholesterol than does either cottonseed oil or lard oil." "Accumulation of cholesterol in the liver was greatest with lard oil and least with wheat germ oil. Liver glycogen storage was least disrupted in the wheat germ oil group and most reduced in the lard oil group." "The low accountability of cholesterol in the wheat germ oil group (C) indicates either that these animals were able to compensate for ingested cholesterol by lack of cholesterol synthesis or that they were capable of degrading and excreting the excess cholesterol." The summary is taken from the publication:

> The effects of 1 per cent cholesterol in the diet as modified by various oil carriers were tested on size groups of mature New Zealand white rabbits. Feeding trials were maintained for sixty-day periods at the end of which blood samples and vital organs were taken for analysis. The tissues were rated histologically for degree of damage, and chemically analyzed for cholesterol concentration.
>
> The group that received lard oil as the cholesterol carrier had the most rapid increase in blood cholesterol concentration, and the

---

* Permission was granted to include the following statement from this remarkably thorough study. In press.

highest final concentration. This group also had the greatest degree of organ damage (heart, liver, spleen, lung, adrenal, kidney, aorta). Wheat germ oil (6%) resulted in the lowest level of blood cholesterol and the lowest amount of organ damage. Cottonseed oil (6%) resulted in blood cholesterol concentrations and organ damage intermediate between those of lard oil and wheat germ oil. Replacement of one-sixth of the lard oil with cottonseed oil and octacosanol or with wheat germ oil reduced the rate of damage and the final blood cholesterol concentration. Results indicate an active principle, probably a combination of polyunsaturated fatty acids, and octacosanol that aid in the degradation and elimination of excess cholesterol.

Addendum II

Review of Biochemical Studies with Wheat Germ Oil and Octacosanol

George Wolf, George J. Wright and B. Connor Johnson

CURETON'S studies revealed improvements in heart response by ingestion of wheat germ oil.[1] Levin reported the discovery that octacosanol isolated from wheat germ oil, and synthesized, showed physiological response.[2] Studies by Cureton using Navy personnel revealed a significant improvement in endurance using octacosanol in controlled studies.[3] Marinetti and Stotz isolated a long-chain fatty alcohol from pig heart cytochrome C reductase, an essential enzyme of the heart mechanism.[4] George Wolf postulated that octacosanol might be involved in the lipid fraction of cytochrome C reductase.

The unsaponifiable fat fraction was prepared from pig heart fat in the manner used by Marinetti. It was then subjected to the same procedures that were used in isolating octacosanol. It was found to have high androgenic activity, the measurement used in evaluating octacosanol.[2] Wolf carried out studies that indicated the fatty acid fraction of cytochrome C reductase might be an ether compound in which octacosanol was the fat ingredient. Unfortunately, Wolf did not continue this promising study.

Work was planned to demonstrate the physiological effect of octacosanol in the diet of animals. This work was done by George Wright, a graduate student at the University of Illinois, under the direction of B. Connor Johnson. First he measured an *in vitro* effect, using livers from rats maintained on a control diet containing no added octacosanol; second, on the same diet containing two levels of added octacosanol, 24 and 50 μg per gram of diet. Third, an experimental group was fed the same diet with the addition of 3% wheat germ oil.

The *in vitro* technique involved incubating an homogenate of the livers in a phosphate buffer with the inclusion of $Mg++$ and

300

nicotinamide under 95% oxygen and 5% carbon dioxide for three hours in a Dubnoff metabolic shaker. The criterion for activity was the measurement of C^{14} incorporated into the fatty acid fraction of the liver lipids, from the labeled acetate in the buffer mixture.

Level of octacosanol in diet (micrograms/gram)	0	24	50	3% WGO
Activity (decompositions/ minute/milligram)	107.8	313.7	978.4	489.4

A second experiment was done using forty animals. The animals were forced to swim for long periods. They were sacrificed and livers processed and evaluated as indicated above.

Level octacosanol in diet (micrograms/gram)	0	25	50	75
Activity (decomposition/minute/milligram)	53.5	237.8	107.1	99.6

Statistical evaluation of both experiments showed the results as significant.

The surprising result that the activity was reduced sharply with increased dosage of octacosanol may be due to the self-limiting physiological effects of the compound. The same effect was found by Levin and Ershoff when high levels of wheat germ oil (10%) were used in the animal diet in a swimming experiment (unpublished).

Such an effect would be expected for an enzyme mechanism involving the heart muscle.

The next experiment involved determination of basal metabolic rate in rats by the Haldane procedure. The results follow:

Treatment[*]	R. Q.	kcal/hour	kcal/M²/hour
0 γ/gm	.733	1.5742	38.39
	.718	1.606	38.24
	.753	1.669	38.28
	.736	1.628	37.42
	.727	1.610	39.56
24 γ/gm	.737	1.8625	44.03
	.722	1.4478	33.67
	.744	1.764	41.22
	.760	1.859	44.69

Octacosanol seems to profoundly affect the BMR of the rat. One animal in the treated group is affected in exactly the oppo-

---

[*] All determinations were made in the post-absorptive state.

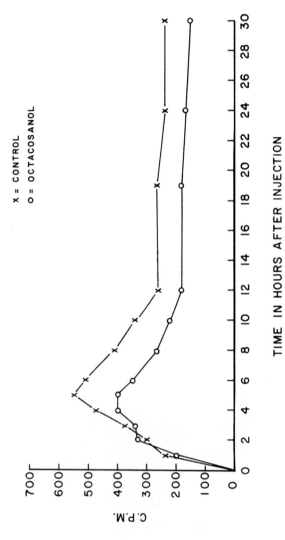

Figure 78-B. Average results-I^{131} uptake studies.

site direction to the same degree as the others. This may be explained by assuming that this animal was below the others in tolerance to the octacosanol and the depressing effect seen in the second experiment was reflected in this animal. The controls are remarkably consistent. It must be concluded that some very basic mechanism is being affected to cause the magnitude of change noted in this experiment.

An experiment was carried out to determine the iodine uptake in the thyroid gland of rats utilizing I^{131} and direct counting techniques. The same rats used in the basal metabolic studies were used in this experiment. Twenty μc of I^{131} were injected intraperitoneally into ten rats and the accumulation and disappearance of I^{131} by the thyroid gland was measured. The average results are given in Figure 78-B.

It is intriguing that iodine uptake can be affected by octacosanol. Do these findings imply that a food ingredient lacking in the average diet is essential to adequate metabolism?

"General conclusions: It can now be stated with certainty that octacosanol exerts a profound effect on the metabolic machinery of the rat when present at low levels in the diet."

This quoted conclusion by George Wright and B. Connor Johnson, written in 1959, is confirmed by Cureton's impressive studies in subsequent years. Unfortunately, Wolf and Wright's studies were not pursued. Their work, if carried to completion, may reveal significant factors in unrefined vegetable oils that protect the heart mechanism.

When whole grains were removed from our diet, the oil went out with the grain. We eat refined vegetable oils. The plant sterols that protect us against accumulation of cholesterol, the long chain alcohols (octacosanol) are largely removed in refining. A paper by Gier and Marion (in press) reviewed in Addendum II in this publication shows that wheat germ oil and octacosanol have a positive effect on cholesterol retention in rabbits.

REFERENCES

1. Cureton, T. K., and Pohndorf, R. H.: Influence of wheat germ oil as a dietary supplement in a program of conditioning exercises with middle-aged subjects, *Res. Quart.*, 26:391-407, 1955.

2. Levin, Ezra: Effects of octacosanol on chick comb growth, *Proc. Exp. Biol. Med.*, 112:331-334, 1963.
3. Cureton, T. K. *et al.:* Improvements in Fitness Associated with U. S. Navy Training in Underwater Swimming and Dietary Supplements, (unpublished report on file at the University of Illinois).
4. Marinetti, G. V., and Stotz, E.: Chemical studies on a pig heart muscle lipid which stimulates the enzymic reduction of cytochrome C, *J. Amer. Chem. Soc.*, 80:402, 1958.

Part Two

Experiment 1

The Effect of Wheat Germ Oil on Physical Fitness

WILLIAM A. FORR[*]

THE purposes of this study were to determine if whole, fresh, capsulated wheat germ oil (VioBin brand) would have any systematic effect upon various physical fitness tests when administered to adult male subjects, and to compare the effects, if any, with those obtained from an equal amount of synthetic alpha tocopherol acetate (300 mg per week) and with corn oil similarly taken in capsules in a double blind experiment, over twelve weeks of feeding.

SUBJECTS

Young college men, 17-26 years of age were used; the volunteers were matched in three groups: (Matching was checked by means and sigmas, and no significant difference.)

Group I, Fraternity Group: N = 8 in each group, by rank order matching,

A—Av. 21.3 yrs. CV Av. (SS) 376.3/8 = 47.03 Differences be-
B—Av. 21.2 yrs. CV Av. (SS) 376.8/8 = 47.1 tween means
C—Av. 21.7 yrs. CV Av. (SS) 374.9/8 = 46.8 are statistically
insignificant.

Group II, Swimming Group: N = 9 in each group

Differences be-
a—Av. 18.1 yrs. CV Av. (SS) 445/9   = 49.4 tween means
b—Av. 19.0 yrs. CV Av. (SS) 456.6/9 = 50.7 are statistically
c—Av. 19.5 yrs. CV Av. (SS) 454.6/9 = 50.5 insignificant.

Group III, Case Studies (extra group)
x—Av. 31.6 yrs. (N = 9)

---

[*] Urbana, M.S. in Physical Education, University of Illinois, 1950, p. 100. (Sponsor: T. K. Cureton; Advisors: Prof. Connor Johnson, Dr. Norris L. Brookens, M.D.)

The subjects were in regular physical education classes, three times per week, all of the fraternity group lived together and ate on a common table. The swimming group also attended a class in beginning swimming three times per week, and the fraternity group took required physical education classes, three times per week. There were no athletes included who were members of a team during the twelve weeks of the experiment. The P. Ed. classes were fifty minutes per day, three times per week.

RESEARCH METHODS

The matching of the groups was done by averaging the standard scores (SS) on three tests: a) the heartograph area, b) Schneider index and c) five-minute step test. The men were matched by threes and in rank order, and the matching was proved statistically, using the F ratio.

FINDINGS

The other tests of weight, basal metabolism, heartograph, Schneider test, vital capacity, strength, C-VJ-D test and Harvard step test did not show significant differences. The effect of WGO on the total body reaction time tests is impressive, and the T-wave has a significant difference in terms of the $S.E._{meas.}$, which equals 0.44 mm of amplitude of the T-wave, so the difference shown of 2.387 in favor of the WGO group is to be taken seriously. The T test here (ratio of $D/S.E._{meas.}$ is probably best, as it has been shown in the study that the range of the small sam-

TABLE XLII

FRATERNITY SAMPLE

Comparison of Group A(syn. E) Versus Group B (WGO) Fraternity Sample

Tests (only those with some significant difference)	Group A N = 8 (syn. E)	Group B N = 8 (WGO)	D	t (for 5% level t = 2.145)
Visual Reaction Response (sec.) ...	−0.005	−0.020	+0.015	19.25
Auditory Reaction Response (sec.) .	+0.006	−0.015	+0.021	6.12
Visual and Auditory Reaction Response (sec.)	+0.005	−0.008	+0.014	8.75
ECG (T-wave, highest) (mm)	−0.037	+2.350	+2.387	0.25

ples is only about one-third of the range of a large sample, indicating that the *t*-test is not fairly applied here. The T-wave difference is also similarly shown in other studies. So, at least, for the *sample in hand* there is a real T-wave change. The S.E.meas. for the total body reaction time test was determined as ±0.002.

MATERIALS USED FOR FEEDING

1. Placeboes of refined corn oil (same number and size as WGO capsules)
2. Synthetic vitamin E (alpha tocopherol acetate* in capsules) (300 mg/2 weeks)
3. VioBin wheat germ oil, fresh, in 3 mm capsules (0.377 mg of E per capsule × 96 × 3/week = 106.5/week)

The groups were matched in each class, i.e. *fraternity group,* matched groups A, B and C; *swimming group,* matched groups a, b and c.

The experiment continued twelve weeks with testing on all tests at 0, 4, 8, 12 weeks. All data were plotted. The feeding procedure was "double blind" in that the experimenter did not know what was in each capsule, as capsules X, Y and Z were given to the subjects by matched groups, and nothing was told the subjects about the contents of the bottles of capsules, except that it was a nutritional experiment. Neither did the experimenter test the subjects, as the laboratory staff was used, thirteen expert examiners, to give the ten tests: Weight Analysis, Basal Metabolism, Electrocardiogram, Heartograph, Schneider Index, Vital Capacity, Strength Test (dynamometers), Larson's Chin-Vertical Jump-Dip Test, Five-Minute Harvard Step Test, Garrett-Cureton Vertical Jump Reaction Time Test. All of these tests are described in Cureton's *Physical Fitness Appraisal and Guidance, Physical Fitness of Champion Athletes,* or in *Endurance of Young Men* (Cureton, *et al.*).

---

* The capsules of synthetic vitamin E and refined corn oil were furnished by the Hoffmann-La Roche Co., through Dr. E. L. Severinghaus, M.D. The content was checked by Professor Connor Johnson, of the Animal Nutrition Laboratory, University of Illinois. Dr. N. P. Brookens was wholly responsible for putting the capsules in bottles X, Y, Z and the name for each bottle was withheld from all others.

The capsules were of the same color, identical in size and shape. All testing was done in the Physical Fitness Research Laboratory in the spring of 1949. The statistics applied to the data included the means and S.D.'s of all groups, differences between the means, and significance of the difference between the means, using Fisher's *t* test, and the 5 per cent level of confidence being accepted. The D/S.E. meas. was also used on the T-wave differences.

It is shown in Table XLIII that the corn oil has lowered the reaction times more than the synthetic vitamin E, and that the differences obtained are statistically significant.

It is shown in Table XLIV that wheat germ oil has lowered the auditory reaction time more than group C on corn oil, but as a whole in the visual and combined reaction times there is a very small difference, statistically insignificant between wheat germ oil and corn oil. The various other tests were dropped out

TABLE XLIII

COMPARISON OF GROUP A (SYN. E) VERSUS GROUP C

(Fraternity Controls on Corn Oil)

Tests (only those with some significant difference)	Group A N = 8 (syn. E)	Group C N = 8 (corn oil)	D	t (5% level t = 2.145)
Visual Reaction Response (secs.)	−0.005	−0.022	+0.017	6.80
Auditory Reaction Response (secs.) ...	+0.006	−0.006	+0.012	4.14
Visual and Auditory Response (sec.) ..	+0.005	−0.011	+0.016	7.72

TABLE XLIV

COMPARISON OF GROUP B (WGO) VERSUS GROUP C

(Fraternity Controls on Corn Oil)

Tests (only those with some significant difference)	Group B N = 8 (WGO)	Group C N = 8 (corn oil)	D	t (5% level t = 2.145)
Visual Reaction Response (sec.)	−0.020	−0.022	+0.002	0.80
Auditory Reaction Response (sec.) ...	−0.015	−0.006	−0.009	4.35
Visual and Auditory Response (sec.)	−0.009	−0.011	+0.002	1.305

TABLE XLV

COMPARISON OF GROUP A (SYN. E) VERSUS GROUP B (CO),
SWIMMING SAMPLE

Tests (only those with some significant difference)	Group A N = 9 (Syn. E)	Group C N = 9 (Corn Oil)	D	t (for 5% level t = 2.131)
Visual Reaction Response (sec.)	+0.019	+0.012	+0.007	9.61
Auditory Reaction Response (sec.)	+0.068	+0.029	+0.039	3.84
Visual and Auditory Response (sec.)	+0.068	+0.013	+0.055	4.96
ECG (mm) T-wave, highest	+0.006	+1.200	−1.194	0.24

in the comparisons on these two tables because there were no other real differences of any account.

Here again it is shown in Table XLV that corn oil is consistently better in speeding up the visual, auditory and combined reaction times than is synthetic vitamin E. Also, we see that group C taking corn oil has increased the T-wave of the ECG more than synthetic vitamin E.

Again, it is shown in Table XLVII that synthetic vitamin E has depressed the brachial pulse wave (heartograph) compared to the effect of WGO, and that this difference is statistically significant. It is also clear that the effect of swimming has been to slow the visual, auditory and combined reaction times. The effect of synthetic E as compared with WGO is inconsistent, although in the auditory and combined reaction times, the slowing up is less in the synthetic vitamin E group C.

TABLE XLVI

COMPARISON OF GROUP B (WGO) VERSUS GROUP C (Corn Oil),
SWIMMING SAMPLE

Tests (only those with some significant difference)	Group B N = 9 (WGO)	Group C N = 9 (Corn Oil)	D	t (for 5% level t = 2.12)
Heartograph area (sq. cm.)	−0.005	−0.050	+0.055	5.88
Visual Reaction Response (sec.)	+0.036	+0.012	+0.024	1.151
Auditory Reaction Response (sec.)	+0.053	+0.029	+0.024	13.3
Visual and Auditory Reaction Response (sec.)	+0.026	+0.013	+0.013	6.84

RESULTS IN THE SWIMMING CLASS

The second group of students in this experiment were not from the fraternity house but were members of a beginning swimming class about a mile away from the fraternity, and the members came from all colleges of the university. The results are shown in Tables XLV and XLVI.

It is shown in Table XLV that the swimming has probably slowed the reaction times, compared with those who did not swim. The WGO group slowed relatively less than group A on synthetic E, except in one visual response test. Synthetic vitamin E also appears to have depressed the area of the brachial pulse wave test a bit. Again the WGO has raised the T-wave of the ECG by enough to be equal to 2.294/0.44 S.E.$_{meas.}$ = 5.1, which is again the best measure to take here. The t test is not a valid test with this sample. On the heartograph test the synthetic vitamin E has a depressive effect, whereas, the WGO has a slightly augmenting effect. Several other studies also show that WGO has a positive effect on the brachial pulse wave, and on the velocity/t component of the BCG (Dempsey).

CONCLUSIONS

It is shown that group B taking wheat germ oil capsules lowered the three total body reaction time tests more than in group A taking synthetic vitamin E, and that these differences were

TABLE XLVII

COMPARISON OF GROUP B (WGO) VERSUS GROUP A (syn. E), SWIMMING SAMPLE

Tests (only those with some significant difference)	Group A N = 9 (syn. E)	Group B N = 9 (WGO)	D	t
Heartograph area (sq. cm.)	−0.06	+0.005	−0.065	1.39
ECG (mm) T-wave, highest	+0.006	+2.300	+2.294	+0.22*
Visual Reaction Response (sec.)	+0.019	+0.036	−0.017	2.638
Auditory Reaction Response (sec.)	+0.088	+0.053	+0.015	2.34
Visual and Auditory Response (sec.)	+0.068	+0.026	+0.042	3.79

* D/$s_{.E. meas.}$ was also computed.

consistent in all three sets of tests, and all were statistically significant by the *t* test.

The tests of weight, and weight components (bone, muscle, fat) were not affected significantly, and were dropped from the summary tables. This was also true of all other tests not in the tables: basal metabolism, heartograph, Schneider index, vital capacity, strength, C-VJ-Dip test and the five-minute step test.

The ECG test (highest T-wave) was influenced very much by the WGO in group B compared to group A taking synthetic vitamin E. The difference in this case is not fairly evaluated by the *t* test in view of the skewness in the data, the sigmas of this distribution being only one-third as large as a large distribution. Therefore, by the $D/S.E._{meas.}$ computed from the actual retests, the ratio T is $2.387/0.44 = 5.44$. This T evaluated by the normal curve, assuming the deviations to be randomly distributed, is significantly better than .01 level of reliability. The control group C (taking corn oil) gained 12.7 per cent, whereas, group B (taking WGO) gained 23.8 per cent and group A (taking synthetic E) gained zero per cent.

Both the synthetic vitamin E (alpha tocopherol acetate) group and the WGO group lowered the basal metabolic rate but the effect of the WGO was relatively greater (24 SS in the swimming group and 45 SS in the fraternity group, compared to 15 SS in the swimming group and 0.5 SS in the fraternity group) in effect than the synthetic vitamin E.

In the visual reaction test the WGO group B and the group C taking corn oil improved by speeding up the time of these reaction tests, compared to the control groups A on synthetic vitamin E and this occurred in *both* the fraternity and swimming groups, the subjects being completely independent of each other.

Experiment 2

The Effects of Training and a Dietary Supplement on Breath Holding at Ground Level and at an Altitude (10,000 Feet Simulated Altitude in a United States Air Force Decompression Chamber)

Glen E. Harvison[*]

PURPOSE

THE purposes of this study[*] were a) to determine if training an individual improves the breath-holding ability or gives more resistance to oxygen depletion of the arterial blood by an anoxia photometer method at ground level and also at altitude; b) to determine if the addition of a dietary supplement of wheat germ oil (VioBin brand, 20 × 3 minims, daily for five days per week) would affect the breath-holding time and/or oxygen depletion (%) during breath holding; c) whether the dietary supplement has any effect at ground level or at altitude.

Six graduate students (23-30 years of age) and three control subjects (who did not change their mode of living) were the subjects of the test.

RESEARCH METHODS

The experiment was conducted in an atmospherically controlled chamber in the Engineering College at the University of Illinois, constant temperature (F) of 75 and 50 per cent relative humidity. The pretraining period was one of adjustment to the chamber and a study was made of the reliability of the tests, November to mid-February, 1950-51. The best of these tests were taken as T_1 (pretraining). The physical conditioning program was run from mid-February to mid-May, when tests were given again and called T_2 (post-training). In the second stage

---

[*] Urbana, M.S. in Physical Education, University of Illinois, 1951, p. 59. (Sponsor: T. K. Cureton.)

each subject was placed on his physical training program, mainly running plus some other exercises, five days per week, for twelve weeks, then T_2 tests were given. In the third stage the physical training continued on the same schedule but the dietary supplements (VioBin wheat germ oil, 20×3 minim capsules) were taken at the end of each day's workout, and this continued for six weeks. The workouts were held at the same level of intensity, an hour per day until T_3 tests were taken.

Breath holding was measured by the use of a stop watch and each subject held his breath against a 20 mm Hg Flarimeter tube to eliminate faking and to standardize the pressure. Before the breath holding test, the Coleman anoxia photometer was standardized on the ear lobe of the subject and the indicating needle was watched carefully throughout the breath-holding to note the percentage drop from 100. Each subject was tested at ground level and at altitude one week apart.

The means of each group, six men in the experimental and control groups, tested at ground level and also at altitude, were determined, together with the mean difference (average of the differences from the mean) for the oxygen depletion test at ground level and at altitude, and the breath-holding time at ground level and at altitude.

CONCLUSIONS

No significant changes were produced in the breath-holding scores due to training at ground level and at a simulated altitude of 10,000 feet.

No significant changes were produced in the breath-holding scores due to the addition of a dietary supplement of WGO (VioBin) to the program of training at ground level or at a simulated altitude of 10,000 feet.

No significant changes were produced in the breath-holding scores due to the combined effects of training plus a wheat germ oil supplement at ground level and at a simulated altitude of 10,000 feet.

The difference in real values and in mean percentage differences for breath holding at ground level and at altitude are included in Table XLVIII.

TABLE XLVIII

EFFECT OF TRAINING VERSUS EFFECT OF WGO ON
BREATH HOLDING AT GROUND LEVEL AND AT
10,000 FEET ALTITUDE

Conditions	Pretraining	Post-training	Mean diff.	Mean per cent diff.	t*
A. Ground level	M_1 = 119.17	M_2 = 146.33	+27.16	+22.79	1.59
10,000 feet altitude	91.00	108.17	+17.17	+18.86	0.54
	Post-training	*Post-dietary*			
B. Ground level	M_2 = 146.33	M_3 = 148.50	+2.17	+1.48	0.23
10,000 feet altitude	108.17	103.33	−4.84	−4.47	−.52
	Pre-training	*Post-dietary*			
C. Ground level	M_1 119.17	148.50	+29.33	+24.61	0.42
10,000 feet altitude	91.00	103.33	+12.33	+13.55	1.96

* Significant at 5 degrees of freedom: 10% level = 2.015; 5% level = 2.57; 2% level = 3.385 (Fisher, *Statistical Methods for Research Workers*, Table IV for t.)

Considering the statistical significance for the use of WGO to increase breath-holding time, the result is borderline and better than the reliability level of .20 and almost good at the .10 level (t = 1.96 versus standard of 2.015), this from pretraining to post-dietary.

The percentage gains show a small positive gain during the stage of training with WGO taken every day of training (Table XLVIII) at ground level where the gain is 1.48 per cent; but at an altitude there was a loss of −4.47 per cent, with statistical insignificance for both.

The effects of the physical training produced one significant change, i.e. significant shift in the oxygen depletion due to the training at ground level (t = 3.546), a mean drop of 6.08 points on the anoxia photometer scale (+121.6%) attributable to the physical training.

There was no significant change attributable to the addition of the WGO supplement at ground level or at 10,000 feet simulated altitude.

The change attributable to the combined effect of training and the addition of the dietary supplement of WGO was significant at the .06 level, pretraining versus post-dietary at ground level

($t = 2.370$). The change at altitude was not statistically significant ($t = 1.027$).

Systematic physical training of the type done in this experiment (one hour per day of strenuous work) will produce changes in the oxygen depletion as measured by the anoxia photometer (Coleman) at ground level at the 2 per cent level of reliability ($t = 3.546$).

While there were measured advantages of 7.75% and 3.0% in oxygen depletion at ground level and at 10,000 feet altitude, respectively, due to the addition of the WGO to the training these differences were not statistically significant.

Statistical significance at the 10 per cent level was obtained for the combined effect of training with the WGO supplement ($t = 2.37$).

DISCUSSION

Breath-holding may depend considerably upon *willpower,* and the effects obtained. Although positive effects in terms of percentage of improvement at ground level due to training, and also due to the training plus the WGO supplement, no real effect of the WGO can be claimed, as these differences could possibly be explained by a willpower effect. Also, since the oxygen stored in the myoglobin is probably the principal reserve being tapped during breath holding, other than the turnover of the circulation, the intake of WGO does not seem to affect this reserve.

Experiment 3

Variations on a Bicycle Ergometer Test with Altitude, Training and a Dietary Supplement

WILLIAM A. SMILEY*

THE purposes of this study were as follows:

To determine the variations in ground level and altitude tests before and after a period of training.

To determine the effects of a dietary supplement of wheat germ oil on a bicycle ergometer test.

To determine the relationships between the bicycle ergometer riding time and other cardiorespiratory tests.

METHOD

The experimental single group type of research was used in this study. Statistics and graphs were used in presenting the data. Only graphs were used in relationship studies to show the trends.

Six experimental subjects and three nonexercising controls were used. They were all first tested at stage A (pretraining). The subjects then went through a ten-week training period and were retested at stage B (post-training). The controls were also tested at stage B. The controls were tested after the dietary stage but other controls were available in the work of Forr (1950) covering the effect of taking placeboes but no exercise in the Spring period. The experimental subjects then entered a six-week period in which 20 × 3-minim capsules of VioBin wheat germ oil were administered (7 days per week) and the training was continued. At the end of the six weeks, they were retested at stage C (postdietary stage).

The Illinois bicycle ergometer is the Hellebrandt electrodynamic brake type. The work rate used for this study was 18,659 foot-pounds per minute. This was achieved by riding at 76 r.p.m.,

* Urbana, M.S. Thesis, Physical Education, University of Illinois, 1951, p. 90.

TABLE XLIX

EFFECT OF TRAINING VERSUS EFFECT OF WGO ON DEPLETION OF
OXYGEN AS MEASURED ON THE ANOXIA PHOTOMETER AT GROUND
LEVEL AND AT 10,000 FEET OF SIMULATED ALTITUDE

Conditions	Pretraining	Post-training	Mean Diff.	Mean Per Cent Diff.	t
A. Ground level	M_1 = 5.0	M_2 = 11.08	+6.08	+121.60	3.546
10,000 feet altitude	11.75	14.17	+2.42	+ 20.6	.851
	Post-training	*Post-dietary*			
B. Ground level	M_2 = 11.08	M_3 = 12.75	+1.67	+ 15.07	.493
10,000 feet altitude	14.17	14.75	+ .58	+ 4.90	.290
	Pre-training	*Post-dietary*			
C. Ground level	M_1 = 5.07	M_3 = 12.75	+7.75	+150.0	2.37
10,000 feet altitude	11.75	14.75	+3.0	+ 25.53	1.03

* Significance at 10 per cent level = 2.051; 5 per cent level = 2.571; 2 per cent
level = 3.363

5½ volts, ridden at least twice for each stage at both ground level
and the simulated altitude of 10,000 feet. The best (longest) ride
for each phase was used in the presentation of data.

RESULTS

The following results were obtained:
1. The mean riding time for stage B was 27 per cent better
   than stage A at ground level (not significant at .05 level);
   stage B was 63 per cent better than stage A at an altitude
   (significant <.02).
2. The mean riding time for stage C was 18 per cent better
   than stage B at ground level (significant at .01 level);
   stage C was 10 per cent better than stage B at an altitude
   (not significant at .05).
3. The mean riding time for stage C was 50 per cent better
   than stage A at ground level (significant at .02 level);
   stage C was 79 per cent better than stage A at an altitude
   (significant <.01).
4. The mean riding times for all stages at ground level were
   better than at an altitude; 52 per cent (significant <.01),
   22 per cent (significant <.02), and 28 per cent (significant
   at .05 level) respectively for stages A, B and C.

TABLE L

ANALYSIS OF STATISTICAL DATA SUBJECTS

Mean Differences Between the Stages in All-out Bicycle Ride Time
(Minutes and Seconds)

T_1 Stage A	T_2 Stage B	T_3 Stage C	Diff.	Per Cent Diff.	t	P	Degrees of Freedom
A. At Ground Level:							
4:03	5:09	—	1:06	27	2.092	.10 insignificant	5
—	5:09	6:05	0:56	18	7.225	.01 significant	5
4:03	—	6:05	2:02	50	3.650	.02 significant	5
B. At 10,000 Feet Simulated Altitude:							
2:27	4:00	—	1:33	63	3.968	.02 significant	5
—	4:00	4:24	0:24	10	1.738	.20 insignificant	5
2:27	—	4:24	1:57	79	4.625	.01 significant	5

Mean Differences Between Ground Level and Altitude

	Ground level	Altitude	Diff.	Per Cent Diff.	t	P	Degrees of Freedom
Stage A	4:03	2:27	1:36	52	4.456	.01 significant	5
Stage B	5:09	4:00	1:09	22	3.584	.02 significant	5
Stage C	6:05	4:24	1:41	28	2.734	.05 significant	5

5. The controls were not significantly changed at .05 level in any respect.

CONCLUSIONS

The following conclusions were reached:

1. As it is to be expected, training has a great effect on the riding time of a bicycle ergometer. T_1 to T_2 was twelve weeks long until a plateau was reached.

2. Whole, fresh VioBin wheat germ oil added daily 20 × 3 minim capsules apparently caused a further gain in bicycle ride time.

3. With endurance work, severe stress is noticeable at 10,000 feet, as shown by the poorer bicycle ergometer times at altitude.

4. The cardiovascular tests in Experiments 4, 5 and 6 show similar trends at ground level but this effect is overshad-

owed at altitude by the severe stress, although the group on WGO withstood the stress better.

5. There does seem to be a relationship between the bicycle ergometer ride times and the body weight of the rider before training is introduced. After training, there still is a tendency toward a relationship, but it is not as great.

Experiment 4

Variations of the Progressive Pulse Ratio with Altitude, Training and Wheat Germ Oil

Jack V. Toohey*

PURPOSE

IT was the purpose of this study to accomplish the following objectives:

1. Determine the normal fluctuations of the progressive pulse ratio at ground level and altitude before and after a period of training of twelve weeks.

2. Determine the variations in the ground level and altitude pulse ratio tests after the feeding of a dietary supplement, wheat germ oil, for six additional weeks while continuing the same training program.

3. Show the relationship of training and wheat germ oil to the progressive pulse ratio, separating one effect from the other.

Six experimental subjects and three control subjects were used.

RESEARCH METHODS

The method of research utilized in this study was the experimental type method of research.

The test used was the progressive pulse ratio performed with 12, 18, 24, 30 and 36 squats per minute. The criteria used for measurement and comparison were as follows: a) the angle of inclination and b) the average pulse ratio.

The three testing stages of this experiment were as follows: a) The pretraining stage (four weeks), b) the post-training (twelve weeks in interval training, 600 yards $\times$ 6) and c) the postdietary stage (six weeks) during which WGO was fed.

The six experimental subjects and the four control subjects

---

* Urbana, M.S. Thesis, Physical Education, University of Illinois, 1951, p. 103. (Sponsor: T. K. Cureton.)

were each given at least two tests at ground level and altitude at each of the three stages of testing. During the training stage, these experimental subjects underwent a strenuous conditioning program and after reaching a relative plateau of performance, the testing stage began. The control group did none of the physical training. The experimental group was then fed wheat germ oil (20 × 3 minims, 7 days per week) and retested after six weeks.

CONCLUSIONS

The altitude environment of 10,000 feet produced no significant changes in the progressive pulse ratios of either the experimental or control group.

The training stage produced no significant variations in the progressive pulse ratio.

The dietary stage produced no significant variations in the progressive pulse ratio.

The combined effects of the training stage and the dietary stage produced significant variations in the progressive pulse ratio of the experimental group at ground level:

1. The change (improvement) in the average pulse ratio was significant at the 2 per cent level (.02).
2. The change (improvement) in the angle of inclination was significant at the 2 per cent level (.02).

The combined effects of the training stage and the dietary stage improved the mean value of the average pulse ratio at altitude and this variation was significant at the 2 per cent level.

When the experimental group on WGO showed trends toward altered cardiac response, it was in favor of more efficient heart action.

The experimental group on WGO as a whole lowered (improved) the mean value of the average pulse ratio from .32 to .19 of a point or 5.6 per cent for ground level post-training. The mean value of the angle of inclination was lowered (improved) from 20.5 degrees to 16 degrees or 28.1 per cent change.

The experimental group taking WGO, as a whole, lowered (improved) the mean value of the average pulse ratio from .42 to .22 of a point or 8.26 per cent for altitude post-training. The mean value of the angle of inclination was lowered (improved) from 24 degrees to 17 degrees or 47.1 per cent.

At an altitude postdietary, the experimental group, as a whole, lowered (improved) the mean value of the average pulse ratio from .22 to .14 of a point or 3.6 per cent. The mean value of the angle of inclination is lowered (improved) from 17 degrees to 14 degrees or 17.6 per cent.

At ground level postdietary, the experimental group, as a whole, lowered (improved) the mean of the average pulse ratio from .19 to .16 of a point or 1.37 per cent.

DISCUSSION

There are certain pertinent findings in this study. For example, during the training stage the average pulse ratio is improved by 5 per cent at ground level and 8.26 per cent at altitude; during the postdietary state, the average pulse ratio is improved by 3.6 per cent at altitude and 1.47 per cent at ground level while continuing the same program. It must be taken into consideration that while the percentage gains during the dietary stage are smaller than those achieved during the training, they may be equally significant. It must be realized that any additional lowering in the pulse ratio after the group had reached a plateau of physical fitness is difficult to achieve, and even slight positive trends should not be minimized.

Experiment 5

The Effect of Physical Training and a Dietary Supplement on the Six-Item Schneider Test at Ground Level and at an Altitude of 10,000 Feet

CHARLES H. WHITE[*]

PURPOSE

THE purpose of this study was to determine the effect of various types of physical conditioning on the six-item Schneider test at ground level and at an altitude of 10,000 feet.

METHODS OF RESEARCH

There were ten graduate students used as subjects for this experiment. The subjects were subdivided into two groups (control and experimental); six subjects composed the experimental group; four subjects composed the control group. The total experiment was divided into three stages: a) pretraining; b) post-training; and c) postdietary.

During the pretraining stage of the experiment all subjects were given the Schneider test at ground level and also at 10,000 feet simulated altitude.

During the post-training stage the six experimental subjects embarked on a ten-week training program. The minimum training periods were from three to five times per week for one hour a day. The training patterns varied with each subject, relative to that subject's background and knowledge of conditioning work. Only the experimental subjects were retested at the conclusion of this stage at ground level and at 10,000 feet altitude.

During the dietary stage the experimental subjects were given dosages of wheat germ oil (20 × 3 minims, 7 days per week) while they continued their training for an additional

[*] Unpublished Master's Thesis, University of Illinois, 1951, p. 95. (Sponsor: T. K. Cureton.)

325

six weeks. Upon completion of this stage, both the experimental and control group subjects were retested at ground level and at 10,000 feet altitude.

RESULTS

The Schneider test scores for individual, and for experimental group, mean scores between stage one and two are graphically shown. The Schneider test score changes, recorded between stage two and stage three for individuals and the mean scores of the experimental group, have been graphically shown also. The changes recorded in the initial and final stages of the experiment for the control group have been graphically shown (Fig. 65).

CONCLUSIONS

The ground level mean score of the experimental group during pretraining (T_1) was 16.8; after training, the mean score of this group was (at T_2) 16.3 with twelve weeks intervening. There was a decrease of .5 of a point—a minor change indicative of comparable physical condition for the groups in the initial and post-training stages of the experiment.

The ground level mean score of the experimental group at the postdietary stage (T_3) was 18.5. The mean difference between the post-training (16.3) and postdietary (18.5) was 2.2 ± 0.52 S.E. This represents an increase of 13.5 per cent and shows good cardiovascular improvement in this six-week period (significance >.01).

The altitude mean score of the experimental group during pretraining (T_1 stage) was 15. The postdietary (T_2 stage) mean score was 16.3 which represents an increase of 1.3 ± 0.52 S.E. raw scores or 7.9 per cent (significance >.05).

The altitude mean score difference between post-training (16.3) and postdietary (17.7) was an increase of 1.4 ± 0.4 raw scores or 8.0 per cent increase after adding the WGO (significance >.01).

The control group mean Schneider test scores were almost the same in both stages of the experiment. This was true both at ground level and at altitude. The score being 14.5 at ground level during pretraining and 14.0 during postdietary. The mean Schneider test score at altitude during pretraining was 13.5 and during postdietary, it was 13.7.

DISCUSSION

Endurance running of the type participated in by subject W. S. seems to improve a normal subject's Schneider test score at ground level and at the altitude of 10,000 feet.

Endurance game activity of the type participated in by subject S. S. seems to improve a normal subject's Schneider test score at ground level and at an altitude of 10,000 feet.

Trends seem to indicate a decrease in time taken for pulse rate to return to standing normal during the training and dietary stages of the experiment at ground level and at the altitude of 10,000 feet.

Using the Schneider test score as an indication of cardiovascular fitness, trends indicate superior vagus tone condition during the dietary stage more than in any other stage at ground level, due to slowing of the pulse rate.

Using the Schneider test score as an indication of cardiovascular fitness, trends indicate superior cardiovascular condition at altitude during the dietary stage more than in any other stage, this improvement being due to the effect of the six weeks of WGO feeding, quite likely, but this is not irrefutably proved. The author does not believe that this additional gain was due to the physical training as neither the intensity nor duration of it were increased.

Experiment 6

The Influence of Training upon the Aerobic and Anaerobic Variables

Richard V. Ganslen[*]

PURPOSE

THIS experiment was conducted to evaluate the oxygen intake and oxygen debt tests as they are influenced by hard endurance training; and a secondary purpose is to provide data to correlate with experiments done at the same time and which used the same subjects as T_1, T_2 and T_3 stages of testing.

RESEARCH METHODS

Six experimental subjects were used in a longitudinal type experiment[*] involving preliminary testing for reliability (four weeks), T_1 systematic strenuous exercise for 1 hour per day involving repetitious 600-yard runs, practice on the bicycle ergometer, basketball, handball, swimming and taking tests (twelve weeks) with testing at T_2; and after reaching a demonstrable plateau (checked by all-out bicycle rides on the Kelso-Hellebrandt Ergometer Bicycle, 72 r.p.m. (cf. data in Exp. 2, 3, 4, 5, 10 and 11); then the feeding was begun of 20 × 3 minim capsules of VioBin whole, fresh wheat germ oil. The research design was that of a single group, trained to a plateau; and then while taking WGO daily at the end of the physical workouts and continuing on the same program for six additional weeks to see if additional gains occurred in the all-out bicycle rides for time or in other tests being used. Several experimenters were involved, the same

---

Note: Ganslen carried out the work on O_2 intake and debt only at ground level but the correlative work on altitude was carried out in a later experiment by Ernest D. Michael (cf. pp. 66-70 in Cureton: *The Physiological Effects of Exercise Programs on Adults*, Springfield, Illinois, Charles C Thomas, 1969).

[*] Urbana, Ph.D. thesis, Physical Education, University of Illinois, 1953, p. 98. (Sponsor: T. K. Cureton.)

testers always giving the same tests on which they had in the pre-training period demonstrated competence. The correlative experiments, on the same subjects as this one, are done by Harvison (Exp. 2), Smiley (Exp. 3), Toohey (Exp. 4), White (Exp. 5), Constantino (Exp. 9), Susic (Exp. 10) and one additional one on different subjects by Maley (Exp. 11).

Normally, from long experience in observing and plotting training curves, such a curve will rise sharply at first, then level off, and finally will turn downward. If the work is harder than the men can adapt to, the turn down may be because of gradual exhaustion; but if the work is relatively easy, it may turn downward because of relatively less effort as the men adjust to the work. (Cf. C. D. Fulton: Progressive Changes in the Heartometer Pulse Wave Tracings During a Season of Basketball, Urbana, M.S. thesis, Physical Education, 1951, p. 89, Sponsor, T. K. Cureton) Fulton's study, as an example, was known to this group. All-out bicycle rides, the amplitude of the precordial T-wave of the ECG and the amplitude of the heartograph were all used to indicate when the plateau had been reached.

Substances Fed

Only the WGO capsules were used, taken at the end of the work, daily, each subject taking 140 capsules per week. No placebo substances were used, as the controls were nonexercising subjects who were laboratory assistants.

Weather Conditions

These were controlled by giving all tests in the Atmospheric Environment Laboratory in the Department of Mechanical Engineering, 76 F, 50 per cent relative humidity.

Exercise Taken

The exercise was strenuous, with all subjects plateauing after twelve weeks of work on the tests selected for checking this. The hard workouts lasted an hour per day, five days per week—the activities not being all the same but fully recorded and listed in the diary record of each subject.

Laboratory Methodology

The laboratory methodology was followed as based upon the following source books: a) C. F. Consolazio, R. E. Johnson and E. Marek, *Metabolic Methods*, St. Louis, C. V. Mosby and Co., 1945; b) *Harvard Laboratory Methods for Assessment of Metabolic and Nutritive Condition*, 1945; c) T. E. Carpenter's *Tables, Factors and Formulas for Computing Respiratory Exchanges and Biological Transformations of Energy*, Washington, D. C.: Smithsonian Institution, 1948; and Cureton, *Physical Fitness Appraisal and Guidance* (1947) and *Physical Fitness of Champion Athletes* (1951).

The ergometer bicycle has been described elsewhere but it was adequately standardized and calibrated (cf. L. E. A. Kelso and F. A. Hellebrandt, The recording electrodynamic brake bicycle ergometer, *J. Lab. Clin. Med.*, 19:1105-1113, 1934).

All personal anthropometric data as to height, weight and age of all subjects and controls are to be found in the Appendix of the original thesis (Chap. IV). The subjects were all graduate students in Physical Education and somewhat better in physical ability than average. One was working long hours at night, which also accounts for his lower physical condition. Even though these subjects were relatively homogenous, they too had observable individual differences.

RESULTS

In the four-week period previous to the beginning of the physical training, at T_1 and T_1, the subjects were double tested and thoroughly adjusted to all of the tests and equipment, and consistency of the retest trials observed. The relatively wide variations of the O_2 debt test was noted.

From T_1 to T_2, in the twelve-week period of physical training and taking of the dietary supplements of WGO there were changes in the O_2 intake from 26.86 to 33.51 cc/min/kg, a gain of 6.65 (or 26.77%), and this difference was found to be statistically significant ($t = 2.96 > .05$ level; $\sigma_{md} = 0.430$). This effect is due mainly to the training as no dietary supplements of WGO were given in this period. These data are in L/minute to rule out the apparent change which may have been affected by a weight

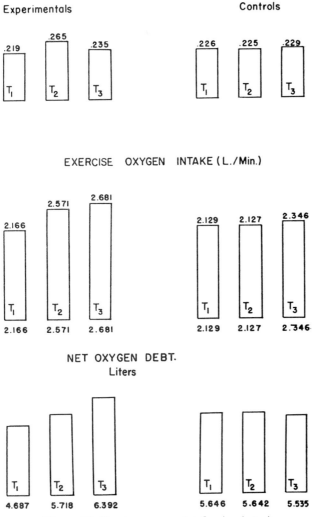

Experimentals   Controls

EXERCISE OXYGEN INTAKE (L./Min.)

NET OXYGEN DEBT.
Liters

Figure 79. Resting oxygen intake (cc/min.)

shift was a change from 2.166 to 2.571 L/minute, a gain of 0.405 (or 16.93%).

The changes in resting O_2 intake, rate of O_2 debt build-up, calorific cost of the exercise, RQ's at rest and during exercise and recovery did not change significantly in the same twelve weeks of training plus taking of the WGO supplements.

The changes during the six-week period from T_2 to T_3, when the WGO supplement was added daily to the normal diet, apparently increased the O_2 intake during the all-out ergometer bicycle ride from 2.571 to 2.681 L/minute, a gain of 0.110 L/minute (or 4.26%), which gain is not statistically significant ($\sigma_{md} =$ 0.881). In this period the ergometer bicycle ride time increased 56 seconds, possibly due to the psychological challenge of beating the previously known time, or possibly to the influence of the WGO effect. The improved ride time was correlated with an improvement of 1.859 cc/min/kg, which was statistically insignificant; and also associated with an increase in net O_2 debt from 5.718 to 6.372 L (D = 0.107), a gain of 0.0674 L (or 12.92%). The σ_{md} for the experimental subjects was 0.633 L and for the control subjects 0.427 L. The gain in O_2 debt is appreciable, although because of the large variable errors was computed to be insignificant. This, however, does not completely settle the issue. During the same period the RQ's of the experimental subjects changed from 0.922 to 0.866 to 0.922 from T_1, to T_2 to T_3, respectively. This shift in RQ indicated improved metabolic efficiency, whereas, the control subjects increased from 0.922 to 0.925 to 0.940, respectively.

The experimental subjects had clearly reached a plateau after twelve weeks of training plus the four weeks in the pretesting period. Reference to Exp. 9 (Constantino) shows the plateau reached in terms of the brachial pulse wave (Fig. 79, Part I) shows some economy developed also in the SMR.

DISCUSSION

This experiment is not foolproof, and the improvement in riding time and the slight parallel gain in O_2 intake and appreciable gain in O_2 debt may have been related to the intake of WGO, so the result is inconclusive. It has been shown in other works that the energy of such violent work may be attributable to the O_2 debt accounting for approximately one-third of the energy. It is still a question as to whether WGO had anything to do with this.

The Effects of Training and a Dietary Supplement (WGO) on Muscle Symmetry and Fat Distribution of Adult Males

WALTER E. STORM[*]

PURPOSE

THE question was whether the taking of 20 of the 3-minim capsules of whole, fresh (VioBin) wheat germ oil, daily, for six weeks would change the total fat index or the distribution of fat in the bodies of middle-aged males, or affect muscle symmetry.

RESEARCH METHODS

The data were collected by measuring eight experimental subjects on a physical training program, at T_1 (before training) and after six weeks of training at a mixed calisthenics and jogging

[*] Urbana: M.S. Thesis, Physical Education, University of Illinois, 1952, p. 43. (Sponsor: T. K. Cureton.)

TABLE LI

CONTROL SUBJECTS

Mean Differences between the Stages

	Stage A	Stage C	Diff.	Per Cent Diff.	t	P	Degrees of Freedom
Ground level	3:22	6:17	2:55	87	1.012	.60 insignificant	2
Altitude	3:33	4:03	0:30	14	1.277	.40 insignificant	2

Mean Differences between Ground Level and Altitude

	Ground Level	Altitude	Diff.	Per Cent Diff.	t	P	Degrees of Freedom
Stage A	3:22	3:33	−0:11	−05	0.378	.80 insignificant	2
Stage B	6:17	4:03	2:14	30	0.606	.80 insignificant	2

333

and games program* to remeasure them (at T_2); and also do like-wise for the control group ($N = 8$) which was also in the same training but *not* taking wheat germ oil, but took cottonseed oil placeboes. The design was two matched parallel groups continuing on the training program for six weeks from T_1 to T_2. The placeboes of cottonseed oil were similar in shape and color and size, 20 per day six-minim size. The vitamin E in the VioBin WGO and the cottonseed oil was assumed to be about the same, 0.427 mg per capsule. Three environmental controls were available also who did not take the training but did take the measurements. The anthropometrical measurements made for bone, muscle and fat were made by Cureton's method (Cureton's *Physical Fitness Appraisal and Guidance*, St. Louis, C. V. Mosby and Co., 1947). From the T_1 and T_2 data, the means, standard deviations and S.E.$_{meas.}$ were calculated, and also the Fisher t for significance of difference between means.

RESULTS

The actual weight change of the experimental (WGO) group was an average loss of -0.41 lb, compared to a gain of $+1.072$ lb as an average for the placebo group; eight men were in each group.

The control group ($N = 3$) gained an average of 0.41 lb, taking neither the exercise, nor the dietary supplements of any kind.

Neither the experimental (WGO) group nor the placebo group

---

* The program of exercise was one hour per day (mixed and not exactly the same).

TABLE LII

MATCHING OF THE EXPERIMENTAL (WGO) GROUP AND THE PLACEBO GROUP

Experimental Versus Placebo at T_1	Mean Experimental Group	Mean Placebo Group	Diff.	md	"t"
Weight	49.5	53.5	4.0	7.99	.500
Muscle Girth Index	52.4	56.7	4.3	9.08	.474
Adipose Index	49.2	51.5	2.3	10.07	.228
Center of Gravity	37.	33.1	−4.9	9.87	.395
Weight Residual	56.3	54.4	−1.9	9.67	.196

Note: In this comparison none of the "t"s were significant.

TABLE LIII

DIFFERENCES BETWEEN THE EXPERIMENTAL (WGO) GROUP, THE
PLACEBO GROUP AND ENVIRONMENTAL CONTROL GROUPS T_1 TO T_2

(Initial testing period (T_1) to final testing period (T_2) in SS)

Experimental (N = 8)	Mean T_1	Mean T_2	Diff.	σ_{md}	"t"
Weight	49.6	48.7	− .9	1.903	.4729
Muscle Girth Index	52.5	51.6	− .9	3.897	.231
Adipose Index	49.2	58.1	8.9	7.928	.8908
Center of Gravity	37.	35.7	− 1.3	7.224	.1799
Weight Residual	56.3	52.1	− 4.2	4.034	.6933

None of the changes were significant.

Placebo (N = 8)	Mean T_1	Mean T_2	Diff.	σ_{md}	"t"
Weight	53.5	53.6	.1	2.125	.4705
Muscle Girth Index	56.7	60.7	4.0	6.029	.663
Adipose Index	51.5	50.5	− 1.0	3.668	.3861
Center of Gravity	33.1	27.	− 6.1	2.841	2.147
Weight Residual	54.4	43.6	−10.8	9.527	1.1336

None of the changes were significant, except the center of gravity, which is correlated with a loss in strength.

Control (N = 3)	Mean T_1	Mean T_2	Diff.	σ_{md}	"t"
Weight	59.	57.3	− 1.7	1.008	1.686
Muscle Girth Index	62.	61.87	− 0.1	.665	.0188
Adipose Index	47.3	57.7	10.4	3.905	2.663
Center of Gravity	25.7	43.	17.3	11.466	1.508
Weight Residual	77.6	74.3	− 3.3	7.056	.468

None of the changes were significant, except the controls, who, as graduate assistants, must have been more active than the men in the program. Because of this, they are invalidated as controls.

made statistically significant differences in weight or any of the other critical measures, with all t's insignificant, so the differences between groups were not tested statistically (Table LII).

At T_2 the placebo group on the same physical exercise program had gained more in weight, muscle and fat than the WGO experimental group. But the weight residual dropped (in SS) more than the experimental (WGO) group, which drop was associated with a drop in the SS rating of the center of gravity test of the placebo group, usually related to a loss of strength in the back and legs. Since these strength tests have been shown in other experiments to be helped by WGO taken as a supplement, this may have been a factor in these advantages, relatively, of the WGO group over the placebo group.

From T_1 to T_2 there was a gain in SS of the experimental (WGO) group compared to the placebo group by reducing more fat than the placebo group, which gained slightly in fat, resulting in a drop in the SS (Table LIII).

Experiment 8

An Experimental Study of the Effects of Training and Dietary Supplements on Motor Fitness Test Items of Adult Men

ELDON W. ARMER[*]

PURPOSE

TO determine if wheat germ oil, used as a supplement to the diet of middle-aged adults will cause an improvement in certain motor fitness test items over and above the physical training practice itself. The physical training was a voluntary program, the men being in various handball, calisthenics, walking, tennis, swimming and jogging work (estimated at 100 calories per day level, three days per week).

RESEARCH METHODS

Three groups of middle-aged men were used, two of which were matched on the basis of five cardiovascular tests by the composite standard scores (progressive pulse ratio, Schneider index, five-minute step test, electrocardiogram, T and R-wave amplitudes, and area under the heartograph wave). These two groups were composed of nine men each, paired as closely as possible in age and in the composite cardiovascular index. A control (inactive) group of five subjects was also used as a check on environmental changes in weather conditions during the longitudinal time of the experiment.

The experimental group (WGO) took 20×3 minim capsules of whole, fresh VioBin wheat germ oil, seven days per week for six weeks. These were made available in a week's supply at the laboratory (140 capsules) each Monday, in an unlabelled envelope. Each capsule of WGO contained 0.427 International units of vitamin E.

[*] Urbana, Illinois, M.S. Thesis, Physical Education, 1952, p. 59. (Sponsored by T. K. Cureton and Wayne Van Huss, University of Illinois Library, Urbana.)

The placebo group (PLACEBO) of nine men took identically appearing capsules of cottonseed oil with an equivalent amount of vitamin E in it as was contained in the WGO capsules, made available in a similar manner without the men knowing the contents. Each placebo capsule contained 169.736 mg of d-alpha-tocopherol acetate from vegetable oils equivalent to 0.427 International units of vitamin E.

Two series of tests were given. At the start of the experiment T_1 (initial tests) were given all men and these data were used for matching the WGO group and the placebo group. The tests included: Chinning, dipping, right grip strength, left grip strength, back lift, leg lift, speed agility run, vertical jump, visual reaction time, audio reaction time, combined audiovisual reaction time. From these data certain other combinations were computed.

It was planned that this experiment would last four months but an unfortunate delay occurred after the initial tests had been given due to the unexpected delay in receiving the placeboes from the pharmaceutical firm. The feeding period was only six weeks long.

Throughout the experiment the subjects did not know what supplements they were taking, but they were told that they were taking "vitamins," and both the WGO group and the placebo group were told the same. The capsules were made up in the laboratory by a medical doctor and were given to the experimenter in envelopes labelled A and B but otherwise unidentified.

RESULTS

All differences between the WGO group and the placebo group were found to be insignificant except *average reaction time* ($t = 2.6412$, significance 5% level) and visual total body reaction time ($t = 3.1997$, significance at 1% level). The WGO group improved from 54.3 to 60.4 SS and the placebo group improved from 48.1 to 49.7 SS on visual reaction time. The average reaction time improved for the WGO group from 54.8 to 63.7 SS and the placebo group improved from 48 to 53.7 SS. The control group did not change significantly, averaging an SS gain of 1.7 SS.

Considering the relative gains made by the WGO group and

the gains made by the placebo group on cottonseed oil placeboes containing an equivalent amount of vitamin E to the WGO:

GAINS OF STATISTICAL SIGNIFICANCE DUE TO TRAINING

Experimental group taking (WGO)	*Placebo group (taking CS oil and vitamin E)*
Agility run (5% level)	Back lift strength (5% level)
Average reaction time (5% level)	Average reaction time (5% level)
Visual reaction time (5% level)	Total strength (5% level)
Audio reaction time (5% level)	Audio reaction time (5% level)
Audio visual reaction time (5% level)	Audio visual reaction time (1% level)

It is a true finding that the advantage is significantly with wheat germ oil in the visual reaction time group ($t = 3.1997$, 1% level).

Several other experiments have shown that cottonseed oil has shown some advantages for strength and reaction time. It is not, therefore, a true placebo (Cf. Fig. 1, Chapter I). Differences may have been sharper on devitaminized lard.

Experiment 9

The Effects of Training with a Dietary Supplement on the Heartograph at Ground Level and Altitude

HENRY FRANKLIN CONSTANTINO[*]

PURPOSE

THE purpose of this experiment was to investigate the effects of physical training and wheat germ oil (VioBin) on the cardiovascular system as measured by the heartograph.

METHODS OF RESEARCH

Six experimental and four control subjects were used in tests as offered by the Cameron heartometer to determine the effects of training and wheat germ oil at ground level and at 10,000 feet altitude. The results were determined after the completion of three stages: a) (T_1) Ground level and altitude heartographs were taken to determine their consistency from week to week. b) (T_2) Ground level and altitude heartographs were taken on the subjects upon reaching a plateau of physical fitness resulting from a period of endurance-type activities. c) (T_3) Ground level and altitude heartographs were taken on the subjects who maintained a plateau of physical fitness after the addition of wheat germ oil (20 capsules, daily) to their normal diet. The total experiment was ten months in duration.

Graphical analysis of each individual subject and average trends for each group were developed for purposes of comparison. The standard error of measurement technique was utilized to find the critical ratio of the experimental sample and to test reliability of changes reported by the measurement of the heartograph.

---

* Urbana, M.S. thesis, Physical Education, University of Illinois, 1952, p. 76. (Sponsor, Professor T. K. Cureton.)

RESULTS

At ground level the area of the brachial pulse wave showed an increase from .52 sq. cm (81 SS %) to .64 sq. cm (97.5 SS %) during the pretraining (T_1) stage, to the post-training (T_2) stage— a gain of .12 sq. cm with a critical ratio of 3.87. Upon the addition of wheat germ oil (Stages II to III) to the diets of the experimental subjects, no appreciable change (.01 cm) was noted. The increase of .12 sq. cm from Stage I to Stage II is shown as an increase in cardiovascular fitness.

Significant gains in the area of the brachial pulse wave from .37 (60 SS %) to .51 sq. cm (80 SS %), a critical ratio of 6.67, was shown at an altitude from the pretraining (T_1) stage to the post-training (T_2 stage. Upon the addition of wheat germ oil, however, the experimental subjects reported a mean loss of .01 sq. cm, a critical ratio of .48, indicating that after the subjects had reached a plateau of fitness due to physical training, additional training and/or wheat germ oil, failed to improve their cardiovascular fitness. It was believed that the experimental subjects had functionally well equipped cardiovascular systems from the start of the experiment and the T_1 measurements verified this. The post-training (T_2) stage upon the addition of wheat germ oil, altitude for the experimental subjects showed considerable increases in the area of the brachial pulse wave, indicating the maintenance of a high stroke volume, therefore, showing that cardiovascular fitness was increased by the training not only at ground level when the subjects were tested in a rested state but also at an altitude when they were under physiological stress.

The systolic and diastolic pulse wave amplitudes (vertical measurements of the heartograph) also showed significant gains from the pretraining (T_1) to the post-training (T_2) stages of experimentation indicating increases in cardiovascular fitness.

At ground level there was a significant gain in the systolic pulse wave amplitude of the experimental subjects from the pretraining (T_1) stage to the post-training (T_2) stage of 1.74 (82 SS %) to 1.91 cm (91 SS %), respectively, or, a .17 cm increase, with a critical ratio of 3.40. The post-training (T_2) to postdietary (T_3) training stages of experimentation show a contrasting sig-

nificant loss from 1.91 (91 SS %) to 1.76 cm (83 SS %), or, a minus
.15 cm with a critical ratio of 3.00. This measurement, indicating
the magnitude of myocardial action due to the contraction of the
ventricles, was increased with training but after the wheat germ
oil diet a considerable decrease was noted. This leads one to believe that one or two of the subjects began to grow stale toward
the end of the experiment and slacked off a little in their training,
or, the wheat germ oil was responsible for decreasing the contracting force of the ventricles of the subjects thereby accounting
for the decrease in systolic amplitudes during this stage.

The systolic pulse wave amplitude, at altitude, showed a gain
from Stage I (1.21 cm) to Stage II (1.50 cm) of .29 cm, or, 16.5
SS %, with a critical ratio of 5.27. Stages II to III produced a mean
loss of .03 cm and a critical ratio of .54.

The diastolic pulse wave amplitude, at ground level, gained
from .83 (83 SS %) to .98 cm (98 SS %) in the pretraining (T_1) to
post-training (T_2) stages of experimentation, again due to the
physical training, with a critical ratio of 3.66. From the post-
training (T_2) to postdietary (T_3) training stages a mean loss of
.05 cm (5 SS %) was found showing an insignificant critical ratio
of 1.22.

A gain from .62 (62 SS %) to .78 cm (78 SS %) was found in
the pretraining (T_1) to post-training (T_2) stages at an altitude
for the diastolic pulse wave amplitude. This increase, showing
a critical ratio of 4.44, again indicates an improved cardiovascular
condition due to physical training. In the T_2 to T_3 stage, there
was a gain from .78 (78 SS %) to .80 cm (80 SS %), with a critical
ratio of .56.

The diastolic surge failed to show any significant increases or
decreases in cardiovascular fitness as a result of physical training and/or the wheat germ oil.

At ground level the diastolic surge did not change from Stage
I (26 cm or 88 SS %) to Stage II. Physical training and wheat
germ oil seems to have lowered this measurement .06 cm or 8
SS % from Stage II to Stage III.

Insignificant critical ratios were found after measuring the
obliquity angle both at ground level and altitude. A critical ratio
of 1.97 was found at ground level from pretraining (T_1) to post-

training (T_2) stages. During this time an increase of .70 degree $(-10 \text{ SS } \%)$ was found indicating a slight loss in cardiovascular fitness. An additional increase of .30 degree was found from Stage II to Stage III, hardly enough to be of any significance.

At an altitude the obliquity angle decreased from 22.6 degrees $(60 \text{ SS } \%)$ to 22.2 degrees $(65 \text{ SS } \%)$ from Stage I to Stage II, or a gain of .4 degrees, with a critical ratio of 1.05. This change is also insignificant. From Stage II to Stage III an increase of .5 degree was found, with an insignificant critical ratio of 1.31.

Physical training lowered the ground level sitting pulse rate during the T_1 to T_2 stages from 73 to 60 beats per minute, with a significant critical ratio of 5.88. This decrease in pulse rate is regarded as an increase in cardiovascular fitness. From Stages II to III the pulse rate remained the same.

At an altitude the sitting pulse rate was lowered slightly from 71 to 70 beats per minute, with a critical ratio of .61. With continued training and the addition of wheat germ oil the pulse rate lowered from 70 to 67 beats per minute, with a critical ratio of 1.83. This change is also insignificant. Since the ground level (T_1) pulse rates had leveled off, the influence of wheat germ oil could be slightly favorable in improving the physical fitness at altitude.

CONCLUSIONS

Ten weeks of physical training significantly improved the brachial pulse wave up to the peak of performance at ground level and altitude.

An additional six weeks of physical training plus a dietary supplement did not significantly affect the brachial pulse wave either at ground level or altitude.

The data in this experiment shows and vividly confirms that the subjects hit a plateau of fitness, represented by the brachial pulse wave, and then leveled off for the duration of the experiment.

Since the brachial pulse wave area was used to determine the plateau after twelve weeks of training, it would not be expected to change unless the intensity of the program changed. This phenomenon also suggests that the improvements due to WGO are nervous and nutritive in nature and not circulatory.

The Effects of Training and Dietary Supplement on the T-Wave of the ECG at Ground Level and at 10,000 Feet Altitude

STEVE SUSIC

THE purpose of this experiment* was to study the effects of training and dietary supplement on the T-wave at ground level and at 10,000 feet altitude.

Six graduate students acted as the experimental subjects and three doctorate candidates acted as the control group.

RESEARCH METHODS

Study was divided into three phases: pretraining (T_1), training (T_2) and training plus dietary supplement (T_3). Two ECG measurements were taken in the quiet lying state at ground level and 10,000 feet altitude in each of the training stages.

CONCLUSIONS

Training at ground level for twelve weeks made insignificant changes in relation to T-wave (highest precordial) of the electrocardiogram.

Training for six weeks plus dietary supplement was significant in increases from T_2 to T_3 within the experimental group and of the experimental group over the control group in terms of $D/_{\text{S.E. meas.}}$

Training with tests at an altitude showed a significant increase from T_1 to T_2 in the T-wave of the experimental group but not from T_2 to T_3, possibly the severity of the stress depressed the T-wave.

Training and dietary supplement with tests at altitude showed an insignificant increase of the T-wave, of the experimental group

---

* Urbana, M.S. thesis, Physical Education, University of Illinois, 1953, p. 53. (Sponsor: T. K. Cureton.)

from T_2 to T_3, but a significant increase was shown at T_3, the experimental group over T_2 of the control group. Significant increases on tests at altitude were also shown in the T_2 and T_3 tests corresponding to stages of training of experimental group over the control group.

The indications are that training and also training plus simultaneous feeding of VioBin wheat germ oil have a significant effect on the T-wave.

DISCUSSION

It appeared that twelve weeks of physical training (as in Experiments 2, 3, 4, 5 and 6) did not raise the T-wave in the highest precordial T-wave of the electrocardiogram as much as the same physical training with the addition of WGO, daily at the end of the work. Twelve weeks is enough to plateau the measures, and the additional gain was not expected. Since the Schneider test behaved similarly, the gain is attributed to the WGO in order to make the improvement in the third stage of six weeks statistically significant at ground level but not at an altitude, inasmuch as the stress was so great it overshadowed the effect of the WGO.

Experiment 11

The Effects of Training and a Dietary Supplement on the Cardiovascular Fitness of Adult Men

Arthur F. Maley

PURPOSE

THE purpose of this experiment* was to determine the effects of training and a dietary supplement of VioBin wheat Germ oil and synthetic vitamin E (alpha tocopherol acetate) on the cardiovascular tests of adult men (26-60 years of age), and to separate the effects of the dietary substances from that of training.

RESEARCH METHODS

Two groups of nine men each were used, matched against each other in the composite standard score of five cardiovascular tests (Av.), five-step (Cureton) pulse ratio test, ECG T and R waves, Cameron heartograph (Av. SS), Schneider index and five-minute Harvard step test. It was proven by paired case matching with systematic rotation, and comparison of means and sigmas, that the groups were well matched on the composite CV criterion and the t was insignificant on every single test item, showing that at T_1 the experimental and placebo groups were well matched. Then, all men were put into the same physical training program, one hour per day of mixed calisthenics, swimming and games at will, without instructional leadership or led drills. Men played volleyball, handball or basketball 1-2 times per week, but if they did not do this, then they did calisthenics, jogged or swam, five days per week. A roll check was maintained, only to see that they participated.

MATERIALS FED

Five days per week from March 17, 1952 until April 25, 1952, for six weeks, the experimental group was fed 20 × 6 capsules of

---

* Urbana, M.S. thesis, Physical Education, University of Illinois, 1952, p. 36. (Sponsor: T. K. Cureton.)

WGO in the double blind way, while the placebo group took the equivalent amount of vitamin E (0.43 I.U. per capsule in cotton-seed oil). The capsules were indistinguishable from each other, the bottles labelled A and B only. Four months of the exercise programs had been taken before the T_1 tests were taken and the feeding begun. This long delay was due to the late arrival of the placeboes, so after the men had adapted well to the program, the WGO and placeboes were added in the T_1 to T_3 period.

From T_1 to T_2, a time of four months, there was a significant positive difference on the heartograph measure (Av. of SS, Cureton method, The Cameron heartometer in industrial medicine, *J. Ass. Phys. Ment. Rehab.*, 21:No. 4, 112-121, 1967; and Cureton, *Physical Fitness Appraisal and Guidance*, pp. 232-280, 1947). This gain was due to training adaptations and not to feeding of supplements or placeboes.

It is shown in Table LIV that in the last six weeks of the experiment, as the feeding of the WGO and placeboes with practice continued, there was a deterioration of the Harvard Step Test SS and also in the Electrocardiograph (Av. of R and T waves in SS of the highest precordial lead), but the heartograph SS gained insignificantly. This table is given to show that these measures had reached a plateau.

Thus, it is demonstrated that the men had reached a plateau

TABLE LIV

COMPARISON OF THE EXPERIMENTAL (WGO) GROUP WITH THE CONTROL GROUP, BEFORE ANY SUPPLEMENTS WERE GIVEN, T_1 TO T_2, FOUR MONTHS ACTIVE

(Two Matched Groups, 9 Middle-Aged Men in Each)

Tests	T_1 Mean of Experimental (WGO) Group	T_2 Mean of Placebo Group, Vitamin E in Cottonseed Oil	D (in SS)	md	t
Heartograph (Av. of SS)	49.78	53.29	3.51	2.20	14.248
Electrocardiograph (Av. of R and T SS)	60.22	50.28	−9.94	6.08	1.637
5-Minute Harvard Step Test	44.00	43.61	−0.39	2.80	1.251

Note: Period of feeding the supplements and the placeboes (six weeks).

by the heartograph, ECG and Harvard step test in four months of rather casual participation.

RESULTS

At T_2, after four months of physical training and the composite CV battery as a whole had made insignificant change, it was decided to deal with each individual item and concentrate upon three tests, namely, the heartograph test, the ECG test (Av. of

TABLE LV

COMPARISON OF TESTS, T_2 TO T_3, AFTER ADDING THE FEEDING OF THE WGO SUPPLEMENT AND ALSO ADDING THE PLACEBOES

Tests	T_2 Mean of Experimental (WGO) Group	T_3 Mean of Placebo Group	D	md	t
Heartograph (Av. of SS)	51.88	53.29	1.41	6.31	0.222
Electrocardiograph (Av of R and T SS)	46.67	44.67	−1.90	4.76	0.420
5-Minute Harvard Step Test	50.14	48.22	−1.82	3.45	0.562

TABLE LVI

INITIAL TESTS—TESTING OF THE MATCHING OF THE EXPERIMENTAL (WGO) GROUP WITH THE PLACEBO (Vitamin E) GROUP

Tests	T_1 Mean of the Experimental (WGO) Group	T_1 Mean of the Placebo Cottonseed Oil + Vitamin E Group	D	md	t
Heartograph (Av. of SS)	49.72	49.00	−0.72	5.09	0.132
Electrocardiograph (Av. of T and R waves in highest precordial lead)	60.22	58.66	−1.96	9.52	0.164
Schneider Index	55.56	58.89	3.33	5.77	0.576
5-Minute Step Test	44.00	40.33	3.67	7.58	0.484
Progressive Pulse Ratio Test (Cureton)	41.56	46.89	5.33	8.27	0.645
Average Standard Scores on 5 CV Tests	50.55	50.44	− .11	xxx	insignificant

TABLE LVII

EXPERIMENTAL VERSUS PLACEBO GROUPS ON THREE
CARDIOVASCULAR TESTS AT T_2

Tests	T_2 *Experimental (WGO) Group*	T_2 *Placebo Cottonseed Oil and Vitamin E Group*	*D*	*md*	*t*
Heartograph (Av. SS)	53.26	51.88	−1.38	7.28	0.189
Electrocardiograph (Av of T and R SS Scores)	50.28	46.67	−5.51	9.46	3.434 (Significant > .01)
5-Minute Step Test	43.67	58.22	14.65	6.82	0.961

R and T precordial waves), and the five-minute Harvard step test in the period of feeding (Table LVII). A significant difference is shown at T_2 for the ECG test, whereas, it did not exist at T_1, associated with adaptations to the training as there was no feeding in this period.

CONCLUSIONS

The comparison of the two groups at T_1 showed that the groups were satisfactorily matched, as the t's between groups were statistically insignificant for all items (Table LIII).

After four months of preliminary physical training, from T_1 to T_2, the brachial pulse wave was shown to have improved from 49.78 to 53.29 SS, a significant improvement ($t = 14.248$). No other change was of importance, as the Harvard step test changed very slightly, and the T-wave (highest precordial lead) deteriorated from 60.22 to 50.28, this difference of −9.94 SS was not quite significant at the .05 level ($t = 1.637$).

In the critical period for the testing of the supplement of WGO, T_2 to T_3, with exercise continued on the same basis but with WGO added daily after the exercise, the heartograph amplitude had improved even further, 1.41 SS (insignificant change, $t = 0.222$); and the ECG (Av. of R and T waves, in SS) had reduced from 46.67 to 44.67 SS (insignificant change, $t = 0.420$); and the Harvard step test had reduced from 50.14 to 48.22 SS (insignificant change, $t = 0.562$). The overall conclusion here is that the subjects were fully adapted to the work, which was rather casual without leadership or goals, so no further significant changes came about in the six-week test period in which the WGO supplement was used.

DISCUSSION

There was a noticeable drop in the T-wave (highest precordial lead) from T_1 50.28 SS to 46.47 SS in the T_1 to T_2 period of four months when the men were active but not on the WGO supplement; and there was a further decrease in the same measurement from 50.14 to 48.22 SS. The first drop −9.46 was statistically significant ($t = 3.43$) but the second drop was *not* significant, a further drop of 2.0 SS. This trend downward is unexplained.

It is clear that the group had become fully adapted to what they were doing for exercise and were taking it easy, without a leader or goals to meet. It is the impression after watching men under stress take wheat germ oil and those not under stress take WGO, that the WGO assists men more when they are under great stress.

Experiment 12

The Effects of Wheat Germ Oil on the Cardiovascular Fitness of Varsity Wrestlers

WILLIAM J. VOHASKA

PURPOSE

THE purpose of this experiment* was to find whether the supplementary feeding of wheat germ oil made any difference in the cardiovascular criterion on which the two groups were matched.

SUBJECTS

During a regular varsity wrestling season the entire squad of University of Illinois wrestlers was tested on a composite six-item cardiovascular test and then matched into two halves. One of these halves was given a dietary supplement of wheat germ oil in capsules and the other was given a placebo in capsules containing cottonseed oil (CSO).

RESEARCH METHODS

The six test items used were as follows: a) Schneider index, b) heartometer, c) ECG (av. of the SS for T-wave and R-wave), d) breath holding after a one-minute step test, e) Harvard five-minute step test and f) all-out treadmill run, 10 miles per hour, 8.6 per cent grade. These five tests were given, scored in raw scores and standard scores, then the standard scores were added together.

Capsules of a similar nature were fed daily, each subject taking twenty of the 3-minim capsules, seven days per week. The supplementary feeding extended for only four weeks, these being after the wrestling season was well under way, the last two weeks in February and the first two weeks in March. The whole pro-

---

* Urbana, M.S. thesis, Physical Education, University of Illinois, 1954, p. 43. (Sponsor: T. K. Cureton.)

gram extended over two weeks from the second week in January until the third week in March. The first and last weeks were used for testing and no feeding was done during this period. (It had been planned to feed the capsules for eight weeks but the place-boes arrived late, so the feeding was done for only four weeks.) There were eleven participants in each group.

The college men did calisthenics, some distance running, conditioning exercises (push-ups, chinning, rope climbing, bridging, and other special exercises); they also practiced wrestling and wrestled in tournaments.

Analysis of variance showed that for three treatments on the T_1 series of test scores that $F = 1.516$, hence the groups were matched closely enough. The two-tailed Fisher "t" was used to evaluate the differences.

RESULTS

The experimental group on WGO improved in the cardiovascular composite index from an average of 282.55 to 336.18, a gain of 22.50 or 7.97 per cent ($t = 2.295$). Correspondingly, the matched group on placeboes did not change significantly ($t = 1.342$) from 302.36 to 332.27. No other changes were significantly different between the WGO group and the C.S.O. control group.

Among the tests used, the all-out treadmill run (7 mi./hr., 8.6% grade) was the only test to change significantly, the change being from 26.67 SS to 35.89 SS, a change of 6.72 SS ($t = 1.953$, significant at the 0.037 level, $N = 10$) this in the control group on nothing; the groups on WGO and cottonseed oil placeboes making insignificant changes, although both improved.

The heartograph, five-minute step test, and breath holding tests had decreased slightly, indicating that some of the athletes were showing "competitive fatigue" near the end of the season.

DISCUSSION

Since it is known that physical fitness tests usually improve in the preseason training, and level off after competition begins, it is clear that toward the end of the season not much improvement could be expected. It is even more surprising that a composite cardiovascular gain could be obtained, related to the dietary supplements. The composite cardiovascular index appeared to summate the effect better than any single CV test.

Experiment 13

Influence of Wheat Germ Oil as a Dietary Supplement in a Program of Conditioning Exercises with Middle-Aged Subjects

Thomas K. Cureton and Richard H. Pohndorf

THIS study* was a staff experiment carried out in 1953 as a follow-up to several preliminary experiments by graduate students at the University of Illinois, School of Physical Education. The studies were carried out in the Physical Fitness Research Laboratory. The preliminary studies as well as the staff experiment of 1953 and the reversal experiment of 1954 all showed some advantage for supplementary feedings of wheat germ oil (WGO) administered during or immediately following physical conditioning periods of conditioning exercises and swimming in an indoor pool with water temperature 74-76 F. The subjects were adult men, 26-60 years of age, mainly sedentary, volunteers from the nonphysical education staff.

The WGO capsules (20 capsules per day, 3 minims each, and each containing 175 mg of WGO and 0.44 mg of mixed tocopherol) were fed for eight weeks in connection with the progressive physical training experiment. Two groups of eight men each were matched in treadmill-running time, the brachial pulse wave and age. Two other inactive control groups of five men each were tested at the beginning (T_1) and at the end (T_2) of the eight-week period. The group results show significant advantage for the experimental subjects who took WGO over those who did not in both performance (willpower dominated) tests and in naive (nonwillpower) tests. (Cf. Figs. 10 and 11)

Note: Acknowledgment is given to Richard H. Pohndorf, instructor in physical education; also to the consultants on the study: Connor Johnson, Ph.D., professor of animal nutrition; Norris L. Brookens, M.D., Ph.D., physician at the Carle Clinic, Urbana; Colin R. Blyth, associate professor of mathematical statistics; and to our staff physician who assisted with medical examinations.

* Reprinted from *The Research Quarterly,* 26:4, December, 1955, pp. 391-407. Copyright, 1955, by the American Association for Health, Physical Education, and Recreation, National Education Association.

The physiological advantage is shown in terms of running endurance in "all-out" treadmill runs, T-wave of the ECG (CR_{IV-V} lead), lower systolic blood pressure, the Schneider index and the Illinois total body reaction-time test in response to light, sound and combined signals. Individual differences in response are shown and some of the factors which cause such variations are identified.

Announcement was first made in October, 1954 of the discovery of the value of wheat germ oil (hereafter called WGO) as an ergogenic aid to men trying to improve their physical fitness in a physical training course.[3, 4, 5] This first report was based upon various experiments extending from 1949 through 1952 carried out by graduate students working under the supervision of the writer. This further report is an experiment carried out in 1953 with the aid of certain staff personnel.

The first experiment as a student thesis was carried out in 1949 by William A. Forr[17] on six groups of college students, three groups of eight in a fraternity house and three other groups of nine each in basic swimming. He found significant changes in the T-wave (highest in Lead $CR_{IV \text{ or } V}$) of the electrocardiogram (ECG) and also in the Illinois vertical jump reaction-time test which favored WGO over the effect of vitamin E capsules (150 mg/week) and corn oil capsules of equal calorific content. The WGO was calculated to match the synthetic vitamin E (alpha tocopherol acetate). The control groups were considered to be those taking the corn oil capsules. None of the subjects knew what they were taking and the administration of the capsules was carefully supervised.

Again in 1950-51, advantage was shown for a group of six men who were fed WGO capsules (20 capsules, 3 minims each, containing 175 mg of WGO and 0.44 mg of tocopherol) daily in connection with a strenuous physical conditioning experiment in which hard endurance training (four times a week) and a weekly "all-out" ergometer bicycle test ride was given both at ground level and at 10,000 feet of simulated altitude in a decompression chamber. After twelve weeks of preliminary training and testing, the men were given the dietary supplement. Instead of holding their position even on the plateau which they had established in the last three weeks of the training period, the men improved, four of them in a rather extraordinary manner, contrary to the usual experience of men in hard training showing evidence of terminal fatigue (staleness). Each one of the graduate students participating in this work wrote up the results on one test item. The significant results are available in the theses of Smiley,[32] who showed advantages in the bicycle "all-out" ride test; Susic,[35] who showed significant changes in the T-wave of the ECG; and White,[37] who showed advantages in the Schneider test. These preliminary experiments awakened considerable interest and further studies were arranged.

In 1952 three experiments were conducted. One of these by Storm,[34] checked the effect which the WGO feeding had with respect to its possible tendency to fatten middle-aged men and to increase their weight. Three groups of eight men each were matched, one group was fed WGO, another was fed cottonseed oil placebos, and these were compared with the third which had no exercise or dietary supplement. While taking 20 of the 3-minim capsules per day, the WGO group showed an insignificant change in weight which averaged less than ±2.0 pounds. This group also lost adipose tissue from 140 mm (49.2 SS) to 124 mm (58.1 SS), by Cureton's composite of six measurements with calipers on the cheeks, abdomen, waist, Gluteal fold, front and rear thigh. The group on cottonseed oil capsules remained about the same, 137 mm to 138 mm (51.5 SS to 50.1 SS). Both of these groups took the same exercise program for twelve weeks. The third group which took no exercise or supplementary feeding changed from 144 mm (47.3 SS) to 125 mm (57.7 SS). The WGO group closely paralleled the control group.

Two studies were conducted on athletic teams by Marx[28] and by Vohaska,[36] using the varsity swimming and wrestling teams, respectively. The same pattern of feeding 20 capsules (3 minims) per day was used for the WGO experimental group. The experimental group was contrasted with a matched group of men taking capsules of cottonseed oil containing equivalent amounts of vitamin E (2.5 mg of alpha tocopherol acetate per gram of cottonseed oil) to that in the WGO. The supplementary feeding was for four weeks only. These experiments produced significant changes in several of the test variables but only the wrestling team groups were differentiated by the WGO and only in one test, namely, the brachial pulse wave. A type of fatigue called by us "competitive fatigue" developed in some of the men on both of these teams which tended to depress the results on the final series of tests, thus minimizing the changes.

In 1955, the work on the wrestling team was repeated with similar results, with trends in the right direction for improvement favoring both wheat germ oil in one group and wheat germ in another matched group, both contrasted with a control group on cottonseed oil placebos. Some advantage showed with respect to treadmill run time, T-wave of the ECG, systolic amplitude of the brachial pulse wave and the Schneider test. However, the same type of "competitive fatigue" showed in some of the men, supported by subjective reports of lassitude, loss of sleep and minor injuries. Even in spite of some gains, the cardiovascular tests were lower on the final (T_2) series of tests than they would have been if the pressure had not been so great toward the end of the season. Thus, the changes obtained were minimized, and we concluded that these types of competitive sports are not very suitable to show the effects of a dietary supplement. In spite of these difficulties, the WGO was judged to be helpful.

Further research was needed and was carried on in the form of the experiment now to be described. The present experiment was carried out in 1953 with the work being done on two groups of middle-aged men with eight men in each group, and also two other groups of men classed as environmental controls. One of the latter was on the same dosage of WGO and the other took nothing; both were inactive compared to the experimental subjects. While the men competed against their own test scores, there was no competition against opponents; furthermore, the work was carefully graduated with every precaution taken to prevent the men from working too hard at first.

EXPERIMENTAL DESIGN

The problem was to determine whether WGO capsules, administered as a dietary supplement for eight weeks in connection with a course in physical conditioning, would significantly differentiate the experimental WGO group from another matched group on equal size and equal calorie content placebos of devitaminized lard, with both groups taking the same program of exercise.

The tests used were the following: a) all-out treadmill run, b) brachial pulse wave (sphygmogram), c) Illinois vertical jump reaction-time test, d) T-wave of the ECG, e) standing systolic blood pressure, f) Schneider test and g) basal metabolic rate (by regular oxygen consumption procedure).

The sixteen experimental subjects were tested (T_1 = initial test) in the last week of May and the first two weeks in June, with the tests given to each man individually by appointment. They were retested in the second week of August. The weather conditions were fairly comparable. At the final test (T_2) some of the men were busy preparing examinations to finish the summer session. If anything, the added anxiety would have hurt the cardiovascular tests. The inactive environmental controls were divided into two groups, one which took WGO and the other took no dietary supplement.

After the T_1 series of tests the sixteen experimental subjects were paired man for man by age and by the time on the all-out treadmill run, just as closely as this would permit. The two resulting groups of this matching were not significantly different from each other. Some good men and some poor men were in both groups. The capsules of WGO and the devitaminized lard placebos were of identical size (6 minims). The men were not told what they were taking, except "just vitamins."

The attendance at the exercise sessions averaged four periods per week and an attendance roll was kept. The participation was about equal in terms of number of periods for the two experimental groups. In the workouts on the pool deck and in the water the men were intermixed at random. A leader set the exercises and the men did the best they could to follow them for twenty-five minutes, then there was a five-minute break for showers, followed by swimming for another 20-25 minutes. The pace could not always be controlled in the exercises or in the swimming, but the men kept busy at exercise to the extent that they could tolerate it. The leader was either Cureton or Pohndorf.

After the first month of gradually progressive work, a series of test exercises were introduced and two or three of these were done every day after 15-20 minutes of warm-up work. In the sixth and seventh weeks, some similar test exercises were added in the pool. Scores were put down for all of the test exercises and it is judged that the motivation to improve was high.

No attempt was made to control the diet of any of the subjects except that all of the experimental subjects were told to eat moderately, to reduce their intake of fried foods, but otherwise to eat normally. This is all of the control that seemed wise with normal university personnel, carrying on their regular duties and home life day by day.

While the two experimental groups were fairly closely matched in age and ability, the WGO group averaging 41.4 years and 3.44 minutes for the run on the treadmill against 36.5 years and 3.34 minutes for the lard placebo group, the two groups of environmental controls who did not exercise in the program were not well matched. One of these was composed of five men, mainly younger laboratory graduate assistants; the other of five older men who were mainly interested in just taking the tests. No attempt was made to control their eating or living habits in any way. None were in competitive sports. In the main they were quite sedentary, especially the older men.

RESULTS

The treadmill run involved exertion of voluntary willpower, whereas the latter did not involve any willpower. It is interesting that the results are much the same. This indicates that the gains[*]

---

[*] The results shown are computed in terms of:

1. Raw score percentages, wherein per cent change $= \dfrac{T_2 - T_1}{T_1} \times 100$

2. Standard Scores (SS), based upon tables from 0 to 100, equal increments of variability with $1 \text{ SS} = \dfrac{6 \times \sigma}{100}$

3. Fisher's "t" tables for small samples.

4. Standard errors of measurement from retest data:
   Reliability of a single case, wherein, interpretation is limited to the subjects in the experiment and not in the universal sample,

were not due to fluctuations of willpower (psychological) changes but were mainly circulatory changes and neuromuscular condition changes. The basic data are not shown at all. In Table LVIII the results are shown only in terms of significance, computed case by case in relationship to the standard errors of measurement. This method shows only whether the individuals changed who were in the experiment and no generalizations about reliability of other samples can be made.

Treadmill Run Results

The WGO actively exercised group (A) composed of eight men averaging 41.4 years of age improved from 3.44 to 5.14 minutes, or 51.5% (18.0 SS) on the all-out treadmill-run test. The comparable group (B) taking lard placebos improved from 3.34 to 4.06 minutes, the men averaging 36.5 years of age. Both of

---

$$s = \sqrt{\frac{d^2}{2N}}$$ d – deviation between T_{1a} and restest T_{1b}

$$t = \sqrt{\frac{T_2 - T_1}{s \sqrt{2N}}}$$ N = number of paired retests included

or in the case of just one set of retests, T_1 and T_2 with N = 1; t = D/s $\sqrt{2}$

Explanation: Assume for any given individual that the item measured is normally distributed. If X and Y are two measurement observations on the same individual, retests being taken within a few days of each other, then,

$d_1 = X_1 - Y_1$ and the mean of all such d's is 0.

variance $r^2 = 2 \sigma^2$

when mean is 0, we may estimate r^2 not by $\Sigma (x_1 - x_2)^2/N-1$ with d.f. = N-1 but by the slightly better estimate $\Sigma d^2/N$ with d.f. = n,

therefore, n = 1, $\sigma^2 = r^2/2$ or $s^2 = \sqrt{\frac{\Sigma d^2}{2n}}$ and s = $\sqrt{\frac{\Sigma d^2}{2n}}$

See page 40 in Gulliksen's *Theory of Mental Tests*, 1950, for more complete derivation. This describes measurement errors and enables us to say whether differences are significant in the sense that they could not be caused by measurement errors.

Single case differences like this, then, are significant if they exceed 2.04 in absolute value, meaning that there are less than 5 chances in 100 of the differences being due to the measurement error.

Significance of the group changes were determined by D/ $\sqrt{165}$ > 2.04 for 5% level of confidence and applied to the two groups of 8, and > 2.75 for 1% level of confidence.

TABLE LVIII

EFFECT OF WHEAT GERM OIL SUPPLEMENT ON THE TREADMILL RUN

N	Group		Avg. Age	T_1 Avg. Raw Score	SS	T_2 Avg. Raw Score	SS	D Avg. Raw Score	D SS	Criterion 5 Per Cent Significance Level	Obtained Group Significance
8	A	Exercise plus WGO	41.4	3.44	51.4	5.14	69.4	1.70	18.0	2.04	8.71
8	B	Exercise plus Placebos	36.5	3.34	50.5	4.06	58.0	0.72	7.5	2.04	3.63
5	C	Inactive plus WGO	36.2	1.90	45.0	2.00	47.6	0.10	2.6	2.04	1.00
5	D	Inactive plus Placeboes	32.0	2.05	47.4	2.05	48.4	0	1.0	2.04	0

these groups made a significant change ($t_A = 8.71$ and $t_B = 3.63$).
These two groups were also significantly different in the gains
that they made ($t_{AB} = 3.59$). The five inactive controls on WGO
improved from 1.90 to 2.00 minutes, an insignificant gain ($t = 1.00$); also, the five inactive controls on placebos failed to gain
(2.05 minutes to 2.05 minutes). The exercised group on WGO
differed significantly from the control group which remained inactive but took WGO ($t_{AC} = 4.62$); whereas the exercised group
on placebos was not significantly different from the inactive control group on placebos ($t_{AD} = 1.95$). Thus, by group means the
advantage of WGO stands out sharply. All changes are shown in
Table LVIII.

Because certain individuals responded to the WGO very definitely and others did not, it was decided to make a test of each
and every case, using the test of significance for an individual
case, using $D/s\sqrt{2}$ for the obtained t value. The results are shown
in Table LIX in terms of the number of individuals who made
significant changes, those who changed in the right direction,
those who did not change, and those who lost. The results again
show that seven out of eight subjects in group A improved, with
four making a significant change. In group B five out of eight
made an improvement but only three made a significant change.
This table does not show the magnitude of the changes and, of
course, is not as satisfactory as Table LVIII. The two tables en-
force the recognition that both the endurance exercise program
and the wheat germ oil were significant factors in the improvements made.

TABLE LIX*

TABULATION OF INDIVIDUAL CHANGES (NUMBER OF INDIVIDUALS)

N	Group	Significant Gain	Gain	No Gain	Loss	Significant Loss
8	A	4	3	0	1	0
8	B	3	2	1	2	0
5	C	0	4	0	1	0
5	D	0	4	0	1	0

* *Statistical Note, Table LIX:* The s was computed from retest data for each
item. The criterion of significance was $D/s\sqrt{2N}$ for each individual case, two degrees of freedom based on T_1 and T_2. *Cf.* Helen M. Walker and Joseph Lev,
Statistical Inference, pp.151-160, New York: Holt, 1953.

An important test was made by running the same program in the summer of 1954 in which the men were reversed as to taking WGO or taking placebos. Eight men gained 11.62 minutes while on WGO compared to the same men gaining only 1.99 minutes while on placebos; the average gain was 1.45 compared to 0.24 minutes. Out of eight reversals available, six men made their peak time on WGO, one man tied, and one man did a bit less well. The latter was in superb condition and had been in the exercise program for several years. These data are most revealing and only space prevents laying the detailed case record out in full.

Brachial Pulse Wave Results

The actively exercised group A taking WGO improved from 0.359 sq. cm. to 0.550 sq. cm., a gain of 50.4% (21.3 SS), a significant change ($t_A = 6.63$). The other matched group on exercise and placebos (B) changed from 0.359 sq. cm. to 0.400 sq. cm., an insignificant change ($t_B = 1.51$). There was also a significant difference between groups A and B ($t = 2.49$). The control group (C), composed of five men averaging 36.2 years of age, were fed WGO over the same eight-week period and deteriorated from an average of 0.514 sq. cm. to 0.468 sq. cm., a loss of 6.2 SS (or 8.94% in raw score per cent). This change was insignificant ($t_C = 1.26$). The other control group (C), inactive and taking placebos, also deteriorated from 0.349 to 0.299 sq. cm., a loss of 6.1 SS (or 14.32% in raw score per cent). This change was insignificant ($t_D = 1.62$). There was no significant difference between the exercised group on placebos (B) and the inactive group on placebos (D), ($t = 1.60$), but the exercised group improved from 0.359 to 0.400 sq. cm. while the inactive group changed from 0.349 to 0.299 sq. cm., a loss rather than a gain. These results again show the apparent value of the WGO. The results are as striking in this "naive" test as they were in the case of the all-out treadmill run.

The data from the reversal in which men on WGO were changed over to placebos and vice versa, from 1953 to 1954, both summer experiments being run under the same conditions, show that six out of twelve men improved more on WGO than they did on placebos; four men improved more on placebos; and two were the same. The average gain of the six men on WGO was 0.209 sq. cm. compared to 0.112 sq. cm. for the four men on placebos, showing that those who gain improve unusually compared to men on placebos.

The systolic amplitude of the brachial pulse wave gave similar results. The exercised WGO group gained from 1.32 to 1.76 cm, a raw score per cent gain of 33.5 per cent (16.9 SS). This is a significant gain at the 1 per cent level (t = 3.20). The exercise group on placebos gained from 1.35 to 1.39 cm, a 2.96 per cent gain (t = 0.33)—an insignificant gain. The inactive WGO control group gained from 1.41 to 1.47 cm (4.26%); and the inactive group of controls on placebos changed from 1.24 to 1.15 cm (a loss of 7.24%), also insignificant (t = 0.62).

The Vertical Jump Reaction-Time Test Results

Of the three tests given in this area, the combined light and sound signal test gave the best results, this being the only test to give a significant difference. The group which exercised and took WGO gained from an average of 0.360 to 0.334, a gain of 0.026 seconds, equivalent to 8.9 SS (t = 2.60). The exercised group on placebos gained from 0.336 to 0.329, or a gain of 0.007 seconds, an insignificant gain equivalent to 2.6 SS (t = 0.69). The inactive control group which took WGO changed from 0.293 to 0.295, a loss of 0.002 seconds, equivalent to 1.4 SS. The inactive group on placebos did not change.

The visual reaction times improved a little from 0.384 to 0.358 for group A on exercise and wheat germ oil, a gain of 4.17 per cent (6.06 SS), but this group was not significantly different from any other group. The inactive group on WGO improved 8.50 SS, but the gain was insignificant. The exercised group on placebos improved 1.17 SS and the control group on placebos improved 3.67 SS—both insignificant changes.

The auditory reaction time gained from 0.353 to 0.329 seconds, equivalent to 6.80 per cent (7.9 SS), but the change was insignificant. The inactive group on WGO gained 5.88 SS, and the inactive group on placebos gained 8.0 SS. The exercised group on placebos gained 1.9 SS, an insignificant change.

Swimming has been shown to slow these reaction times in

some other experiments at the University of Illinois. It is possible that the use of swimming with these groups depressed the results.

Results with the T-wave (CR$_{IV-V}$ lead) of the ECG

The trend of evidence favors the exercised group which took WGO, as the mean gain of this group was from 9.84 mm to 11.04 mm, a gain of 12.20 per cent (8.3 SS)—a significant change (t = 3.13). The exercised group on placebos also made a significant change from 11.06 to 12.07 mm, a 9.13 per cent gain (5.9 SS) (t = 2.80). These two groups, A and B, were insignificantly different, so the gains are attributed wholly to exercise. The changes in the control groups and between the control groups were insignificant. Of the inactive controls on WGO, one man gained from 15.5 to 22.7 mm, a gain of 7.2 mm and an improvement of 46.5 per cent equivalent to 87 SS. This illustrates the type of effect which is considered extraordinary. Among seven inactive controls on placebos, only two men gained as much as a millimeter. One of these was a swimming instructor who changed from 7.2 to 9.8 mm, a control who was not as inactive as he was supposed to be, working five days a week teaching swimming. A second subject gained from 4.3 to 7.0 mm, but this subject was unusually low to begin with and the exercise improved him in an extraordinary manner. A third subject in this group of controls lost from 11.7 to 9.6 mm, probably because he was genuinely sedentary, working the entire period as a statistical clerk. Various other experiments at the University of Illinois laboratory have shown that endurance exercise will usually improve the height of the T-wave in the C$_{IV-V}$ lead.

Systolic Blood Pressure (Standing) Results

The group which exercised and took the WGO reduced the blood pressure from an average of 120.75 mm Hg to 114.5 mm Hg, a gain of 5.18 per cent in raw scores (7.4 SS). This mean difference is statistically significant at the 5 per cent level of confidence (t = 2.25). The blood pressure rose from 118.4 to 123.0 mm Hg for the control group which took WGO, an insignificant change of 5.2 SS in the opposite direction. The changes in the active group on placebos and the inactive group on placebos were both insignificant, changes of 1.0 SS and 4.8 SS, respectively.

Changes in standing diastolic blood pressure were all statistically insignificant.

Results with the Schneider Index

The group which exercised and took WGO improved from 12.75 to 15.0 in the Schneider index. This gain of 2.25 points is equivalent to 17.65 per cent (9.7 SS). This was a significant change at the 5 per cent level of confidence ($t = 2.33$). No other group made a significant change. The matched group which exercised and took placebos changed from 13.87 to 14.12, an average gain of 0.25 points; the inactive controls which took the wheat germ oil changed from 14.4 to 13.6, a loss of 0.8 points; and the inactive control group improved from 9.8 to 10.1, a gain of 0.3 points.

Basal Metabolic Rate Results

The group which exercised and took WGO changed from −10.43 to −8.68 per cent in basal metabolic rate, an average gain of 16.78 per cent (7.00 SS). This was an insignificant change. The matched group on exercise and placebos changed from an average of −18.42 per cent to −7.80 per cent, a gain of 57.6 per cent in raw score per cent and 10.62 per cent in basal metabolic rate, a change equivalent to 10.60 SS but insignificant ($t = 1.43$). The inactive group on WGO changed from −16.94 per cent to −13.66 per cent, or a gain of 19.37 per cent in BMR in raw score per cent units, equivalent to 3.25 SS. The control group on placebos changed from 5.50 per cent to 0.69 per cent, a loss of 87.5 per cent in raw score per cent and 4.81 per cent in basal metabolic rate, equivalent to 5 SS. All of these measurements were based upon the usual oxygen intake, corrected to standard conditions, using a Sanborn metabolator. Relatively, these changes tend to show that there is a trend for exercise to raise the metabolic rate.

DISCUSSION OF CONFIRMATION WORK

The gains in treadmill-run times seem to indicate real gains in favor of WGO. When these gains were obtained in connection with the preliminary experiments they were thought to be due to the influence of training, but as various experiments have been conducted of diverse pattern and some of the experiments repeated, it is certain that some of the gain should be accredited to WGO. The support for this is not only in the advantages shown in the matched group experiment of 1953, but also in the 1954 follow-up experiment in which the men were reversed. The fact that the gains are significant in willpower performances like the treadmill run and reaction-time vertical jump and that they were also significant in the naive tests like the brachial pulse wave area, brachial pulse wave systolic amplitude, T-wave of the ECG and standing systolic blood pressure would certainly seem to be a strong case.

When we had obtained such favorable evidence on human subjects in 1953 and 1954, the president of the VioBin Corporation, Mr. Ezra Levin, arranged to have the experiment checked by Dr. Benjamin Ershoff, of the Department of Biochemistry and Nutrition, at the University of Southern California. He chose to simulate and repeat the work on guinea pigs, swum to exhaustion with weights tied to their legs in a barrel of water. Each one was carefully timed. In groups and on several contrasting diets, the results always favored the WGO diet. Since this work was published after our paper was written and reported to the American Physiological Society, the reference to Ershoff and Levin's work is given below in a footnote.*

----

* B. H. Ershoff, and E. Levin: Beneficial effect of an unidentified factor in wheat germ oil on the swimming performance of guinea pigs, *Federation Proceedings*, 14:431-32, March, 1955.

Male guinea pigs ranging from 250 to 300 gm in body weight were fed ad libitum highly purified rations containing all known nutrients but differing in the amount and source of dietary fat. Corn oil or wheat germ oil was incorporated in the diet at levels of 2 per cent, 5 per cent, or 10 per cent of the ration. A control group was fed a natural food ration (Purina Rabbit Pellets) supplemented daily with ascorbic acid. After twenty-eight days of feeding, swimming tests were conducted on all guinea pigs. A weight equal to 2.5 per cent of the animal's body weight was attached to each of the hind legs. Animals were placed in a barrel, filled to a depth of 18 inches with water. The water temperature was maintained at 37 C. All the animals fed the natural food ration drowned within ten minutes. From 25 per cent to 33.3 per cent of the guinea pigs fed the corn oil ration swam for 60 minutes, at which time the swimming tests were termi-

In view of the studies already reported on the value of the T-wave (CR_{IV-V} lead) to predict endurance[3, 5, 9, 29, 38] and the similar work on the value of the brachial pulse wave as standardized by Cureton,[7, 12, 37] it is logical to expect the improvement to show in these tests if the gain appeared in the treadmill run. The previous work showed good relationships of the naive tests to the all-out treadmill-running performance. Then it was not much of a surprise to find all of these relationships going together in this present work. It is plain to us that many debilitated subjects have T_{IV-V} waves as low as 2 to 3 mm and most of these can hardly walk on the treadmill; the average of the University of Illinois students is 9.5 mm; the Olympic swimming and diving men averaged 17.0 mm; a collection of top track and field stars averaged 15.9 mm; John Marshall measured 18.7 mm in our laboratory and shortly afterward broke five world's records in swimming races from 200 to 600 yards; then finally Roger Bannister, first to break the four-minute mile standard, was predicted to accomplish this feat after our work on him in the University of London's Royal Free College of Medicine, in 1952, when we found his T-wave to be 27.5 mm. Many of our other experiments have shown the gain in this important measurement as associated with improvements in endurance.

It is illogical to attribute the gains in endurance to synthetic vitamin E or to the natural vitamin E in WGO. Since each of the 3-minim capsules contained only 0.44 mg of mixed tocopherols, at the most 21.1 mg could have been accounted for, whereas the normal diet contains from 30 to 100 mg per day. The results point to some unidentified factor in wheat germ oil which is also partially contained in corn oil. So far, direct biochemical assays have failed to find any hormones in the oil which is classed

---

nated. In contrast to the above groups, over 60 per cent of the guinea pigs fed the wheat germ oil containing rations were still swimming after 60 minutes. Diets containing 2 per cent wheat germ oil were as effective as rations containing 10 per cent wheat germ oil in promoting swimming performance. Increasing the tocopherol content of the corn oil containing rations by the addition of 1 gm of a tocopherol acetate/kilogram of diet was without significant effect on swimming performance. In contrast to findings in the guinea pig, weanling rats fed purified rations containing wheat germ oil for 28 days did not swim longer than those fed diets containing corn oil.

wholly as a food. One report indicates that the WGO produces "hormone-like" effects in which the combs of chickens grow faster and the gonads increase in weight.[27]

It is interesting to see that some subjects are helped so much in endurance, or in tests which are correlated with endurance, whereas others are very little affected. This type of variation has been reported by Embden, Grafe and Schmitz[15] in their study of the effect of phosphoric acid upon muscular work capacity of their subjects, wherein subject *Schr.* made a clear-cut increase, whereas subject *Hoe.* did not. Such individual variations have also been shown by Droese[11] in his study of the effect of dextrose plus vitamin B_1, wherein it is explained that persons whose vitamin B_1 stores are adequate to handle extra sugar at high temperature differ from those whose vitamin stores are inadequate to handle the same sugar. In our own work in Susic's[35] experiment in which men were trained for ten weeks on a hard endurance-type program, one subject, W.S., of slight body build improved from 13.35 to 13.85 mm in the ECG T-wave (CR_{IV-V} lead) but after administration of WGO for the last six weeks of the experiment raised this measure to 22.65 mm. This gain is not only contrary to what occurs in hard training as a number of our subjects have shown staleness and lost amplitude in that state, but the amount of the gain is not paralleled in ordinary training experiments to our knowledge. In this same experiment, subject H.C., of excellent athletic build, changed from 9.00 mm in the ten weeks of preliminary training, to 10.75 mm, then after six weeks of taking the WGO, measured 10.35 mm, showing practically no effect. Such individual differences force the study of each and every case.

It is clear in our work that the men who began their training in the experiment at a high level of physical fitness, brought about by previous training, did not improve as much in the continued training. A man like our subject *Rae* even lost a bit, probably owing to overtraining. These individual variations complicate the experiment. It is impossible to know the exact level of need or tolerance for WGO and to start all men from the same relative level. As long as we take a random sample of men from all walks of life great differences will be found in the way they respond. In the light of this, the group mean differences are seen to be minimized results. Any average which includes some men who cannot respond will lower the level of response for some who had a great need or who were able to utilize and respond to the effects of WGO. We came to the computation of significance for change in each and every subject.

Table LIX shows an example of the results of such work but even this table does not show what happened in detail to every man. The basic data are not published but they are on file in our department—data which show the changes for each man in detail. These are the data which seem to us to be most valuable. We have no better way than trying each man to see if he will respond to the WGO after a period of training long enough to have the plateau established. While changes of significance are shown for the group data in treadmill-run time, brachial pulse wave, combined light and sound vertical jump reaction time, T-wave of the ECG, systolic blood pressure, and Schneider index, some individuals are strongly affected while others are not. Trends in the right direction for improvement are shown in basal metabolism (to raise it), in reaction to light and sound signals in the total body reaction time test, and in several of the combination cardiovascular tests like the Barach index. Several of these latter items are not reported in full.

Two other effects seem of importance. One of these is to note the effect of wheat germ or WGO on a group of men who have been relatively confined and who are not in good condition for endurance or cardiovascular condition. One such group of workers were studied who were employed in an automobile plant. We used them as a group of controls. It was a mistake not to match them carefully with our experimental groups because they made significant improvements in heartograph area and amplitude, all of the reaction times, and in some of the other quiet cardiovascular tests when put on WGO or wheat germ supplementation, but they did not improve in the treadmill run. The nutritive supplements appear to be helpful to the cardiovascular measures and neurological speed but these phases must be studied more carefully.

Workers in physical fitness (physical education, performance physiology, and sports medicine) have long striven to discover food supplements which will increase physical performance. Long documentary reviews of this line of research have been provided by Hellebrandt and Karpovich,[18] P. V. Karpovich,[23] Austin Henschel[20, 21] and Ancel Keys.[25] While a few studies using performance criteria have been reported in the literature,* we do not seem to find a study which has shown the effects in a parallel way in both the willpower exertions (treadmill run) and the naive tests (brachial pulse wave and T-wave). It seems very important to have both sets of tests in any such experiment.

Few studies have produced favorable evidence for improved physical performance which has remained uncontradicted, holding in mind the studies of vitamin B_1,[10, 11, 20, 21, 22, 23] B-complex,[14] B_{12},[30] the gelatin studies,[24, 27] alcohol,[1] caffeine,[16] the basic (alkaline) diets,[10] and ascorbic acid.[30] However, a fault seems to be present in most of these feeding experiments, namely, too short a time for the dietary supplement to act. In some studies, only two or three days have been allowed;[23] in others, as long as a week;[23] and only five to six weeks in important United States Army ration studies.[26] We also believe that the mixing of WGO with other types of food in the stomach may minimize its utilization or destroy some of its value. To feed it on an empty stomach just before or just after exercise seems to increase its effect as borne out in our own experiments.

CONCLUSIONS

The following conclusions have been drawn for the work reported:

Wheat germ oil (WGO) was found to be a valuable food supplement which helped the endurance of middle-aged men to run the all-out treadmill-run test, and produced significant gains over a matched group which took the same course of conditioning exercises for eight weeks.

The significant gains in running endurance were paralleled by significant gains in nonwillpower (naive) tests, such as: the brachial pulse wave of the upper arm (heartograph area and

---

* See references: 1, 2, 10, 11, 14, 15, 16, 22, 24, 26, 30, 31.

systolic amplitude), the T-wave (CR_{IV-V} lead) of the ECG, systolic blood pressure (to lower it) and the Schneider index. These appear to be important cardiovascular effects.

Significant gains have been found in the speed reaction of the total body (using the Illinois total body reaction time test), and near significant findings on light and sound reactions which are in the right direction and favor the groups which have taken WGO.

Trends for the basal metabolic rate to rise (oxygen consumption tests) are noted which are more attributable to the type of exercise taken as shown in other experiments in our series. WGO did not depress the BMR as much as vitamin E is known to do but produced a slight relative rise. The group on exercise and swimming with placeboes of devitaminized lard raised the BMR about 11 per cent in per cent BMR units, equivalent to 57.6 raw score per cent, whereas the control groups changed very slightly or not at all.

Individual sensitivity to WGO enforces the recognition of studying the reactions case by case rather than wholly in terms of group mean changes. These computations, using standards for significance for each individual change, in relation to the standard errors of measurement ($s\sqrt{2}$), show significant gains for the subjects on WGO in all-out treadmill running as well as in the nonperformance tests of cardiovascular condition.

REFERENCES

1. Asmussen, E. and Böje, O.: The effect of alcohol and some drugs on the capacity for work, *Acta Physiol. Scand.*, 15:109, 1948.
2. Barborka, B. J., Foltz, E. E. and Ivy, A. C.: Relationship between vitamin B-complex intake and work output in trained subjects, *J.A.M.A.*, 122:717-720, July 10, 1943.
3. Cureton, T. K.: Effect of wheat germ oil and vitamin E on normal human subjects in physical training programs, *Amer. J. Physiol.*, 179:628, Dec., 1954.
4. Cureton, T. K.: Exercise, wheat germ oil for middle aged men, *Science News Letter*, 66:216, Oct. 2, 1954.
5. Cureton, T. K.: Wheat germ oil, the wonder fuel, *Scholastic Coach*, 24:36-37, 67-68, March, 1955.
6. Cureton, T. K.: *Physical Fitness of Champion Athletes*. Treadmill tests of maximal physical efficiency. Urbana, University of Illinois Press, 1951, pp. 314-350.

7. Cureton, T. K.: *Ibid.*, pp. 228-254: The Brachial Pulse Wave of Cardio-vascular Condition.

8. Cureton, T. K.: *Ibid.*, pp. 94-102: Vertical Jump Reaction Times of Champion Athletes.

9. Cureton, T. K.: Review of research to determine cardiovascular condition (1941-1950), *Proc. Amer. Ass. Health* (56th National Convention, Detroit, Research Section), pp. 167-177, Washington, D. C. The Association, 1201 Sixteenth St., N.W., 1951.

10. Cureton, T. K.: Diet related to success in competitive swimming, *Beach and Pool*, 7:335, Nov., 1933; also, 8:10, Jan., 1934.

11. Droese, W.: Die Hebung der Leistungfahigkeit Durch B_1 und die Erkennung Einer B_1-Hypovitaminose, *Arbeitsphysiologie*, 11:338-360, 1941.

12. Dupain, G. Z.: Specific diets and athletic performance, *Res. Quart.*, 10:33-40 (Dec. 1939).

13. Editorial: "Care and Feeding of Athletes," *Newsweek*, p. 102 (Mar. 23, 1953).

14. Eganā, E., Johnson, R. E., Bloomfield, E., Brouha, L., Meikeljohn, A. P., Tittenberger, J., Darling, R. C., Heath, C., Graybiel, A. and Consolazio, F.: The effects of diet deficient in the vitamin B-complex on sedentery men, *Amer. J. Physiol.*, 137:731, 1942.

15. Embden, Gustav, Grafe, Edward and Schmitz, Ernst: About the increase in productivity through phosphate supply, *Zeitschrift für Physiologische Chemie*, 113:67-107, 1921.

16. Foltz, E. E., Ivy, A. C. and Barborka, B. J.: The use of double work periods in the study of fatigue and the influence of caffeine on recovery, *Amer. J. Physiol.*, 136:79-85, March, 1942.

17. Forr, W. A.: *The Effect of Wheat Germ Oil and Vitamin E on Physical Fitness*, unpublished M.S. thesis, Physical Education, University of Illinois, 1950, 92 pp.

18. Hellebrandt, F. A. and Karpovich, P. V.: Fitness, fatigue and recuperation, *War Medicine*, 1:745-768, Nov., 1941.

20. Henry, F. M.: Influence of athletic training on the resting cardiovascular system, *Res. Quart.* 25:28-41, March, 1954.

20. Henschel, Austin: Diet and muscular fatigue, *Res. Quart.* 8:280-285, Oct., 1942.

21. Henschel, Austin: Vitamins and physical performance, *The Journal-Lancet* (Minneapolis), 63:355-357, Nov., 1943.

22. Karpovich, P. V. and Millman, N.: Vitamin B_1 and physical endurance, *New Eng. J. Med.*, 226:881-882, May 28, 1942.

23. Karpovich, P. V.: Ergogenic aids in work and sport, *Supp. Res. Quart.*, 12:432-450, May, 1941.

24. Kaczmarek, R. M.: Effect of gelatin on the work output of male athletes, non athletes and girl subjects, *Res. Quart.*, 11:109-119, Dec., 1940.

25. Keys, Ancel: Physical performance in relation to diet, *Fed. Proc.*, 2:164-187, Sept., 1943.

26. Keys, Ancel and Henschel, A. F.: Vitamin supplementation of U. S. Army rations in relation to fatigue and the ability to do muscular work, *J. Nutr.*, 23:259-269, March, 1942.

27. Levin, Ezra, Burns, John F. and Collins, V. K.: Estrogenic, androgenic and gonandotrophic activity in wheat germ oil, *Endocrinology*, 49:289-301, Sept., 1951.

28. Marx, Elizer I.: *The Effect of a Dietary Supplement on Varsity Swimmers*, unpublished M.S. thesis, Physical Education, University of Illinois, 1952, 40 pp.

29. Massey, B. H.: *Prediction of All-Out Treadmill Running from Electrocardiograph Measurements*, unpublished M.S. thesis, Physical Education, University of Illinois, 1947, 102 pp.

30. Montoye, H. J., Spata, P. J., Pinckney, Virgil and Brown, L.: Effects of vitamin B_{12} supplementation on physical fitness and growth of young boys, *J. Appl. Physiol.*, 7:589-592, May, 1955.

31. Robinson, S. and Harmon, P. M.: Effects of training and of gelatin on muscular work, *Amer. J. Physiol.*, 133:161-169, May, 1941.

32. Smiley, William A.: *Variation in a Bicycle Ergometer Test Due to Physical Training and a Dietary Supplement*, unpublished M.S. thesis, Physical Education, University of Illinois, 1951, 91 pp.

33. Staton, Wesley M.: The influence of ascorbic acid in minimizing post-exercise muscle soreness in young men, *Res. Quart.*, 23:356-360, Oct., 1952.

34. Storm, Walter N.: *The Effects of Training and a Dietary Supplement on Muscle Symmetry and Fat Distribution of Adult Males*, unpublished M.S. thesis, Physical Education, University of Illinois, 1952, 43 pp.

35. Susic, S.: *Effect of Training and a Dietary Supplement on the T-wave of the Electrocardiogram at Ground Level and at 10,000 Feet Simulated Altitude*, unpublished M.S. thesis, Physical Education, University of Illinois, 1953, 55 pp.

36. Vohaska, William J.: *The Effects of Wheat Germ Oil on the Cardiovascular Fitness of Varsity Wrestlers*, unpublished M.S. thesis, Physical Education, University of Illinois, 1952, 43 pp.

37. White, C. H.: *The Effect of Physical Training and a Dietary Supplement on the Schneider Index at Ground Level and at 10,000 Feet Simulated Altitude*, unpublished M.S. thesis, Physical Education, University of Illinois, 1951, 96 pp.

38. Willet, Albert E.: *The Prediction of Treadmill Running from Heartometer Measurements*, unpublished M.S. thesis, Physical Education, University of Illinois, 1948, 73 pp.
Electrocardiogram, *Res. Quart.*, 24:475-490, Dec., 1953.

39. Wolf, J. Grove: Effects of Posture and Muscular Exercise on the Electrocardiogram, *Res. Quart.*, 24:475-490, 24:475-490, Dec., 1953.

Experiment 14

The Effects of Dietary Supplements (WGO) and Various Athletic Programs Upon Strength

THEODORE W. CONNER[*]

PURPOSE

THE purpose of this experiment was to see if dietary supplements of VioBin wheat germ oil, octacosanol or Kretchmer wheat germ added to the daily diet will improve strength; and also to observe the differential value of four physical activity programs upon young boys.

RESEARCH METHODS

The study was carried out on four groups of boys, 7-13 years of age, inclusively, who were normal participants in the Sports Fitness School of the University of Illinois (part of the summer session for eight weeks). Sixty-eight boys were available for the study. The first and last weeks were used for testing, in which dynamometer strength was part of the total program of testing required. The six weeks in-between the T_1 and T_2 testing periods were used for exercising the boys and also instructing them in basic gymnastics, swimming, track and field and team games. In addition to these activities, a fifty-minute period was available four afternoons per week (Monday, Tuesday, Wednesday and Thursday) from 4:00 PM to 4:50 PM for *endurance work*. It was this last period of hard work, continuous for thirty minutes at least, which was utilized for this experiment, in the summer of 1957.

The strength tests were the usual dynamometer strengths of hand grips (right and left), back lift and leg press, administered by experienced examiners. The techniques and equipment are de-

---

[*] Urbana, M.S. thesis, Physical Education, University of Illinois, 1958, p. 53. (Sponsor: T. K. Cureton.)

374

scribed in Cureton's *Physical Fitness Appraisal and Guidance* and in his *Physical Fitness Workbook* (3rd ed.).

The boys were classified into four groups according to paired matching in groups of four, by age, weight and strength, using an empirical system from the heaviest and strongest four to the weakest four, then randomly the boys were alternately assigned with systematic reversal of order until all four groups were established. The 600-yard run was also run in the pre-experiment period. Then each group was led by an instructor in the particular activity drawn by the group by random draw, and the group continued on that particular activity throughout the six week program until they were finally tested. The four groups were classified as: a) circuit training—running 220 yards and then doing a muscular exercise (as demonstrated by the instructor: push-ups, sit-ups, side leg-raisings, V-sit, etc.) continuing the entire thirty minutes with this alternation, b) muscular endurance exercises—as led by an instructor: running in place, all of the ones mentioned in (a) and lifting the body in various ways repetitiously, c) interval training—consisted of running 440 yards, walking 600 yards, and repeating this the entire period, d) steeplechase—following a leader over various obstacles, jumping, climbing, dodging and continuous running for the thirty minutes.

MATERIALS FED

The supplements taken in a brief rest period at 3:15 PM were labelled red, white, blue and green. What the capsules contained was not explained except that it was "vitaminization." After all testing was done, the code was broken—red was Kretchmer wheat germ (1.5 oz. per day), white was VioBin WGO capsules, blue was octacosanol crystals (VioBin) and the green was lecithin oil capsules. The boys took 15×3 capsules in three groups and one group took the 1½ oz. of wheat germ in paper cups, mixed and washed down with ½ pint of 2 per cent of fat milk. All boys in all groups used the milk.

RESULTS

The results are shown in Tables LXI, LXII, LXIII, and LXVI, for the strength tests, which also show how the boys were grouped.

Table LXIV shows the groupings by *total proportional strength* (the sum of the four tests) and Table LXV shows the same test results and groupings for *strength body weight* (1 lb/lb). The t test was used to test the differences between T_1 and T_2 for each of the strength tests, and also each of the programs of conditioning: all t's were statistically insignificant for hand grip strengths, right and left; but amongst the four physical conditioning methods, the only groups to show statistical significance were the muscular endurance group (left hand only), t = 2.14 (significance .05 level); back strength in the steeplechase group ($t =$ 2.49, significance at .05 level).

All results for the dietary supplement groups were statistically insignificant except the placebo group (lecithin oil) where the right hand grip improved from 33.44 to 40.38 SS, a difference of 6.94 SS ($t = 2.54$, significance at .05 level); also, the octacosanol group improved significantly in the leg strength ($t = 2.22$); and the wheat germ group improved significantly on the back lift ($t = 2.39$).

DISCUSSION

More cases were needed in this study but all were used who were available and could be controlled. The octacosanol fed group improved relatively more on the leg strength, back strength and strength per pound of body weight. The Kretchmer wheat germ group made the greatest improvements in the left grip strength and in total strength.

Some interference resulted from two broken arms in the high jumping practice and four boys could not complete the tests. This produced slight irregularities in the matching of the groups and imbalanced the numbers.

TABLE LX
RIGHT-HAND TABULATION SHEET
Raw Scores

Circuit	T_1	T_2	M. Endurance	T_1	T_2	Interval	T_1	T_2	Steeple	T_1	T_2		T_1	T_2
Wheat Germ														
P.T.	34	34	S.F.	26	27	K.K.	25	27	J.D.	30	38	Total	513	582
F.E.	16	16	J.S.	28	21	L.S.	45	38	J.H.	26	40	M	28.50	32.33
C.H.	28	29	G.S.	Incomplete		J.C.	12	13	T.S.	48	39	σ		11.01
M.B.	26	30	L.S.	36	48	C.D.	30	20	J.D.	30	58			
D.F.	8	12	K.C.	25	56	T.S.	40	36	J.S.	42	42			
W. G. Oil														
R.B.	50	45	T.F.	54	64	R.B.	20	31	T.B.	16	29	Total	488	525
C.T.	34	20	M.P.	40	32	M.N.	32	25	C.D.	Broken arm		M	30.50	32.18
B.L.	18	22	J.M.	26	30	D.H.	42	41	D.W.	29	34	σ		7.93
D.K.	28	28	W.S.	14	30	G.H.	20	22	D.E.	23	30			
S.R.	Incomplete													
Octacosanol														
J.T.	40	42	S.B.	37	34	T.M.	30	36	A.H.	Broken arm		Total	522	542
R.G.	22	23	R.G.	25	32	H.S.	16	24	S.S.	24	27	M	29.00	30.11
R.K.	28	22	D.H.	10	16	R.C.	16	16	J.S.	52	32	σ		7.91
G.G.	22	32	R.F.	20	22	D.S.	26	34	R.G.	38	30			
			J.S.	30	18	D.H.	16	28	T.H.	70	74			
Placeboes														
P.B.	Incomplete		J.K.	32	41	E.Y.	30	31	D.T.	30	36	Total	496	563
P.K.	26	32	D.C.	32	40	M.J.	16	25	J.G.	32	27	M	31.00	35.19
B.W.	36	36	C.S.	32	30	R.R.	22	32	W.A.	26	30	σ		4.30
S.H.	12	26	E.F.	42	38	B.H.	32	31	C.H.	38	42			
R.S.	58	66							B.C.	Incomplete				
Total	486	515	Total	509	579	Total	470	510	Total	554	608			
M	28.59	30.29	M	29.94	34.06	M	26.11	28.33	M	34.63	38.00			
σ	6.22		σ	10.02		σ	6.44		σ	10.75				

TABLE LXI

LEFT HAND TABULATION SHEET

Raw Scores

	Circuit			M. Endurance			Interval			Steeple					
	T_1	T_2		T_1	T_2		T_1	T_2		T_1	T_2			T_1	T_2
Wheat Germ															
P.T.	34	32	S.F.	25	34	K.K.	30	28	J.D.	26	40	Total		454	519
F.E.	14	16	J.S.	20	22	L.S.	40	38	J.H.	21	33	M		25.22	28.83
C.H.	28	17	G.S.	Incomplete		J.C.	14	13	T.S.	48	40	σ			8.44
M.B.	28	31	L.S.	33	35	C.D.	10	18	J.D.	20	38				
D.F.	9	10	K.C.	24	46	T.S.	30	28							
W. G. Oil															
E.B.	38	38	T.F.	51	65	R.E.	22	23	J.S.	40	32	Total		452	489
F.E.	34	24	R.G.	40	25	M.M.	36	24	T.B.	22	21	M		28.25	30.56
C.H.	16	20	J.M.	20	30	D.H.	44	41	G.D.	Broken arm		σ			9.73
M.B.	20	18	W.S.	24	34	G.H.	12	22	D.W.	19	30				
S.R.	Incomplete								D.E.	14	32				
Octacosanol															
J.T.	35	35	S.B.	37	36	T.H.	38	32	A.H.	Broken arm		Total		505	495
R.G.	24	21	R.O.	20	36	H.S.	16	26	S.S.	22	23	M		28.06	27.50
R.K.	34	20	D.H.	16	14	R.C.	16	18	J.S.	38	28	σ			7.58
G.G.	18	28	R.F.	17	20	D.S.	28	26	R.C.	38	29				
			J.S.	24	13	D.H.	20	24	T.K.	64	66				
Placeboes															
P.B.	Incomplete		J.K.	36	39	E.Y.	27	26	D.T.	34	32	Total		487	498
P.K.	30	29	D.C.	26	44	H.J.	19	25	J.G.	34	22	M		30.44	31.13
B.W.	30	30	C.S.	30	32	R.R.	17	20	W.A.	26	24	σ			8.30
S.H.	10	18	E.F.	40	37	B.H.	30	45	C.H.	42	28				
R.S.	56	47							B.C.	Incomplete					
Total	458	434	Total	483	562	Total	449	487	Total	508	518				
M	26.94	25.53	M	28.41	33.06	M	24.94	27.06	M	31.76	32.38				
σ		6.31	σ		9.59	σ		6.67	σ		10.59				

TABLE LXII
LEGS TABULATION SHEET
Raw Scores

	Circuit T_1	T_2		M. Endurance T_1	T_2		Interval T_1	T_2		Steeple T_1	T_2		T_1	T_2
Wheat Germ														
P.T.	190	193	S.F.	145	168	K.K.	255	212	J.D.	170	255	Total	3,472	3,554
F.E.	80	140	J.S.	203	232	L.S.	288	310	J.H.	270	213	M	198.89	197.44
C.H.	165	152	G.S.	Incomplete		J.C.	150	133	T.S.	278	250			
H.B.	230	238	L.S.	240	198	C.D.	108	80	J.D.	170	276	σ	44.77	
D.F.	88	100	K.C.	272	215	T.S.	170	190						
W. G. Oil														
R.B.	290	199	T.F.	318	302	R.E.	260	225	T.S.	182	135	Total	2,953	2,651
C.T.	132	140	M.P.	225	212	M.M.	120	125	T.B.	120	88	M	184.56	165.69
B.L.	92	90	J.H.	218	162	D.H.	307	273	G.D.		Broken arm			
D.K.	133	110	W.S.	142	195	G.M.	70	150	D.W.	114	150	σ	50.68	
S.R.	Incomplete								D.E.	230	540			
Octacosanol														
J.T.	220	205	S.B.	175	230	T.M.	200	172	A.H.		Broken arm	Total	2,930	3,208
R.G.	175	190	R.C.	70	145	H.S.	122	85	S.S.	180	233	M	162.78	178.22
R.K.	110	168	D.H.	170	130	R.C.	160	150	J.S.	200	190			
G.G.	60	90	R.F.	150	140	D.S.	90	150	R.G.	170	155	σ	36.03	
			J.S.	90	130	D.H.	98	105	T.H.	490	540			
Placeboes														
P.B.	Incomplete		J.K.	233	258	E.Y.	250	208	D.T.	270	208	Total	3,099	3,065
P.K.	90	168	D.C.	220	340	H.J.	70	95	J.G.	230	170	M	193.69	191.56
B.W.	210	173	C.S.	272	168	R.R.	72	70	W.A.	130	155			
S.H.	120	145	E.F.	363	232	B.N.	228	300	C.H.	150	115	σ	67.38	
R.S.	191	260							B.G.	Incomplete				
Total	2,576	2,761	Total	3,506	3,457	Total	3,018	3,033	Total	3,354	3,227			
M	151.53	162.41	M	206.24	203.35	M	167.67	168.50	M	209.63	201.69			
σ	40.86		σ	63.04		σ	48.06		σ	59.53				

TABLE LXIII
BACK TABULATION SHEET
Raw Scores

Circuit			M. Endurance			Interval			Steeple				T_1	T_2
	T_1	T_2		T_1	T_2		T_1	T_2		T_1	T_2			
Wheat Germ														
P.T.	160	168	S.F.	108	98	K.K.	160	138	J.D.	152	135	Total	2,598	2,352
F.E.	100	70	J.S.	130	112	L.S.	200	211	J.H.	190	153	M	144.33	130.67
C.H.	115	155	G.S.	Incomplete		J.C.	73	75	T.S.	185	168	σ	21.04	
N.B.	65	60	L.S.	180	193	C.D.	110	45	J.D.	160	140			
D.F.	170	135	K.C.	190	172	T.S.	150	125						
W. G. Oil														
R.B.	220	165	T.F.	272	212	R.E.	160	118	J.S.	183	175	Total	2,237	2,134
C.T.	75	80	J.P.	170	182	M.M.	142	140	T.B.	105	70	M	139.81	133.38
B.L.	92	80	J.M.	118	100	D.H.	198	245	G.D.	Broken arm		σ	33.56	
D.K.	85	100	W.S.	90	130	G.M.	70	100	D.W.	117	147			
S.R.	Incomplete								D.E.	140	90			
Octacosanol														
J.T.	172	138	S.B.	228	200	T.M.	130	150	A.H.	Broken arm		Total	2,320	2,307
R.G.	145	112	R.C.	70	122	R.S.	100	100	S.S.	150	128	M	128.89	128.17
R.K.	100	92	D.H.	90	100	R.C.	100	120	J.S.	175	220	σ	36.15	
G.C.	80	70	R.F.	100	90	D.S.	80	120	R.G.	140	125			
			J.S.	70	110	D.H.	60	80	T.H.	330	230			
Placeboes														
P.B.	Incomplete		J.K.	163	173	E.Y.	150	160	D.T.	170	105	Total	2,245	2,255
P.K.	90	105	D.C.	170	168	M.J.	50	68	J.C.	200	125	M	140.31	140.94
B.W.	150	135	C.S.	160	178	R.R.	80	90	W.A.	115	110	σ	31.38	
S.H.	70	90	E.F.	240	230	B.N.	130	168	C.H.	125	130			
R.S.	182	220							B.C.	Incomplete				
Total	2,071	1,957	Total	2,549	2,569	Total	2,143	2,253	Total	2,637	2,251			
M	121.82	115.12	M	149.94	151.11	M	119.06	125.17	M	164.82	140.69			
σ	27.81		σ	26.96		σ	27.11		σ	35.60				

TABLE LXIV
TOTAL TABULATION SHEET
Raw Scores

	Circuit			M. Endurance			Interval			Steeple				
	T_1	T_2		T_1	T_2		T_1	T_2		T_1	T_2		T_1	T_2
Wheat Germ														
P.T.	318	427	S.F.	304	327	K.K.	470	405	J.D.	378	468	Total	6,801	7,007
F.E.	210	242	J.S.	381	387	L.S.	573	597	J.H.	507	439	M	377.83	389.28
C.H.	336	353	G.S.	Incomplete		J.G.	249	234	T.S.	423	497			
N.B.	454	434	L.S.	489	473	C.D.	258	163	J.D.	380	511	σ	58.78	
D.F.	170	182	K.C.	511	489	T.S.	390	379						
W. G. Oil														
R.B.	598	447	T.F.	595	643	R.E.	462	407	J.S.	447	384	Total	6,050	5,823
C.T.	275	264	M.P.	495	451	M.M.	330	314	T.B.	263	228	M	378.13	363.94
B.L.	218	212	J.M.	382	322	D.H.	591	600	G.D.	Broken arm				
D.K.	266	256	W.S.	270	389	G.M.	172	298	D.W.	279	361	σ	78.49	
S.R.	Incomplete								D.E.	407	247			
Octacosanol														
J.T.	467	420	S.B.	477	500	T.M.	398	390	A.H.	Broken arm		Total	6,267	6,452
R.G.	366	346	R.G.	185	335	H.S.	254	235	S.S.	376	411	M	348.17	358.44
R.K.	272	302	D.H.	286	260	R.C.	292	304	J.S.	465	470			
G.G.	180	220	R.F.	277	272	D.S.	224	330	R.G.	386	339	σ	51.55	
			J.S.	214	171	D.H.	194	237	T.H.	954	910			
Placeboes														
P.B.	Incomplete		J.K.	464	511	E.Y.	457	435	D.T.	504	381	Total	6,317	6,321
P.K.	246	334	D.C.	448	592	M.J.	155	213	J.G.	496	344	M	394.81	395.06
B.W.	426	374	C.S.	494	408	R.R.	191	212	W.A.	297	319			
S.H.	212	279	E.F.	685	537	B.N.	420	544	C.H.	335	315	σ	89.31	
R.S.	487	533							B.C.	Incomplete				
Total	5,501	5,625	Total	6,957	7,067	Total	6,080	6,287	Total	6,897	6,624			
M	323.59	330.88	M	409.24	415.71	M	337.78	349.28	M	431.06	414.00			
σ	58.93		σ	76.85		σ	60.04		σ	83.94				

TABLE LXV

STRENGTH PER POUND OF BODY WEIGHT TABULATION SHEET

Raw Scores

	Circuit T₁	Circuit T₂		M. Endurance T₁	M. Endurance T₂		Interval T₁	Interval T₂		Steeple T₁	Steeple T₂		Total T₁	Total T₂
Wheat Germ														
P.T. 3.88 5.34			S.F. 5.80 5.43			K.K. 6.56 5.66			J.D. 4.65 5.87					
F.E. 4.04 4.67			J.S. 6.20 5.66			L.S. 5.24 5.40			J.H. 5.07 4.48					
C.H. 4.80 5.08			G.S. Incomplete			J.C. 4.17 4.85			T.S. 3.88 4.69					
M.B. 7.12 6.70			L.S. 5.12 4.97			C.D. 4.70 3.00			J.D. 3.44 4.72					
D.F. 3.86 4.12			K.C. 6.33 9.98			T.S. 3.73 3.54								
Total 85.59 90.16 M 4.92 5.01 σ .81														
W. G. Oil														
R.B. 5.98 4.30			T.F. 5.96 6.40			R.E. 5.15 4.52			J.S. 5.38 4.74					
C.T. 4.67 4.66			M.P. 5.03 4.71			M.M. 5.05 4.91			T.B. 4.78 4.15					
B.L. 3.01 2.97			J.M. 6.11 5.20			D.H. 5.91 6.01			G.D. Broken arm					
D.K. 3.00 3.82			W.S. 3.16 4.10			G.M. 2.61 4.66			D.W. 3.96 5.12					
S.R. Incomplete									D.E. 6.49 3.93					
Total 76.25 74.20 M 4.77 4.64 σ 1.08														
Octacosanol														
J.T. 5.42 4.85			S.B. 6.12 6.36			T.M. 5.38 5.31			A.H. Broken arm					
R.G. 5.70 5.32			R.G. 3.03 5.36			H.S. 4.67 4.28			S.S. 5.29 5.68					
R.K. 4.18 4.53			D.H. 4.70 4.37			R.C. 5.58 5.85			J.S. 4.93 4.02					
G.G. 2.85 3.45			R.F. 3.85 3.75			D.S. 3.50 5.24			R.G. 5.07 4.40					
			J.S. 3.43 4.51			D.H. 3.66 4.45			T.H. 7.59 7.55					
Total 84.95 89.28 M 4.72 4.96 σ .82														
Placeboes														
P.B. Incomplete			J.K. 5.50 6.11			E.Y. 6.34 5.59			D.T. 6.47 4.89					
P.K. 3.91 5.32			D.C. 5.06 8.11			M.J. 3.19 4.35			J.C. 5.84 4.07					
B.M. 5.91 5.19			C.S. 5.93 4.30			R.R. 3.30 3.80			W.A. 3.93 4.39					
S.H. 3.85 5.00			E.F. 4.90 3.81			B.H. 3.65 4.61			C.H. 3.45 3.44					
R.S. 3.24 3.34									B.C. Incomplete					
Total 74.47 76.32 M 4.65 4.77 σ 1.27														

Column totals:

	Circuit	M. Endurance	Interval	Steeple
Total	74.42 78.66	86.23 89.13	82.39 86.03	80.22 76.14
M	4.44 4.63	5.07 5.24	4.58 4.78	5.03 4.76
σ	.79	1.15	.92	1.10

TABLE LXVI

RIGHT-HAND TABULATION SHEET

Standard Scores

	Circuit			M. Endurance			Interval			Steeple			Total	
		T₁	T₂		T₁	T₂		T₁	T₂		T₁	T₂		T₁	T₂
Wheat Germ															
	P.T.	39	39	S.F.	25	26	K.K.	24	26	J.D.	32	45	Total	534	641
	F.E.	9	9	J.S.	29	16	L.S.	56	45	J.H.	25	49	M	29.67	35.61
	C.N.	29	30	G.S.	Incomplete		J.C.	1	4	T.S.	62	46	σ	19.38	
	M.B.	25	31	L.S.	46	62	C.D.	31	15	J.D.	32	79			
	D.F.	0	1	K.C.	24	75	T.S.	49	43						
W. G. Oil															
	R.B.	65	56	T.F.	72	89	R.E.	15	34	J.S.	52	52	Total	523	586
	C.T.	39	15	M.P.	49	35	M.M.	35	24	T.B.	9	30	M	32.69	36.63
	B.L.	11	19	J.M.	25	32	D.H.	52	50	G.D.	Broken arm		σ	13.37	
	D.K.	29	29	W.S.	5	31	G.M.	15	19	D.W.	30	39			
	S.R.	Incomplete								D.E.	20	32			
Octacosanol															
	J.T.	49	52	S.B.	43	39	T.M.	31	42	A.H.	Broken arm		Total	545	572
	R.G.	18	20	R.G.	24	35	H.S.	9	21	S.S.	22	27	M	30.28	31.78
	R.K.	29	19	D.H.	0	9	R.C.	9	9	J.S.	69	35	σ	13.17	
	G.G.	18	35	R.F.	15	19	D.S.	25	38	R.G.	45	32			
				J.S.	32	12	D.H.	9	28	T.H.	98	100			
Placeboes															
	P.B.	Incomplete		J.K.	35	50	E.Y.	31	33	D.T.	32	42	Total	535	646
	P.K.	25	35	D.C.	35	49	M.J.	9	24	J.G.	35	26	M	33.44	40.38
	B.W.	41	41	C.S.	35	31	R.R.	19	35	W.A.	25	32	σ	8.94	
	S.H.	2	25	E.F.	52	45	B.N.	35	34	C.H.	45	52			
	R.S.	79	92							B.G.	Incomplete				
	Total	507	548	Total	542	655	Total	455	524	Total	633	718			
	M	29.82	32.24	M	31.88	38.53	M	25.28	29.11	M	39.56	44.88			
	σ	10.46		σ	17.87		σ	10.36		σ	15.92				

TABLE LXVII

LEFT-HAND TABULATION SHEET—STANDARD SCORES

	Circuit			M. Endurance			Interval			Steeple			Total	
	T_1	T_2		T_1	T_2		T_1	T_2		T_1	T_2		T_1	T_2
Wheat Germ														
P.T.	52	48	S.F.	38	52	K.K.	45	42	J.D.	40	60	Total	702	797
F.E.	23	26	J.S.	32	35	L.S.	60	58	J.H.	33	50	M	39.00	44.28
C.H.	43	28	G.S.	Incomplete		J.C.	22	21	T.S.	72	60	σ	12.17	
M.B.	43	48	L.S.	50	53	C.D.	18	29	J.D.	32	58			
D.F.	17	18	K.C.	37	69	T.S.	45	42						
W. G. Oil														
R.B.	58	58	T.F.	76	96	R.E.	35	50	J.S.	60	49	Total	696	750
C.T.	52	37	M.P.	60	39	M.M.	55	38	T.B.	35	33	M	43.50	46.88
B.L.	26	32	J.H.	32	46	D.H.	66	61	C.D.	Broken arm		σ	14.19	
D.K.	32	29	W.S.	37	52	G.M.	20	35	D.W.	30	46			
S.R.	Incomplete								D.E.	22	49			
Octacosanol														
J.T.	53	53	S.B.	56	55	T.H.	56	49	A.H.	Broken arm		Total	767	766
R.G.	37	33	R.G.	32	55	H.S.	26	40	S.S.	34	35	M	42.61	42.55
R.K.	52	32	D.H.	26	23	R.C.	26	29	J.S.	58	44	σ	11.31	
G.G.	29	43	R.F.	17	32	D.S.	42	40	R.G.	58	45			
			J.S.	38	22	D.H.	32	38	T.H.	95	98			
Placeboes														
P.B.	Incomplete		J.K.	55	59	E.Y.	41	40	D.T.	52	49	Total	748	760
P.K.	46	46	D.C.	40	65	M.J.	30	39	J.G.	52	35	M	46.75	47.50
B.W.	18	29	C.S.	46	49	R.R.	28	31	W.A.	40	38	σ	11.87	
S.H.	84	70	E.F.	60	56	B.N.	47	68	C.H.	63	42			
R.S.	46	44							B.C.	Incomplete				
Total	711	674	Total	732	858	Total	694	750	Total	776	791			
M	41.82	39.59	M	43.12	50.47	M	38.56	41.67	M	48.50	49.44			
σ	8.41		σ	13.83		σ	9.31		σ	15.22				

TABLE LXVIII

LEG STRENGTH TABULATION SHEET—STANDARD SCORES

Circuit			M. Endurance			Interval			Steeple			Total		
	T_1	T_2		T_1	T_2		T_1	T_2		T_1	T_2		T_1	T_2
Wheat Germ														
P.T.	54	55	S.F.	38	46	K.K.	77	62	J.D.	47	77	Total	990	1,019
F.H.	15	36	J.S.	59	69	L.S.	88	97	J.H.	83	62	M	55.00	56.61
C.H.	45	41	G.S.	Incomplete		J.C.	40	34	T.S.	84	76	σ	15.76	
P.M.	69	71	L.S.	72	57	C.D.	24	14	J.D.	47	84			
D.F.	18	22	K.C.	83	63	T.S.	47	53						
W. G. Oil														
R.B.	90	57	T.F.	99	94	R.E.	78	66	J.S.	51	34	Total	883	722
C.T.	34	36	M.F.	67	62	M.M.	29	31	T.B.	29	18	M	52.06	45.13
B.L.	19	18	J.M.	64	44	D.H.	96	83	G.D.	Broken arm		σ	17.90	
D.K.	34	26	W.S.	37	55	G.M.	11	39	D.W.	27	39			
S.R.	Incomplete								D.E.	68	20			
Octacosanol														
J.T.	65	60	S.B.	49	68	T.M.	58	47	A.H.	Broken arm		Total	716	810
R.G.	49	54	R.G.	11	38	H.S.	29	16	S.S.	51	69	M	39.78	45.00
R.K.	26	46	D.H.	47	37	R.C.	43	39	J.S.	58	54	σ	11.88	
C.G.	8	18	R.F.	18	33	D.S.	18	39	R.G.	47	42			
			J.S.	18	32	D.K.	21	23	T.H.	100	100			
Placebos														
P.B.	Incomplete		J.K.	69	78	E.Y.	76	61	D.T.	83	61	Total	869	866
P.K.	18	46	D.C.	64	100	M.J.	11	20	J.G.	68	47	M	54.31	54.13
B.W.	61	48	C.S.	83	46	R.R.	12	11	W.A.	33	42	σ	21.49	
S.H.	29	38	E.F.	100	69	B.N.	68	93	C.H.	39	27			
R.S.	55	79							B.C.	Incomplete				
Total	689	751	Total	978	586	Total	826	828	Total	915	852			
M	40.52	44.18	M	56.47	56.12	M	45.89	46.00	M	57.19	53.25			
σ	14.49		σ	19.47		σ	14.26		σ	20.76				

TABLE LXIX

BACK STRENGTH TABULATION SHEET—STANDARD SCORES

Group		Circuit T_1	T_2		M. Endurance T_1	T_2		Interval T_1	T_2		Steeple T_1	T_2
Wheat Germ	P.T.	57	61	S.F.	30	25	K.K.	56	45	J.D.	53	44
	F.E.	26	12	J.S.	41	33	L.S.	76	82	J.H.	71	53
	C.H.	24	54	G.S.	Incomplete		J.C.	13	14	T.S.	69	60
	M.B.	61	44	L.S.	66	73	C.D.	32	0	J.D.	56	46
	D.F.	8	6	K.C.	71	63	T.S.	51	39			
W. G. Oil	B.R.	86	57	T.F.	100	83	R.E.	57	35	J.S.	67	64
	C.T.	13	14	M.P.	63	67	M.M.	43	42	T.B.	29	11
	B.L.	23	17	J.M.	35	26	D.H.	75	99	G.D.	Broken arm	
	D.K.	19	26	W.S.	21	41	G.M.	12	27	D.W.	35	50
	S.R.	Incomplete								D.E.	46	21
Octacosanol	J.T.	63	45	S.B.	90	77	T.M.	41	51	A.H.	Broken arm	
	R.G.	49	33	R.C.	11	37	H.S.	27	27	S.S.	51	40
	R.K.	26	23	D.H.	21	27	R.C.	27	36	J.S.	64	86
	C.C.	16	11	R.F.	27	21	D.S.	16	36	R.G.	46	39
				J.S.	11	32	D.H.	7	16	T.H.	100	91
Placeboes	P.R.	Incomplete		J.K.	57	63	E.Y.	51	56	D.T.	61	29
	P.K.	21	27	D.C.	62	60	M.J.	2	10	J.G.	76	39
	B.W.	51	44	C.S.	56	65	R.R.	16	21	W.A.	34	32
	S.H.	11	31	E.F.	91	97	B.N.	41	60	C.H.	39	41
	R.S.	67	86							B.C.	Incomplete	
	Total	631	751	Total	859	884	Total	643	696	Total	897	746
	M	37.12	34.18	M	50.53	52.00	M	35.72	38.67	M	56.06	46.63
	σ	12.94		σ	11.03		σ	14.13		σ	14.72	

TABLE LXX

TOTAL TABULATION SHEET—STANDARD SCORES

Wheat Germ

Circuit	T_1	T_2	M. Endurance	T_1	T_2	Interval	T_1	T_2	Steeple	T_1	T_2		T_1	T_2
P.T.	37	55	S.F.	34	37	K.K.	63	53	J.D.	47	63	Total	841	897
F.E.	17	23	J.S.	47	48	L.S.	81	85	J.H.	69	57	M	46.72	49.83
C.H.	40	43	G.S.	Incomplete		J.C.	25	39	T.S.	55	67	σ		10.33
M.B.	60	56	L.S.	66	64	C.D.	26	10	J.B.	47	70			
D.F.	8	14	K.C.	70	66	T.S.	49	47						
Total	633	658	Total	884	907	Total	721	762	Total	845	810			
M	37.42	38.71	M	52.00	53.35	M	40.06	42.33	M	52.81	50.63			
σ	10.42		σ	13.53		σ	9.81		σ	14.46				

W. G. Oil

Circuit	T_1	T_2	M. Endurance	T_1	T_2	Interval	T_1	T_2	Steeple	T_1	T_2		T_1	T_2
R.B.	85	57	T.F.	84	93	R.E.	62	51	J.S.	57	47	Total	749	696
C.T.	29	27	M.P.	67	59	M.W.	39	36	T.B.	27	21	M	46.81	43.51
B.L.	19	18	J.M.	48	37	D.H.	84	85	G.D.	Broken arm		σ		12.84
D.K.	28	26	W.S.	27	48	G.M.	12	23	D.W.	30	44			
S.B.	Incomplete								D.E.	51	24			

Octacosanol

Circuit	T_1	T_2	M. Endurance	T_1	T_2	Interval	T_1	T_2	Steeple	T_1	T_2		T_1	T_2
J.T.	62	54	S.B.	63	69	T.M.	50	49	A.H.	Broken arm		Total	702	748
R.C.	45	42	R.C.	13	40	H.S.	25	23	S.S.	47	52	M	39.00	41.56
R.K.	29	34	D.H.	31	26	R.C.	33	34	J.S.	62	63	σ		8.71
S.R.	13	20	R.F.	29	28	D.S.	20	39	R.G.	48	40			
						D.H.	15	23	T.H.	100	100			

Placeboes

Circuit	T_1	T_2	M. Endurance	T_1	T_2	Interval	T_1	T_2	Steeple	T_1	T_2		T_1	T_2
P.B.	Incomplete		J.S.	17	12	E.Y.	60	55	D.T.	69	48	Total	791	796
P.K.	24	39	J.K.	62	70	M.J.	8	18	J.G.	67	41	M	49.44	49.75
B.W.	55	47	D.C.	59	84	R.R.	15	17	W.A.	29	37	σ		15.56
S.H.	17	30	C.S.	67	52	B.W.	54	75	C.R.	40	36			
R.S.	65	73	E.F.	100	74				B.C.	Incomplete				
Total	658		Total	907		Total	762		Total	810				
M	38.71		M	53.35		M	42.33		M	50.63				
σ	10.42		σ	13.53		σ	9.81		σ	14.46				

TABLE LXXI

STRENGTH PER POUND OF BODY WEIGHT TABULATION SHEET—STANDARD SCORES

	Circuit			M. Endurance			Interval			Steeple			Total	
	T_1	T_2		T_1	T_2		T_1	T_2		T_1	T_2		T_1	T_2
Wheat Germ														
P.T.	43	61	S.F.	67	62	K.K.	76	65	J.D.	53	68	Total	1,004	1,025
F.E.	44	53	J.S.	72	65	L.S.	60	62	J.H.	58	50	M	55.78	56.94
C.H.	54	58	G.S.	Incomplete		J.C.	46	55	T.S.	43	53	σ	10.05	
M.B.	83	78	L.S.	58	56	C.D.	53	32	J.D.	37	53			
D.F.	43	46	K.C.	73	69	T.S.	41	39						
W. G. Oil														
R.B.	69	48	T.F.	69	74	R.E.	59	51	J.S.	62	54	Total	863	839
C.T.	53	53	M.P.	57	53	M.M.	57	56	T.B.	54	46	M	53.94	52.44
B.L.	32	31	J.M.	71	60	D.H.	68	70	G.D.	Broken arm		σ	13.58	
D.K.	32	42	W.S.	34	46	G.M.	27	53	D.W.	44	58			
S.R.	Incomplete								D.E.	75	44			
Octacosanol														
J.T.	62	54	S.B.	71	75	T.M.	62	61	A.H.	Broken arm		Total	960	1,016
R.C.	66	61	R.G.	32	61	H.S.	53	48	S.S.	60	65	M	53.33	56.44
R.K.	47	51	D.E.	53	49	R.C.	64	68	J.S.	55	45	σ	10.64	
G.G.	30	38	R.F.	43	41	D.S.	38	60	R.G.	58	49			
			J.S.	37	51	D.H.	40	50	T.H.	89	89			
Placeboes														
P.B.	Incomplete		J.K.	63	71	E.Y.	74	64	D.T.	75	55	Total	842	863
P.K.	43	61	D.C.	58	96	M.J.	34	49	J.G.	67	45	M	52.63	53.94
B.W.	68	59	C.S.	69	48	R.R.	36	42	W.A.	44	49	σ	16.13	
S.H.	42	57	E.F.	56	42	B.N.	40	52	C.H.	38	37			
R.S.	35	36							B.C.	Incomplete				
Total	846	887	Total	983	1,019	Total	928	977	Total	912	820			
M	49.76	52.18	M	57.82	59.94	M	51.56	54.28	M	57.00	53.75			
σ	9.99		σ	14.44		σ	11.53		σ	13.41				

Experiment 15

The Effects of Training and Supplementary Diet on the Cardiovascular Condition of Young Boys

Andre S. Hupé

PURPOSE

THE purpose of this experiment[*] was to investigate the effect of physical training with an endurance component included four days per week and also the differential effect of a dietary supplement on the cardiovascular fitness of young boys.

Data were collected on forty boys participating in the Summer Sports Fitness School at the University of Illinois in the summer of 1957.

RESEARCH METHODS

All boys were tested at the outset (T_1) in the 600-yard run for time and were matched in four groups by this test. In the first week of the school, all boys were tested in the following cardiovascular tests: Schneider test; amplitude of the brachial pulse wave; area of the brachial pulse wave (by planimeter); change in pulse rate, lying to standing; change in pulse pressure, lying to standing; terminal pulse rate after five-minute step test; treadmill run (all-out at 7 mi./hr., 8.6 per cent grade); total recuperation on a five-minute step test. These tests were selected to represent at least five different components of cardiovascular fitness as shown by the factor analysis studies. The separate tests were converted into standard scores and these were averaged into a composite average SS cardiovascular criterion. All boys were measured again in the eighth week. In the middle six weeks a dietary supplement was fed, four capsules of 3-minim size four days per week, at the end of each of these regular program days. The capsules differed in color but none of the boys knew the

---

[*] Urbana, M.S. thesis, Physical Education, 1958, p. 74. (Sponsor: T. K. Cureton.)

contents, and they were taken from bags in the laboratory labelled "dark," "light" (white and red) and also blue and green. The secret of their content was kept throughout the experiment.

Four methods of training for endurance were introduced at the end of each day, after the basic skill instruction program was over (including basic swimming, gymnastics, track and field and games), because previous studies had shown that the stamina of the boys was not increased by the basic skill program, therefore, steeplechase, interval training, circuit training and muscular endurance exercises (on the spot) were introduced for thirty minutes at the end of the day, four days per week.

RESULTS

The results of comparing the four methods of endurance training were as follows: Table LXXII given in standard score per cent of improvement.

TABLE LXXII

RESULTS FROM FOUR METHODS OF ENDURANCE TRAINING

	SS Per Cent	N
Steeplechase training	10.40	5
Interval training	4.07	5
Circuit training	3.13	5
Muscular endurance exercise	2.29	5

The results of the four differential methods of feeding were as follows:

TABLE LXXIII

RESULTS OF WGC, OCTCNL, WGO AND LECITHIN OIL ON
ENDURANCE TRAINING

	SS Per Cent	N
Wheat germ	10.40	5
Wheat germ oil crystals	5.57	5
Wheat germ oil	4.47	5
Lecithin oil placeboes	2.24	5

The steeplechase was shown to give improvement significantly better than circuit training ($t = 3.26$, 1% level); better than muscular endurance exercise ($t = 3.22$, 1% level); better than interval training (t = 3.01, 1% level); and except for steeplechase being the best, the other three methods were not significantly different from each other.

On the composite cardiovascular criterion, the wheat germ (fresh from the factory in June, as guaranteed fresh) was shown to be significantly better than wheat germ oil (t = 2.06, 5% level); wheat germ oil was shown to be better than the lecithin oil placeboes (t = 2.78, 1% level). Wheat germ oil crystals (now known as octacosanol) were better than the placeboes (t = 3.12, 1% level); and wheat germ was shown to be better than the placeboes (t = 3.30%, 1% level).

Both wheat germ and wheat germ oil were shown to affect the brachial pulse, the systolic amplitude being improved 26.15 SS per cent on wheat germ compared to 18.78 SS per cent for octacosanol; whereas, wheat germ oil was best in affecting the area of the brachial pulse wave, this by 28.03 SS per cent compared to wheat germ by 17.10 per cent, octacosanol by 9.74 per cent and the placeboes −19.93 per cent.

The treadmill run gave an advantage to wheat germ by an improvement of 14.69 SS per cent, compared to 8.76 for the placeboes, 7.89 SS per cent for the wheat germ oil and 5.70 SS per cent for the octacosanol.

It should be noted that the 600-yard run was given only once at the beginning and was not given during the last week during this year. This was the only year also that absolutely fresh wheat germ was demanded from the Kretchmer Corporation.

Experiment 16

The Effects of Dietary Supplements and Different Training Methods on Reaction Time and Agility

Kenneth G. Tillman

PURPOSE

THE purpose of this experiment* was to determine what effect different dietary supplements, i.e. wheat germ oil (VioBin brand), octacosanol crystals, and lecithin oil placeboes have on reaction time and agility. Also to determine what effect different training methods have upon the 600-yard run times (endurance), i.e. circuit, muscular endurance repetitions, interval training on the track and the steeplechase (880-yards) have upon the same test measures.

The subjects were young boys from the University of Illinois Sports Fitness School, 7-13 years of age. (Refer to *Improving the Physical Fitness of Boys* by Cureton and Barry for a more complete description of the boys and results from this school.) The seventy-one boys in the 1957 summer school session were divided into four groups by matching on the 600-yard run; and also four groups to take four different training programs for eight weeks: circuit, muscular endurance, interval and steeplechase.

RESEARCH DESIGN

The eight matched groups on T_1 by the 600-yard run time were given an eight-week physical training program composed of four basic instructional classes in gymnastics, swimming, indoor conditioning and posture drills, and outdoor games and track and field activities. A "break" was given at 3:15 PM for rest and feeding of the capsules. Then a thirty-minute endurance drill was given, with each of the four groups carrying out its own program under the leadership of a sports-fitness school instructor. The improvement differences were tested by the "t" test, based upon the differences (D) between the means from T_1 to T_2, cov-

* Urbana: M.S. in Physical Education, University of Illinois, 1958, p. 63.

392

ering six weeks. The tests were 600-yard run time, figure eight agility run test (Illinois test), and the total body reaction time test. The methodologies of testing are carefully described in the literature, and also in the original thesis. (For reliability, the Illinois figure eight agility run = 0.917; the 600-yard run = 0.88; the Garrett-Cureton total body reaction time test = 0.75, 0.68, and 0.72, for visual, auditory and sound stimuli, respectively. The latter are based upon fifteen practice trials and then five trials each which were averaged for final score.)

The results are shown in the following tables.

TABLE LXXIV

AGILITY RUN TIME CHANGES IN FOUR METHODS OF TRAINING

	M_1 Secs. (SS)	M_2 Secs. (SS)	D Secs.	SS Per Cent Diff.	t
A. Circuit training	22.90 (36.7)	22.79 (37.2)	−.11	0.50	.130
B. Muscular endurance	22.12 (43.4)	21.90 (45.6)	−.22	2.22	.636
C. Interval training	22.56 (40.2)	23.02 (35.7)	.46	−4.50	1.480
D. Steeplechase	21.70 (47.9)	21.82 (46.6)	.12	−1.26	.339

The interval training group and the steeplechase training group made a poor showing in time performance from T_1 to T_2. The improvements made by the groups on circuit training and muscular endurance training were not statistically significant.

TABLE LXXV

AGILITY RUN TIME CHANGES IN FOUR METHODS OF FEEDING
DIETARY SUPPLEMENTS

	M_1 Secs. (SS)	M_2 Secs. (SS)	D Secs.	SS Per Cent Diff.	t
A. Wheat germ	22.45 (40.9)	22.72 (39.7)	.27	−1.15	.437
B. Wheat germ oil	22.17 (43.7)	22.15 (43.9)	.02	.26	.061
C. Octacosanol	22.19 (43.3)	22.39 (41.3)	.20	−2.00	.692
D. Placeboes of lecithin oil	22.62 (39.5)	22.60 (39.6)	−.02	− .17	.043

The group on wheat germ and the group on octacosanol as well as the placebo group on lecithin oil showed a loss in time performance between T_1 and T_2 of the agility run. The improvements made on the wheat germ oil group were insignificant.

TABLE LXXVI

AUDITORY REACTION TIME CHANGES IN FOUR METHODS
OF TRAINING

	M_1 Secs. (SS)	M_2 Secs. (SS)	D Secs.	SS Per Cent Diff.	t
A. Circuit training	.375 (68.2)	.334 (83.2)	−.041	15.00	4.178
B. Muscular endurance ...	.344 (76.7)	.327 (83.9)	−.017	7.22	2.357
C. Interval training	.359 (72.0)	.328 (83.0)	−.031	11.00	2.625
D. Steeplechase	.337 (79.5)	.316 (88.1)	−.021	8.66	2.562

The circuit training group had an improvement which was significant at the 1 per cent level of significance on the auditory reaction time test. The other three groups had improvements which were significant at the 5 per cent level of significance.

TABLE LXXVII

AUDITORY REACTION TIME CHANGES IN FOUR METHODS OF
FEEDING DIETARY SUPPLEMENTS

	M_1 Secs. (SS)	M_2 Secs. (SS)	D Secs.	SS Per Cent Diff.	t
A. Wheat germ	.346 (76.9)	.316 (88.5)	−.030	11.63	3.332
B. Wheat germ oil	.354 (73.8)	.337 (80.9)	−.017	7.13	2.187
C. Octacosanol	.369 (67.6)	.328 (82.7)	−.041	15.05	3.257
D. Placeboes of lecithin oil	.349 (76.1)	.327 (83.7)	−.022	7.58	3.225

The wheat germ group, the octacosanol group and the placebo group showed improvements in auditory reaction time which were significant at the 1 per cent level of significance. The wheat germ oil group had an improvement which was significant at the 5 per cent level of significance.

TABLE LXXVIII

VISION REACTION TIME CHANGES IN FOUR METHODS
OF TRAINING

	M_1 Secs. (SS)	M_2 Secs. (SS)	D Secs.	SS Per Cent Diff.	t
A. Circuit training	.382 (72.4)	.347 (83.4)	−.035	10.94	3.799
B. Muscular endurance ...	.367 (75.7)	.333 (85.3)	−.034	9.61	2.496
C. Interval training	.368 (74.2)	.332 (86.0)	−.036	11.77	3.055
D. Steeplechase	.348 (80.7)	.314 (90.1)	−.034	9.46	3.691

The groups on circuit training, interval training and steeple-chase training showed improvement which was significant at the 1 per cent level of significance on the visual reaction time test. The muscular endurance group improvement was significant at the 5 per cent level of significance.

TABLE LXXIX

VISUAL REACTION TIME CHANGES IN FOUR METHODS OF FEEDING
DIETARY SUPPLEMENTS

	M_1 Secs. (SS)	M_2 Secs. (SS)	D Secs.	SS Per Cent Diff.	t
A. Wheat germ	.367 (75.3)	.328 (87.7)	−.039	12.36	4.414
B. Wheat germ oil	.364 (77.1)	.339 (83.8)	−.025	6.66	1.753
C. Octacosanol	.384 (70.9)	.335 (85.2)	−.049	14.26	3.918
D. Placeboes of lecithin oil	.353 (79.2)	.327 (87.0)	−.026	7.76	1.930

The wheat germ group and the octacosanol group had improvements which were significant at the 1 per cent level of significance on the visual reaction time test. The wheat germ oil group and the placebo group did not have significant improvements at the 1 per cent or 5 per cent level of significance.

TABLE LXXX

COMBINED VISUAL AND AUDITORY REACTION TIME CHANGES IN
FOUR METHODS OF TRAINING

	M_1 Secs. (SS)	M_2 Secs. (SS)	D Secs.	SS Per Cent Diff.	t
A. Circuit training	.373 (64.4)	.342 (75.1)	−.031	10.5	2.632
B. Muscular endurance	.355 (69.5)	.323 (80.6)	−.032	11.11	3.912
C. Interval training	.351 (70.9)	.323 (80.7)	−.028	9.72	3.797
D. Steeplechase	.320 (77.5)	.310 (81.0)	−.010	3.53	1.312

The groups on muscular endurance training and interval training had improvements on the combined visual and auditory reaction time test which were significant at the 1 per cent level of significance. The circuit training group had an improvement which was significant at the 5 per cent level of significance. The group on steeplechase training did not have a significant improvement.

TABLE LXXXI

COMBINED VISUAL AND AUDITORY REACTION TIME CHANGES IN
FOUR METHODS OF FEEDING DIETARY SUPPLEMENTS

	M_1 Secs. (SS)	M_2 Secs. (SS)	D Secs.	SS Per Cent Diff.	t
A. Wheat germ	.347 (71.4)	.321 (80.6)	−.026	9.26	3.046
B. Wheat germ oil	.359 (65.7)	.329 (75.9)	−.031	10.2	3.400
C. Octacosanol	.356 (69.1)	.322 (79.8)	−.034	10.77	3.008
D. Placeboes of lecithin oil	.342 (74.5)	.330 (80.1)	−.012	5.52	2.052

All three of the dietary supplement groups, wheat germ, wheat germ oil and wheat germ crystals, improved at the 1 per cent level of significance on the combined visual and auditory reaction time test. The placebo group did not quite show a significant improvement on this test. None of the changes between the four groups were significant.

TABLE LXXXII

Method of Workout	"t" Standard 5 Per Cent	1 Per Cent	Dietary Supplement	"t" Standard 5 Per Cent	1 Per Cent
Circuit	2.110	2.898	Wheat germ cereal	2.101	2.878
Muscular endurance	2.110	2.898	Wheat germ oil	2.145	2.977
Interval training	2.110	2.898	Octacosanol crystals	2.110	2.898
Steeplechase training	2.145	2.977	Lecithin placeboes	2.120	2.921

CONCLUSIONS

The agility run time changes in the four methods of training were not significant. The group on muscular endurance training had a 2.22 standard score per cent improvement ($t = .636$) and the circuit training group had an improvement of 0.50 standard score per cent ($t = .130$). The steeplechase group had a decrease of 1.26 standard score per cent ($t = .339$) and the interval training group had a decrease of 4.50 standard score per cent ($t = 1.480$).

The agility run time changes in the four methods of feeding dietary supplements were not significant. The wheat germ oil group had a 0.26 standard score per cent improvement ($t = .061$)

and the placebo group had a 0.17 standard score per cent improvement ($t = .143$). The wheat germ group had a decrease of 1.15 standard score per cent ($t = .437$) and the octacosanol group had a decrease of 2.00 standard score per cent ($t = .692$).

On the auditory reaction time test, the circuit training group improved at the 1 per cent level of significance and the other three methods of training improved at the 5 per cent level of significance. When these training methods were ranked according to the standard score per cent improvement, circuit training was first with a 15.00 standard score per cent improvement ($t = 4.178$), interval training was next with a 11.00 standard score per cent improvement ($t = 2.625$), next came steeplechase training with a 8.66 standard score per cent improvement ($t = 2.562$) and then muscular endurance training with a 7.22 standard score per cent improvement ($t = 2.357$). None of the differences between groups were significant.

All of the dietary supplement groups and the placebo group made significant gains on the auditory reaction time test. The standard score per cent improvements of 15.05 by the octacosanol group ($t = 3.257$), 11.63 by the wheat germ group ($t = 3.332$), and 7.58 by the placebo group ($t = 3.225$) were significant at the 1 per cent level. The 7.13 standard score per cent improvement ($t = 2.187$) by the group on wheat germ oil was significant at the 5 per cent level of significance. None of the changes between groups were significant.

On the visual reaction time test the groups on circuit training, interval training and steeplechase training had improvements which were significant at the 1 per cent level of significance. The muscular endurance group improvement was significant at the 5 per cent level of significance. The interval training group had a 11.77 standard score per cent improvement ($t = 3.055$), the circuit training group had a standard score per cent improvement of 10.94 ($t = 3.7990$), the group on muscular endurance training had an improvement of 9.61 ($t = 2.496$), and the group on steeplechase training had an improvement of 9.46 ($t = 3.691$). None of the differences between groups were significant.

On the visual reaction time test, the groups on wheat germ and octacosanol had standard score per cent improvements that were significant at the 1 per cent level of significance. The wheat germ oil group and the placebo group did not have significant improvements. The octacosanol group had a 14.26 standard score per cent improvement (t = 3.918), the wheat germ group had a 12.36 standard score per cent improvement (t = 4.414), the placebo group had a 7.76 standard score per cent improvement (t = 1.930), and the wheat germ oil group had a 6.66 standard score per cent improvement (t = 1.7530). None of the differences between groups were significant.

The groups on circuit training, interval training and muscular endurance training all made gains which were significant at the 1 per cent level of significance on the combined visual and auditory reaction time test. The steeplechase group did not have a significant improvement on this test. The standard score per cent improvements were 11.11 (t = 3.912) by the muscular endurance group, 10.5 (t = 2.632) by the circuit training group, 9.72 (t = 3.797) by the group on interval training, and 3.53 (t = 1.312) by the group on steeplechase training. None of the differences between groups were significant.

On the combined visual and auditory reaction time test, all of the groups on dietary supplements had improvements that were significant at the 1 per cent level of significance. The placebo group did not have a significant improvement. The octacosanol group had a standard score per cent improvement of 10.77 (t = 3.008), the group on wheat germ oil had a standard score per cent improvement of 10.2 (t = 3.400), the wheat germ group had a standard score per cent improvement of 9.26 (t = 3.046), and the placebo group had a standard score per cent improvement of 5.52 (t = 2.052). None of the differences between groups were statistically significant.

It was recommended that lecithin oil be dropped as a placebo inasmuch as it apparently affected auditory reaction response time. There were too many groups and too few cases in each group.

Experiment 17

The Influence of Exercise and Diet Supplement (Wheat Germ Oil) on Fitness Changes During Training

JAMES WOOD TUMA

PURPOSE

THE purpose of this experiment° was multiple: a) To develop a success-prediction equation for underwater demolition team candidate selection in terms of certain physiological/ psychological variables; b) To assess the value of wheat germ oil and octacosanol as ergogenic aids to groups under pressure of extreme physical conditioning; c) To compare UDT fitness gains made during a fourteen-week training period with those made in college physical education programs.

Forty-eight beginning UDT Navy candidates were given sixty-three physical tests representing areas of strength, physique, muscular endurance and cardiovascular fitness.

RESEARCH METHODS

The investigation was longitudinal in design. Personality assessment of UDT personnel was determined with the Cattell 16 P. F. Profile. A correlation matrix from initial scores made by the forty-eight subjects on these seventy-nine dependent variables was computed against an independent variable of "pass-fail." Various combinations determined betas selected for establishing a raw score success-prediction regression equation. The forty-eight candidates were divided at commencement of training into three matched groups, A (octacosanol), B (cottonseed oil, control), C (wheat germ oil), by a composite muscular endurance and cardiovascular test battery. Each group was fed daily 60 minims of its assigned diet supplement throughout the fourteen-

---

° Department of Physical Education, University of Illinois, 1959. Ph.D. thesis.

week course (double blind experiment). Fitness changes, T_2-T_1, were determined on individual survivors, within each matched group, and between matched groups.

CONCLUSIONS

Choice of a multiple correlation of R = 0.6070 representing test items of the Navy physical fitness test was selected over sixteen other multiple combinations (R = 0.2827 to R = 0.6825) because of adaptability to shipboard testing, ease of administration and high reliability. The regression equation derived for use with raw score data is as follows:

$$Y_{\text{estimate pass}} = .0124 \text{ (squat jumps)} - .0061 \text{ (push ups)} + .0033 \text{ (sit ups)} + .0051 \text{ (squat thrusts)} + .0565 \text{ (pull ups)} - 0.6805.$$

Based on results of the sample tested, provided presently existing entrance requirements are met, raw scores of 69 squat jumps, 48 push ups, 36 sit ups, 33 squat thrusts (1′ minute), and 10 pull ups estimate a 73.44 per cent chance of completing training. As determined from the Cattell Profile, personality traits of the majority of the active UDT population showed definite aggressiveness, enthusiasm, shyness, bohemianism, and unsureness; none of these factors were sufficiently weighted to be included as success-predictors.

Gains within groups, averaged from fifteen tests (Table LXXXIII) representatively divided between the four areas of fitness considered, revealed a mean gain of 16.36 SS for the octacosanol group; 13.12 SS for the wheat germ oil group; and 7.98 SS for the placebo (control) group. The greater gains made by diet supplemented groups parallel those cited in the literature reviewed. While a between-group nonparametric determination gave no statistical evidence that the lesser attrition of students in Group A (5 remained of 16) and Group C (6 remained of 16) over that of Group B (2 remained of 16) can be wholly attributed to wheat germ oil supplementation, it still remains unexplained that appreciably larger attrition occurred in the placebo (control) group.

Withstanding diet supplementation, time allotted, and objectives desired in UDT and college programs, fitness improvements

TABLE LXXXIII

T₁-T₂ STANDARD SCORES MADE ON FIFTEEN PHYSICAL FITNESS
TESTS TAKEN BY THREE MATCHED UDT GROUPS

Test Measurement	SS_1 SS_2 Group A Wheat Germ Crystal		SS_1 SS_2 Group B Placebo		SS_1 SS_2 Group C Wheat Germ Oil	
1. *Cardiovascular tests*						
a. Heartometer area						
b. Systolic amplitude						
c. Diastolic amplitude						
d. Angle of obliquity	62.7	75.2	46.6	40.7	67.2	72.2
e. Five-minute step test	27.2	70.0	54.5	80.0	50.0	81.0
2. *Strength*						
a. Four-item strength test	71.0	92.0	71.5	87.0	81.3	98.0
b. Strength/pound of body weight	65.6	80.0	75.5	98.0	73.5	90.0
3. *Muscular endurance*						
a. Mile run	39.4	53.0	48.0	55.0	41.0	53.3
b. Squat jumps						
c. Push ups						
d. Squat thrusts						
e. Pull ups	50.1	66.0	52.7	59.9	47.7	64.2
4. *Physique*						
a. Muscle girth	40.2	45.0	35.0	35.0	29.3	38.0
b. Adipose index	49.0	61.0	49.0	56.0	50.3	59.0
c. Weight residual	87.0	97.0	69.5	67.0	92.0	100.0
Total Average SS	54.67	71.03	56.32	64.30	59.03	72.15
Total Average SS Gain		16.36		7.98		13.12

were overwhelmingly in favor of UDT graduates, especially in areas of cardiovascular and muscular endurance gains.

Due to the heavy attrition of the trainees, the drop-outs upset the matching, but for the subjects who survived the course and remained as originally paired, the results favored the octacosanol and WGO groups over the placebo group.

As a selective measure to decrease attrition of UDT candidates, it is recommended that the weighted regression equation evolved be considered for adoption by the United States Navy. Greater fitness gains made by individuals and within groups fed wheat germ supplements definitely indicate further investigation in this direction using larger samplings which are not subject to such heavy attrition.

The Influence of Wheat Germ Oil as a Dietary Supplement in a Training Program of Varsity Track Athletes at the University of Illinois

EDMUND M. BERNAUER AND THOMAS K. CURETON

PURPOSE

THE problem was to determine whether WGO capsules, administered as a dietary supplement for twelve weeks would significantly improve the experimental WGO group over another matched group given placebo capsules of devitaminized lard with both groups taking the same training program.

Twelve varsity trackmen, between the ages 18-20 years served as subjects for this study.[*] The group was selected primarily from those individuals who run repetitious 440's as a matter of routine in practice. Consequently, middle distance and distance runners formed this experimental group. The runners were given the complete battery of tests prior to the diet supplementation and again twelve weeks later at the termination of the outdoor track season. The dietary supplement was fed for twelve weeks.

RESEARCH METHODS

The "matched group" technique was employed as the experimental design. Each group was given an initial battery of cardiovascular tests and a 440 yard running performance test. The athletes had already attained a preseason level of physical condition and, following the initial battery of tests, entered a twelve-week training program which carried them to the termination of the spring track season. One group was fed ten capsules of WGO per day (6 minims size) and each containing 350 mg of WGO and also 0.88 mg each of mixed tocopherol, a natural constituent

---

[*] Physical Fitness Research Laboratory, University of Illinois, Urbana, Illinois, 1958.

of WGO, and the other group was fed 10 capsules per day of devitaminized lard (6 minims size). The WGO capsules are products of the VioBin Corporation, Monticello, Illinois. The individuals were matched on the basis of their 440-yard run performances to $\pm$ 1 second. Six runners were assigned to each group. No attempt was made to control the diet of any of the subjects, but all ate moderately the usual track training diet without abuses or excesses, without smoking or drinking alcohol.

The test battery consisted entirely of measurements taken in the resting post-absorptive state with the exception of the 440-yard run performance. Five basic measurements were obtained, described as follows:

The Cameron heartometer was applied to measure the circulatory dynamic factors observed in the brachial pulse wave, namely: systolic amplitude with a .91 reliability, area under the curve of .86 reliability, pulse pressure which has a $\pm$ 8 mm Hg variation with indirect determinations and heart rate with a .99 reliability. The above reliabilities were determined on ninety-seven young men at the University of Illinois physical fitness research laboratory. The average of three representative waves was recorded. The technique of measurement may be found in Cureton's *Physical Fitness Appraisal and Guidance* (1947).

The Sanborn Viso Cardiette was used to record the electro-cardiographic phenomena manifested by the heart during the phases of contraction and relaxation. The QRS-deflection which has a reliability of .82 and the T-deflection which has a reliability of .87 in the chest leads were measured for this study. The reliabilities were determined in a study made at the University of Illinois Physical Fitness Research Laboratories, of eighty-one normal young male subjects. The average height of three representative waves was recorded in either the fourth or fifth precordial leads. The measurement technique may also be found in *Physical Fitness of Champion Athletes*, pp. 228-254 (1951).

The basal metabolism (BMR) was recorded applying the Sanborn Metabalator. The subject was asked to recline in bed in a quiet, semi-dark room for a period of thirty minutes. Oral temperatures and environmental measurements were recorded to

TABLE LXXXIV

EFFECTS OF VARSITY TRACK TRAINING AND SUPPLEMENTARY FEEDING
UPON SELECTED CARDIOVASCULAR AND ORGANIC MEASURES

Experimental

| Item | Unit | Raw Scores | | | Standard Scores | | | "t" | "t" Matching |
		T_1	T_2	D	T_1	T_2	D	T_2-T_1	T_1(exp.)-T_1(cont.)
Systolic amplitude	cm	1.50	1.63	0.13	69.0	76.2	7.0	1.92*	0.82
Area under curve/surface area		0.254	0.327	0.073	75.3	91.5	16.2	4.66‡	0.78
Area under curve	sq.cm	0.490	0.628	0.138	76.8	92.7	15.9	4.78‡	1.61
Pulse pressure	mm Hg.	46.7	49.8	3.1	49.7	52.5	2.8	0.87	1.07
Heart rate	beats/min.	70.0	70.6	0.6	62.3	61.5	-0.8	0.02	2.06*
T-wave (ECG)	mm	13.4	13.7	0.3	73.0	75.8	2.8	0.55	2.18*
R-wave (ECG)	mm	23.8	29.9	6.1	63.8	85.2	21.4	1.87*	1.19
Basal heat	cal/sq.m/hr.	37.2	39.7	2.5	48.2	54.5	6.3	1.43	2.44†
Per cent BMR	%	-14.0	-6.8	7.2	39.7	46.7	7.0	2.98†	3.48‡
Schneider index	points	13.7	14.0	0.3	54.7	55.8	1.1	0.64	1.86*
Running performance	secs.	56.5	54.3	-2.2	83.0	94.0	11.0	1.39	1.69

N = 6

10df
* = 10 per cent level of confidence
† = 5 per cent level of confidence
‡ = 1 per cent level of confidence

TABLE LXXXV
EFFECTS OF VARSITY TRACK TRAINING AND SUPPLEMENTARY FEEDING UPON SELECTED CARDIOVASCULAR AND ORGANIC MEASURES
Control

Item	Unit	Raw Scores			Standard Scores			"t" T_2-T_1	"t" Matching $T_1(exp.)-T_1(cont.)$
		T_1	T_2	D	T_1	T_2	D		
Systolic amplitude	cm	1.44	1.55	0.11	65.5	71.5	6.0	1.60	0.82
Area under curve/surface area		0.256	0.298	0.042	71.0	83.3	12.3	1.92*	0.78
Area under curve	sq.cms	0.463	0.545	0.082	70.3	82.0	11.7	2.95†	1.61
Pulse pressure	mm Hg.	53.2	54.3	1.1	55.8	58.7	2.9	0.39	1.07
Heart rate	beats/min.	57.2	55.7	-1.5	79.2	81.2	2.0	1.38	2.06*
T-wave (ECG)	mm	10.3	10.3	0	53.5	53.5	0	0.11	2.18*
R-wave (ECG)	mm	23.5	29.0	5.5	42.3	65.7	23.4	3.86‡	1.19
Basal heat	cal/sq.m/hr.	47.3	50.8	3.5	74.0	82.0	8.0	1.84	2.44†
Per cent BMR	%	14.0	7.3	-6.7	67.7	60.3	-7.4	2.09*	3.48‡
Schneider index	points	16.2	15.5	-0.7	65.8	61.7	-4.1	0.47	1.86*
Running performance	secs.	54.5	53.5	-1.0	93.0	98.0	5.0	1.07	1.69

N = 6

10df
* = 10 per cent level of confidence
† = 5 per cent level of confidence
‡ = 1 per cent level of confidence

insure the necessary DuBois standardization during the tests. The reliability .49 is somewhat lower than the other reliability measurements recorded in this study.

The Schneider index is a very general measure of the state of training of the autonomic nervous system. The Cureton revision of the Schneider index was adopted for this study. The total test has a retest reliability of 0.86.

Running performance was determined by timed efforts over 440 yards recorded under meet conditions. No reliability was obtained, but in all cases, a noticeably consistent downward trend was observed in performance times as the season progressed (for 600 yards, $r_{1_1} = 0.41$ to 0.96).

The laboratory routine of the testing program was as follows: Each subject reported to the laboratory at 7:00 AM in a post-absorptive state and immediately reclined in bed for a period of thirty minutes. The room was kept semi-dark and quiet. Following this thirty-minute interval of rest, the subject was given the electrocardiogram, basal metabolism, Schneider and heartograph tests, in that order. The running performance as previously stated was obtained during the varsity track practices in the afternoons at the time of designated time trials.

The data are presented in graphic (cf. Figs. 3, 4 and 5) and tabular form (Tables LXXXIV and LXXXV). Essentially, three different statistical procedures are utilized in presenting the results. The graphs illustrate the standard score changes, while the tables indicate significant changes through "t" value interpretation and the association between the measurement and running performance is determined by Pearson's product moment coefficients of correlations.

RESULTS

The results are summarized in Tables LXXXIV and LXXXV representing the mean differences in the measures and the "t" values for the various changes between the control and experimental groups and also between T_1 and T_2 within the experimental and the control group in standard scores (SS) and per cent differences. The coefficient of correlation between the functional measures and running performance are summarized in Table XCIII. Reliabilities of the changes are in trends of "t" values.

Brachial Pulse Wave

Table XXX indicates a significant difference for the systolic amplitude, area under the curve/surface area and area under the curve in the WGO group compared to the same measures in the control group. The levels of confidence are higher in the WGO group than in the control group. The coefficient of correlation between the areas under the pulse wave and the running performance are 0.55 ± .23 and 0.60 ± .21 with both values being significant at the 10 per cent level of confidence. The T_1-T_2 difference between the control and WGO group was not significantly different. The pulse pressure shows very slight change in both groups ("t" = 0.39 for the control group and 0.87 for the WGO group) and a relatively low coefficient of correlation with the running criterion.

Figure 3 reflects similar trends as outlined in the above paragraph. Standard score per cent improvement favors the WGO group over the control group. The relative magnitude of change is greatest in the brachial pulse wave area measures; followed next by the systolic amplitude and also very small change in pulse pressure.

Heart rate changes were found to be insignificant in both the WGO and the control group. A significant difference ("t" = 2.06) at the 10 per cent level of confidence existed between the control group and the WGO group at the onset of the training program which would have invalidated any changes if they had occurred. However, the coefficient of correlation .60 ± .21 significant at the 10 per cent level of confidence between the heart rate and running performance indicates a fair degree of association.

T-Wave and R-Wave (CR IV-V Lead) of the ECG

The T-wave was not appreciably altered following the twelve-week period of training in either the control or the WGO group. Again the control and WGO group were significantly different at the beginning of the program ("t" = 2.18, 10 per cent level of confidence) thus placing some reservation upon the slight changes that were observed. The coefficient of correlation between the T-wave measure and running performance is +.56 ±

.23 significant at the 10 per cent level of confidence. The SS differences favor the WGO group with 2.8 SS per cent gain compared to a −.7 SS per cent for the control group.

The R-wave was markedly lower following the training; however, in this instance more so in the control group ("t" = 3.86) significant at the 1 per cent level than in the WGO group ("t" = 1.87) significant at the 10 per cent level of confidence. The co-efficient of correlation between the R-wave and the running performance was −0.38 ± 0.29 which was not significant. The SS variations also heavily favor the control group showing 23.4 SS per cent change, while the WGO group recorded at 21.4 SS per cent. This was the largest change observed of the ten measures recorded following the training program and supplementary feeding.

Basal Metabolic Rate

Tables LXXXIV and LXXXV show a "t" value of 2.09 for the control group, 2.98 for the WGO group and 3.48 for the WGO versus control group at the beginning of the training program in per cent BMR. On this item, therefore, the groups were not well matched but a −0.38 ± .29 coefficient of correlation was recorded between Cal./Sq.M./Hr. and running performance. This was not statistically significant. A very low coefficient of correlation (.09 ± .35 without corrections for curvilinearity) was obtained between the per cent BMR and running performance. The SS changes reflect a somewhat different picture. In both the Cal./Sq.M./Hr. and the per cent BMR the WGO group increased 6.3 SS per cent and 7.0 SS per cent, respectively.

Schneider Index

The WGO group shows a "t" of 4.27 which is significant at the 1 per cent level of confidence. The control has a "t" of 0.47 and this is not significant. The initial "t" value between the control and the WGO group was 1.86 (significant at 10 per cent level). The low coefficient of correlation between the Schneider index (.19 ± .32) and running performance indicates that this test does not predict the blood flow in running performance.

Running Performance

Both the WGO group and the control group demonstrate improvement in their running performance. Although neither change is significant, the −2.2 change in seconds for the WGO group and −1.0 control group decrease is of great practical significance. A 0.7 second difference in a 440-yard run would approximate a 5-yard advantage. Viewed individually, there is a general pattern of improvement in each and every athlete following twelve weeks of training.

The overall gain for the control group was 5.44 SS per cent and for the WGO group 8.25 SS per cent.

DISCUSSION

The subjects chosen for this investigation had completed a training period of approximately twelve weeks. Each subject was a varsity track athlete in average or better than average physical condition.

This study verifies the many earlier investigations carried out at the Research Laboratory at the University of Illinois. A very definite trend of improvement is apparent in the organic and functional measures of both the WGO and control groups (refer to Figs. 3, 4 and 5). The WGO group shows significant improvement in the brachial pulse wave results R-wave (of ECG), metabolism and Schneider index. The control group recorded a significant change in the R-wave (of ECG) and in the brachial pulse wave. This lends added evidence to an ever-increasing thesis, supporting the functional value of WGO.

The brachial pulse wave is considered an indirect measure of the stroke volume of the heart. The systolic amplitude may be considered proportional to the contractile force of the heart forcing blood into the systemic vessels, i.e. Ft = Mv.

The WGO group shows a significant change following the supplementary feeding and training, whereas, none was shown in the control group. This agrees with earlier work by Cureton and other investigators at the University of Illinois. The area under the brachial pulse wave is significantly different in both the

WGO and control groups. The area under the wave is considered an indirect measurement of the cardiac output and in agreement with the generally accepted mode of adjustment during endurance training. Since the heart rate has changed only slightly in both groups measured before and after the twelve-week training period, and the pulse pressure shows only a slight change favoring the WGO group (Fig. 3), it is logical to anticipate an increased cardiac output when accompanied by an increase in contractile force. As previously mentioned, the systolic amplitude measures this force and is seen to favor the WGO group (Fig. 3). This is shown in both Fig. 3 and in Table XXX. The WGO group shows a significant change at the one per cent level and the control indicates a significant change at the 5 and 10 per cent level of confidence.

A further bit of evidence to support the premise that the systolic phase of cardiac function is the fundamental adjustment recorded may be seen by the Schneider index. The systolic pressures increased in both groups but more so in the WGO group. The diastolic pressure remained approximately the same. Again the underlying factor appears to be the systolic phase. The Schneider index is a rough measure of the parasympathetic response of the autonomic nervous system to levels of stress. The WGO group shows a significant change and the control group does not.

The fact that all subjects began this training program in a state of fitness considerably above average makes further increases in their fitnesses quite unusual. This same type of effect was noticed in a similar hard training experiment on six young men studied in 1950, when their fitness levels in bicycle riding endurance and in similar cardiovascular measures responded to WGO added to their diet after 12 weeks of continuous training (cf. Exp. 5 and 12).

Experiment 19

Factors Influencing Improvement in the Oxygen Intake of Young Boys

Stanley R. Brown[*]

PURPOSE

THE principal purpose of this experiment was to study boys in the University of Illinois Sports-Fitness School to determine whether the program of sports instruction and endurance would improve the "peak" oxygen intake in the all-out run test, and secondly, to observe if any systematic difference would develop in endurance or oxygen intake capacity between boys taking a Kretchmer wheat germ supplement compared to a matched group of boys not taking it.

RESEARCH METHODS

Twenty-two boys were studied from the 1960 summer school session of the Sports Fitness School, directed by Professor T. K. Cureton and Dr. Frederick B. Roby. The boys were 9-12 years of age. The entire program of the Sports Fitness School was eight weeks, but the twenty boys were tested again after the school had determined to check upon the "fatigue factor" thought to be present in the boys during the last set of tests. The T_1 series was completed the week before the school began, the T_2 series was given in the first week after the school closed, the T_3 series was given after one week of rest and the T_4 series was given after 3-4 weeks of rest. No regular exercise program was conducted after the school closed, but during the eight weeks of the school, the boys took instruction in basic gymnastics, swimming, track and field and group games; they also had a special fifty-minute endurance period from 4:00 to 4:50 PM on four days

---

[*] Urbana, Ph.D. thesis, Physical Education, University of Illinois, 1960, p. 170. (Sponsor: T. K. Cureton.)

411

TABLE LXXXVI

RELIABILITY RESULTS FOR ALL-OUT TREADMILL
RUN AND OXYGEN INTAKE MEASURES

	r_{11}
All-out treadmill run time (secs.)	0.826
Peak O_2 intake	
(L/min)	0.810
(cc/min/kg)	0.798
Gross O_2 intake	
(L)	0.875
(L/min)	0.869
(cc/min/kg)	0.785
(cc/kg)	0.885

of each week (Monday, Tuesday, Wednesday and Thursday). The program was considered fairly strenuous, and averaged four hours per day of physical activity, mixing skill instruction and endurance work.

Reliability testing was completed by the test and retest method, and the results are given in Table LXXXVI (T_2 to T_3, one week apart).

The work was done in the Physical Fitness Research Laboratory, of the University of Illinois, with techniques exactly like those used in Experiments 6 and 13, but using the motor driven treadmill, at 8.6 per cent grade, 7 miles per hour.

RESULTS

The program definitely improved the all-out run time of the boys as shown in Table LXXXVII, and it also improved the oxygen intake capacity:

TABLE LXXXVII

CHANGES IN THE ENTIRE GROUP OF BOYS IN EIGHT WEEKS (N = 20)

Test	T_1	T_2	D	t	T_3	T_4	Units	Per Cent
All-out run time on treadmill	85.32 (57 SS)	103.86 (66 SS)	18.54	4.44	105.71	113.8	secs.	25.0
In run	1.748	1.771	0.023	0.90	1.898	1.913	L/min	1.32
Peak O_2 intake	54.8	69.0	14.2	4.34			cc/kg	35.3

It was found that there was no systematic difference between the wheat germ group and the control group in the all-out treadmill run time.

TABLE LXXXVIII

COMPARATIVE CHANGES BETWEEN THE WHEAT GERM GROUP AND THE CONTROL GROUP ON NOTHING, IN EIGHT WEEKS, IN RUN TIME
(secs.)

Group	N	T_1	T_2	D	Gain in Per Cent	SS (Gain)
Wheat germ group	9	85.2	103.4	18.2	21.5	(57 to 66 = 9 SS)
Control group on nothing	9	85.0	108.0	23.0	27.2	(57 to 69 = 12 SS)
Between groups $t = 0.852$						

After a rest period from the close of the Sports Fitness School on August 6, which averaged forty-one days, twenty of the boys were retested in the all-out treadmill run with "peak" O_2 intake determinations.

TABLE LXXXIX

CHANGES T_3 TO T_4 IN TREADMILL RUN TIME AND PEAK O_2 INTAKE AFTER A REST PERIOD FOLLOWING CLOSE OF S-F SCHOOL

Test	T_3	T_4	D	t	Gain in Per Cent
All-out treadmill run (secs.) ..	104.65	113.80	9.15	1.257	8.77
"Peak" O_2 intake (cc/min/kg) ..	39.1	41.71	2.61	3.13	6.69

CONCLUSIONS

The use of a two ounce wheat germ supplement on four days per week did not make a significant difference in the all-out treadmill run time or in the "peak" oxygen intake between two matched groups of boys, nine in each group, over a period of eight weeks of feeding in the Sports Fitness Summer School.

The Sports Fitness School did improve the twenty boys who were tested at the beginning and at the end of the school period of eight weeks in both the all-out treadmill run time (25%) and the "peak" oxygen intake capacity test—1.32% in L/min. and 35.3% in L/kg, and 6.69% in cc/min/kg.

It was confirmed that after a rest period after the close of the school on August 6, averaging forty-one days, a retest of twenty

The line at 45° is a dividing line between the group which improved and the group which did not improve at T_3. It is not a regression line.

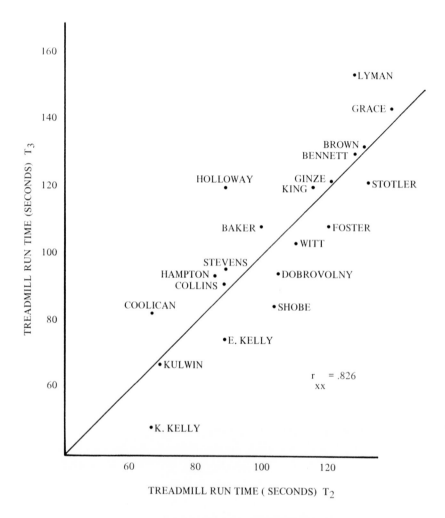

SCATTER DIAGRAM OF CHANGES IN SCORES

USED FOR RELIABILITY COEFFICIENT

TEST – RETEST

Figure 80. Test and retest on all-out treadmill run time ($r = 0.826$) (boys in Brown's Exp. 19).

The line at 45° is a dividing line between the group which improved and the group which did not improve at T3. It is not a regression line.

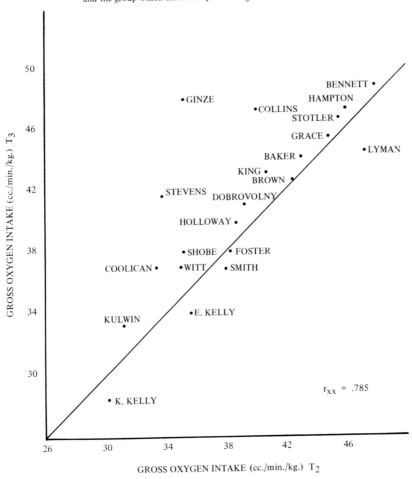

SCATTER DIAGRAM OF CHANGES IN SCORES

USED FOR RELIABILITY COEFFICIENT

TEST – RETEST

Figure 81. Test and retest on gross oxygen intake in all-out treadmill run ($r = 0.785$) (boys in Brown's Exp. 19).

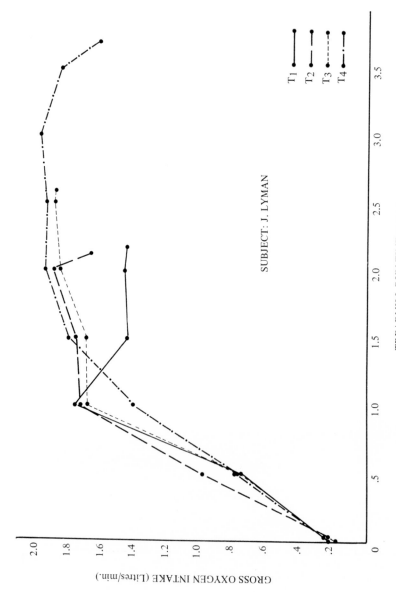

Figure 82. Gross oxygen intake, serial bag results (J. Lyman) in four tests (boy from Brown's Exp. 19).

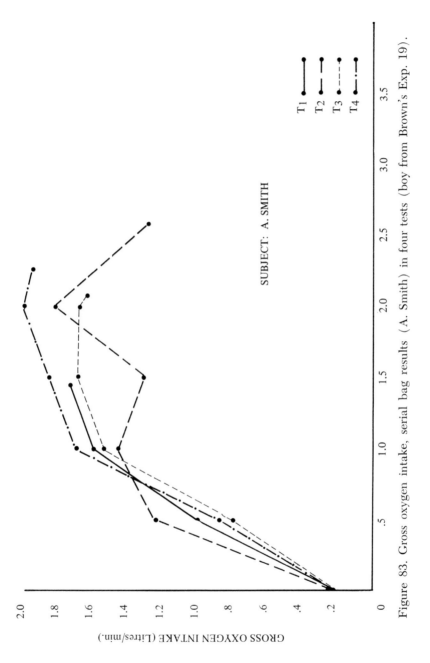

Figure 83. Gross oxygen intake, serial bag results (A. Smith) in four tests (boy from Brown's Exp. 19).

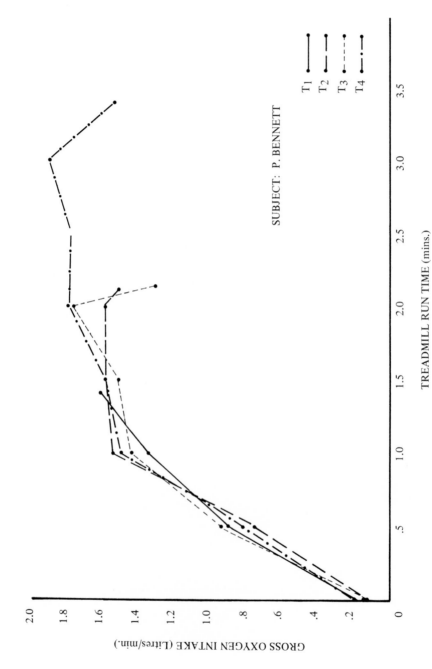

Figure 84. Cross oxygen intake, serial bag results (P. Bennett) in four tests.

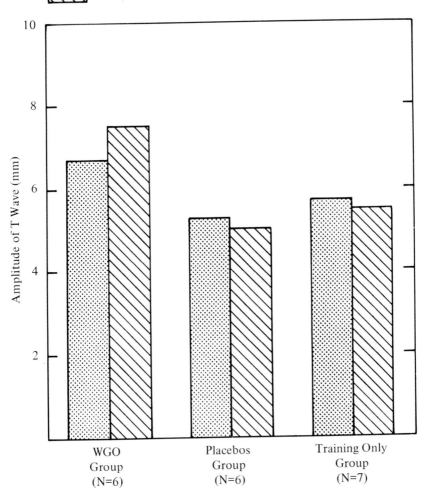

Figure 85. Effect of WGO on T-wave during sixth minute of recovery (Wiley's Exp. 30).

TABLE XC

STATISTICS OBTAINED FROM TEST—RETEST DATA

Variable	Standard Deviation of T_1 Scores S_{T1}	Reliability Coefficient $r_{T_2 T_3}$	Standard Error $S_{T1}\sqrt{1-r_{T_2 T_3}}$	Standard Error of Difference Between Two Scores of One Individual $S_{T1}\sqrt{2}\sqrt{1-r_{T_2 T_3}}$
Treadmill Run Time (secs.)	19.0	.826	7.923	11.203
Gross Oxygen Intake				
(L.)	0.649	.875	0.230	0.325
(L./min.)	0.198	.869	0.0717	0.1014
(cc/min./kg)	4.24	.785	1.966	2.780
(L./kg)	0.0167	.885	0.0057	0.0080
Maximum Oxygen Intake				
(L./min.)	0.230	.810	0.1003	0.1418
(cc/min./kg)	5.10	.798	2.290	3.238

boys demonstrated that there had developed some appreciable fatigue in the last week of the school. This most likely was when group contests were held in the seventh week, this poor showing in tests made during the week the school closed. But in an average of forty-one days after this, the boys were refreshed and did better on the tests. This effect may have been partly psychological as it showed in the all-out run time (8.77%) and somewhat less in the "peak" O_2 intake test (1/min/kg), this being (6.69%).

The groups were proved to be matched by the usual *t*-test method, the differences between the T_3 and T_4 trials, one week apart, being statistically insignificant.

There were certain irregularities which were brought out by an analysis of each and every case. A line was drawn between the boys who improved in the all-out treadmill run and those who did not in the eight weeks of participation. Two of the boys who did not improve were overweight (KK) and (EK). The first of these was 22 lb overweight and was dropped from the comparative data. The second (EK) was 5 lb overweight and gained 13 lb during the course. It was also noted on this same chart that three boys on wheat germ did not improve, whereas, six boys on nothing did not improve; and seven on wheat germ improved and five on no supplement improved. (Figs. 80 and 81)

TABLE XCI

DIFFERENCE BETWEEN VARIANCES OF TEST—RETEST DATA

Hypothesis Tested   H: $\sigma^2_{T2} = \sigma^2_{T3} = \sigma^2$, $\overline{H}$: $\sigma^2_{T2} \neq \sigma^2_{T3} \neq \sigma^2$

N = 21   Degrees of Freedom (N − 2) = 19

Critical Region σ = .05, Two Tail Test

Value of t Necessary to Reject H or Accept $\overline{H}$ = 2.09

Variable	S^2_{T3}	S^2_{T2}	S_{T3}	S_{T2}	r_{T2T3}	Obtained t	Result
Treadmill Run Time (secs.)	645.16	571.21	25.4	23.9	.826	.471	Accept H
Gross Oxygen Intake							
(L.)	0.7379	0.6724	0.859	0.820	.875	.419	Accept H
(L./min.)	0.0462	0.0424	0.215	0.206	.869	.037	Accept H
(cc/min./kg)	28.484	25.888	5.337	5.088	.785	.336	Accept H
(L./kg)	0.00534	0.00462	0.0231	0.0215	.885	.613	Accept H
Maximum Oxygen Intake							
(L./min.)	0.0595	0.0524	0.244	0.229	.810	.472	Accept H
(cc/min./kg)	35.2836	35.8801	5.94	5.99	.798	.471	Accept H

TABLE XCII

STATISTICS OBTAINED FROM RESULTS OF SIX TREADMILL
RUNS DONE BY ONE SUBJECT

Variable	Range	$\bar{x}$	S	S_E
Treadmill Run Time (secs.) .	150-173	163.33	3.95	1.767
Gross Oxygen Intake				
(L)	4.21 - 5.09	4.773	0.3233	0.1446
(L/min.)	1.68 - 1.84	1.755	0.0575	0.0257
(cc/min./kg)	42.4 - 46.2	43.983	1.2876	0.5758
(L/kg)	0.106- 0.126	0.1197	0.0078	0.0035
Maximum Oxygen Intake				
(L/min.)	2.02 - 2.12	2.058	0.0492	0.0220
(cc/min./kg)	50.1 - 53.3	51.62	1.2449	0.5568

TABLE XCIII

ZERO-ORDER CORRELATION COEFFICIENTS-TREADMILL
RUN TIMES WITH OXYGEN INTAKE VARIABLES

Variables Correlated	Correlation T_2	Coefficients T_3
Time of Treadmill Run (secs.) With Gross Oxygen Intake		
(L)	.923	.907
(L/min.)	.495	.402
(L/min./kg)	.579	.677
(L/kg)	.944	.963
Time of Treadmill Run (secs.) With Maximum Oxygen Intake		
(L/min.)	.419	.263
(cc/min./kg)	.465	.603

Experiment 20

Effects of Wheat Germ Oil, Octacosanol and Wheat Germ Versus a Devitaminized Lard Placebo in an Extended Endurance Program with Young Boys

ERIC W. BANISTER AND THOMAS K. CURETON[*]

PURPOSE

THE aim of the study was to compare the possible effects of three dietary supplements versus a placebo in an extended program of physical education and endurance running.

A group of sixty-four boys in the Summer Sports Fitness Experimental School for Boys at the University of Illinois during the summer of 1963 was given a 600-yard run twice on an outdoor track, with two days separating the trials. The boys were paired off into four matched groups by the 600-yard run time and also by age as closely as this could be done. Analysis of variance was used to show that the four groups were matched.

RESEARCH METHODS

Reliability for the all-out run was established by the test and retest method as 0.88. This was very satisfactory and compares favorably with 0.80 obtained by Cureton and Doroschuk in the summer of 1960 with a similar group of boys.

Each of the experimental cases was fed fifteen capsules of the 6-minim size of whole fresh WGO and the same of octacosanol and also of the placeboes (of devitaminized lard), and the other group was fed 1 oz. of wheat germ. On four days per week the feeding was supervised by two inspectors at 3:00 PM Monday, Tuesday, Wednesday and Thursday. Additional feedings of the same amount per day were put up in envelopes and sent home for Friday, Saturday and Sunday. A check was made at every home to see if the boy took his supplements and this was done every

[*] Physical Fitness Research Laboratory, University of Illinois, 1963.

RESULTS

COMPARATIVE IMPROVEMENTS IN THE 600-YARD RUN IN FOUR MATCHED GROUPS
SUPPLEMENTED WITH WHEAT GERM, WHEAT GERM OIL, OCTACOSANOL VERSUS A PLACEBO

Summer, 1963
Standard Score Changes

	I Control*			II Octacosanol†			III Wheat Germ Oil‡			IV Wheat Germ§		
	T_1	T_2	d	T_1	T_2	d	T_1	T_2	d	T_1	T_2	d
	41	57	16	55	84	29	42	56	14	38	35	- 3
	56	64	8	59	66	7	56	73	17	52	69	17
	77	79	2	79	78	- 1	82	84	2	78	87	9
	53	65	12	69	71	2	60	69	9	59	66	7
	64	70	6	59	62	3	56	71	15	59	69	10
	71	82	11	62	61	- 1	71	81	10	60	68	8
	64	69	5	63	65	2	71	71	0	70	74	4
	45	42	- 3	59	63	4	47	61	14	54	70	16
	74	81	7	73	74	1	73	75	2	71	69	- 2
	67	71	4	66	68	2	72	75	3	54	59	5
	60	54	- 6	53	56	3	61	71	10	43	44	1
	41	36	- 5	71	79	8	43	62	19	43	58	15
	67	77	10	71	76	5	73	81	8	73	71	- 2
	70	77	7	74	71	- 3	78	82	4	69	77	8
	55	63	8	35	43	8	41	38	- 3	63	64	1
	78	80	2	63	67	4	75	74	- 1	76	76	0
Σ=983		1067	+98 / -14	1011	1084	78 / - 5	1001	1124	123	962	1056	101 / - 7
			84			73						94
M= 45.2	49.1		3.9	46.5	49.9	3.4	46.0	51.7	5.7	44.3	49.6	4.3
Means of RS=143.06 (secs.)	136.50		- 6.56	141.60	136.20	- 5.40	143.80	134.20	- 9.50	138.95	131.20	- 7.75

* 15 capsules, 6 minims of devitaminized lard with ½ pint milk
† 15 capsules, 6 minims of VioBin octacosanol with ½ pint milk
‡ 15 capsules, 6 minims of VioBin whole wheat germ oil with ½ pint milk
§ 1 ounce Kretschmer's wheat germ, freshly opened, with ½ pint milk

Errors of Measurement (by re-test)

$$S.E._d = \sqrt{\frac{\Sigma d^2}{N\,(N-1)}}$$

$d = T_1 - T_2$ r_{11} for 600 Yd.

$N = 64$ Run = 0.88

$S.E._{dev.} = \pm 1.09$ secs.

Significance (by ratio of D to SE$_d$)

	D	S.E.$_D$	D/SE$_D$
(in favor of WGO, sig. 1% level)	4.1	1.42	2.88
Wheat Germ Oil versus Octacosanol			
Wheat Germ Oil versus Control Placeboes (significant, 5% level)	2.94	1.37	2.14
Octacosanol versus Control Placeboes (insignificant)	−1.16	1.30	−0.79
Wheat Germ versus Octacosanol (insignificant)	2.35	1.42	1.81
Wheat Germ versus Wheat Germ Oil (in favor of Wheat Germ Oil)	−1.75	1.32	−1.29

CONCLUSIONS

Octacosanol is different and inferior in its effect to wheat germ oil. Wheat Germ Oil is superior to Wheat Germ. ($D = -1.75$ secs; $t = -1.29$). Wheat Germ Oil is superior to control placeboes of devitaminized lard. ($D = 2.94$ secs; $t = 2.14$).

Monday morning. The capsules were similar and it was not known for certain what was in the capsules, as they were placed in the custody of the laboratory technician, who labelled them only A, B, C and D. While D was uncamouflaged (WGC) the others were fed double blind. Later, and after the experiment was over, A was identified as placebo, B as octacosanol and C as wheat germ oil. The feedings were continued for six weeks until each boy took his final tests. The two sessions for testing were designated T_1 and T_2 at the start in the first week and in the last week of the program.

Twice each week each boy took tests in the Physical Fitness Research Laboratory. Some exertion was involved. They also took Physical Education class work in a group from 1:30 to 4:00 PM on Monday, Tuesday, Wednesday and Thursday (four classes in succession including swimming, track and field, conditioning exercises and games) and then went to the "milathon." This event was the feature of the year. Each boy was asked to run as far as he could around a large track at the best pace he could maintain for thirty minutes without stopping. A large chart was kept of the laps completed by each boy and this was posted day by day, four days per week. All boys improved their running (cf. Table VIII).

Experiment 21

Improvements in Physical Fitness Associated with a Course of U. S. Navy Underwater Trainees, with and without Dietary Supplements

Thomas K. Cureton[*]

A N evaluation of the United States Navy's program of training for underwater swimmers, at Key West, during one typical course of six weeks, shows muscular, cardiovascular, and fat reduction improvements. The program of intensive physical conditioning, both in and out of the water, totaled about five hours of vigorous exercise per day, five days per week. In addition to swimming, the thirty men took land calisthenics drills, ran on an outdoor track, carried scuba packs weighing about sixty lb, and took many test exercises to virtual exhaustion. Improvements equalled those obtained in wartime university programs but appear to be proportional to time spent, and were better than peacetime programs.

Improvements in the cardiovascular area are considered handicapped and were probably hampered by insufficient sleep and the fatigue which accumulated during the course of the experiment. The time was considered inadequate to make the fullest cardiovascular adjustments. Fatigue showed especially in quiet cardiovascular tests. Changes in fat, both by specific gravity tests and by caliper fat measurements, were significant.

The entire group was subdivided into three matched groups upon the basis of the composite standard scores on five muscular endurance items. The matched groups differed insignificantly in the composite scores and also on each item, matched 10, 10 and

[*] Assisted by: William A. R. Orban, A. J. Barry, E. E. Phillips, E. L. Herden, and P. S. Carhart, staff members of the Physical Fitness Research Laboratory, College of Physical Education, University of Illinois, Urbana, Illinois, at the time of the experiment.

Note: Reprinted from *The Research Quarterly*, 34:4, December, 1963.

10 for feeding dietary supplements; A (10 men, on octacosanol crystals of wheat germ oil), B (10 men on placeboes of cotton-seed oil) and C (10 men, on whole, fresh wheat germ oil). Comparison of the improvements made by these three equivalent groups produced advantages for the octacosanol or WGO in four muscular endurance events (except chinning) and also in strength/weight tested on dynamometers; the level of significance obtained was >0.13 but was <.05. Standard error of measurement calculations showed the groups to have benefited in muscular endurance and strength from the wheat germ oil and/or octacosanol supplementation but not at the irrefutable level of reliability.

The principal aim of the study was the evaluation of the physical fitness status and improvements made during a typical six-weeks course at the United States Navy Underwater Swimmer's School, Key West, Florida. The secondary objective was to discover the possible effects of certain dietary supplements (wheat germ oil and octacosanol) as dietary supplements on the various physical fitness tests used. Daily consultations were held to improve fitness methods.

The program of training was intensive, lasting six weeks from May 6 to June 15, 1956, under the supervision of Commander J. C. Roe. Daily activities included six days per week of basic swimming, land calisthenics, portage of scuba equipment, penalty running and taking various physical tests; the program, as a whole, included about five hours per day of physical exercise. Every morning there were two hours of mask and fin swimming followed by two hours of scuba activities, or skin diving in the open sea, in the afternoon. In addition about three hours of lecture, paper and pencil work, and moving pictures were a required part of the program with various tests interspersed. Great interest centered in the physical fitness of the men, the mental and physical adjustments and the improvements made in the physical fitness tests.

REVIEW OF THE LITERATURE

Reduction of Fat

Changes in fat have been shown to parallel changes in specific gravity and vice versa.[52] Roby[47] was unable to verify the idea of spot reduction of fat. Fat does not change much in statical weight training programs but several studies have shown that it can be reduced in endurance programs.[38, 44, 52, 53]

Improvement of Muscular Endurance

From the beginning of World War II, many studies have reported the improvement of young men in muscular endurance. The best are by Hughes, 1942;[33] Bookwalter, 1943;[2] Johnson, 1943;[34] Wilbur, 1943;[55] Cureton, 1943;[5] Douglas, 1944;[26] Kistler, 1944;[37] Brown, 1944;[4] Cureton and others, 1945;[6] Fordham, 1949;[28] Berrafato, 1949;[1] Nelson, 1949;[45] Nakamura, 1950;[44] Kristufek, 1951;[39] Sigerseth, 1951;[49] Surles, 1952;[51] Joranko, 1953;[35] Kong, 1954;[38] Heusner, 1955;[32] Moore, 1955;[43] Samples, 1959.[48] Most of these studies include some muscular endurance tests, some physique tests, and also some cardiovascular tests. Our review leaves the impression that programs of minimal duration, 1½ hours per week, produced the smallest gains; whereas those with maximal duration, 4-10 hours per week, made greater relative improvement, the advantage being approximately proportional to the added time available.

Improvement of Cardiovascular Fitness

The more important studies are by Cureton,[8, 15, 16, 25] Heusner,[32] Kong,[38] Kristufek,[39] Michael and Gallon,[41] Michael and Cureton,[42] and Reindell.[46]

Endurance studies report greater improvements in cardiovascular fitness than studies of games and recreational activities. Time and intensity are factors in such improvements. The nervous system adjusts best when the dosage is very gradually increased over several months. Such adjustments may, in fact, continue as physiological adaptation over several years. For the purpose of this paper only a gross comparison is presented. Such improvements may also be classified according to each sport or type of activity.

The Use of Dietary Supplements of Vitamins

There are many studies involving the use of vitamins to bolster physical performance.[3] Various types of ergogenic aids have also been used. The results shown in the very extensive review by

Ancel Keys[36] in 1943, which summarized 410 studies, are contradictory, and to quote Keys, "It is difficult to reconcile the opposing reports." From our own review and experience with the testing itself, the difficulty is probably due to a) the great variation in human subjects due to their living habits and psychological states, i.e. biological variability; b) the nature of the activities involved, certain ones being hard to motivate at a maximal level; c) the very great amount of variation in the energy cost level of the various work performances; d) the variable length of time the dietary substances take to act. However, in spite of the difficulty in obtaining Fisher's statistical significance at a level of .05 or .01, the actual amount of improvement may be of some real consequence. Some studies use this system and others only show that the gains are two or three times as great as the σ_d errors of measurement with application only to the group or individuals at hand.

While many of the studies are negative, positive claims have been made by competent investigators for vitamin B_1, vitamin C, glycine and phosphate compounds. The studies cannot be reconciled, as we see it, because the levels of stress that are compared are too different, and the amount and quality of the dietary supplementation is so variable. However, the 1960 report of the International Congress of Sport Medicine,* held in Vienna, devotes forty-two pages to reviewing various studies made in the past few years in Western Europe. Positive claims for the value of supplementation have been put forth to show that vitamins B_1 and C, and phosphate compounds have positive influence on performance. However, these studies have avoided the precision required in meeting the Fisher .05 and .01 levels of virtual irrefutable statistical significance and usually evaluate only the errors of measurement of the group or individual at hand.

Goldman and Ramey[29] point to the enormous quantities of vitamin C used by the body in the face of stress. This is the same position taken by G. H. Bourne,[3] who states that as much as 15 mg of vitamin B_1 is needed to keep up hard work for several

---

* International Congress of Sport Medicine. *Proceedings,* 1960.

hours per day, performed day after day. Henschel[31] reviews the situation but leaves the door open for new work.

Our translation of Yakovlev's work,[57, 58] and review of the research work since 1943, has pointed up the principle adopted by the Russian, Austrian and East German scientists, that "with more work, more vitamins, phosphates and wheat germ oil" is the rule now. Cureton, in his review of this new work, commented upon the Russian emphasis upon wheat germ oil, and vitamins B_1, C, P and K being given to athletes proportionately to the work done.[9] A survey of the coaches made at and just after the Rome Olympic Games showed that a majority of the most successful American coaches recommend vitamin supplements, wheat germ oil, wheat germ and brewer's yeast, and about a fifth of the foreign coaches, especially those from Russia, Australia, and Germany,[14] said that they recommend such supplements.

Wheat Germ Oil and Its Derivatives

The studies of wheat germ oil, vitamin E, and wheat germ began in 1953 at the University of Illinois. The first study, published in 1955, was by Cureton and Pohndorf,[8] on middle aged men. It compared two matched groups of men, who worked out in the same programs for six weeks, with ensuing advantages in time on the all-out treadmill run and the amplitude of the brachial pulse wave for the group which took ten capsules of the 6-minim size of WGO at the end of workout. A confirmation of this advantage was found the next year, after which a paper was read before the American Physiological Society, in Madison, Wisconsin, reporting the results.[7] The small amount of vitamin E in the wheat germ oil dosage was discounted as the significant dietary ingredient. The dietary control was devitaminized lard in identical capsules, with the feeding dosages made up blind by Dr. Brookens. A number of other experiments followed, some of which encountered extreme human variation because of competitive fatigue and emotional conditions, and produced insignificant trends which favored the wheat germ oil and wheat germ only slightly.[11] Still, many teams reported apparent improvements attributable to the dietary supplements.[10, 12, 13] Erchoff and Levin[27] repeated the wheat germ oil experiments on animals at the Western Biological Laboratories and concluded that several groups of guinea pigs, matched in weight, outswam similar groups that were not fed on the wheat germ oil but on standard diet.

Another experiment completed on forty-eight men training for underwater demolition work at the U. S. Marines base, Little Creek, Va., is summarized in the dissertation of Lt. Col. James Tuma.[53] This study was assisted by the Bureau of Medicine and Surgery, U. S. Navy, Washington, D. C. Three groups were matched in muscular endurance after preliminary testing and the same dietary supplements were used as in the Key West experiment. In this fourteen week experiment the results showed an improvement in standard scores of 16.0 as an average for the men on octacosanol crystals, 7.98 for the group on cottonseed oil placeboes and 13.12 for the men on WGO capsules. Because a large number of men dropped out in the placeboes group, the matched group plan broke down, but man for man those on the octacosanol or WGO did better than those on the placeboes.

Parallel with the work on college students,[15, 16, 47] middle aged men,[8] and special individual athletic subjects,[10] work was proceeding in a similar manner with young boys in the University of Illinois Sports Fitness School. In 1959 a report was rendered on four years of work involving young boys in the dietary supplement feeding.[17, 21] In this the octacosanol crystals group improved 10.93 seconds over six weeks of training in the sports activities of the Sports Fitness School. In an endurance period run four times per week for forty minutes, in which the criterion performance was the 600-yard run, the wheat germ oil group improved 8.92 seconds, and the cottonseed oil placebo group improved 3.02 seconds. These were average results for 1955, 1956, 1957 and 1958. These differences were significant >.10 but did not meet the .05 or .01 levels.

PROCEDURE

A squadron of thirty male underwater scuba swimmers was tested by an expert staff during the first five days of the six-week course on a battery of forty-three physical fitness tests:

17 physical tests (including specific gravity and lean body mass)

13 cardiovascular-respiratory tests

13 motor fitness tests

These tests were repeated during the last five days of the course following the five weeks of intensive training. Because of the size of this report, the specific gravity, body water and total body computed fat data are deleted, to be rendered in another study.

Techniques of measurement for all tests shown in the tables were according to Cureton's specifications.* The quiet cardiovascular tests were given in the morning before breakfast (5:00 to 7:00 AM) and the strenuous tests were added before lunch or supper, or later in the evening during the free time of the men. Only one strenuous all-out test-exercise was given each day, in the following order: a) squat jumps, b) push-ups, c) sitting tucks, d) pull ups and e) mile run. In addition, the men took the 466-yard swim for time in the 33⅓ yard pool during two of the regular morning instruction periods. In this event skill differed widely, three men were not able to complete the swim without small life-preservers, which greatly increased the variability and errors of measurement in this event. Nevertheless, the Navy wanted it included and considerable improvements were shown for the three groups in this event.

At the beginning of the program, the U. S. Navy men were given a battery of five land tests, all of the muscular endurance type (chinning, sitting tucks, push-ups, squat jumps and mile run).[6] They were then ranked according to the average of standard scores on these five tests. These scores ranged from 101.7 to 26.2 on the University of Illinois Muscular Endurance tables for young men, with the mean of the thirty men averaging 50.46. Three matched groups, designated as A, B and C, were formed by division in varying order from this ranking. The groups varied insignificantly from each other as tested by the analysis of variance technique, with the following F values: Average standard

---

* See references: 18, 19, 20, 22, 23, 24, 25.

score of 5 items, F = 0.128; mile run, F = 0.304; sitting tucks, F = 0.199; squat jumps, F = 0.181; chinning, F = 0.882; push-ups, F = 0.273. The t test for significance of the difference between the means of the five muscular endurance items was also used, and further upheld the equalization of the several groups: $t_{AB} = 0.91$, $t_{AC} = 0.58$, $t_{BC} = 0.85$.

The daily supplementary feeding was in terms of ten capsules (6 minims each), designated A, B and C. These were fed at the morning muster under the supervision of the medical officer at the base, he was the only person who knew exactly what the capsules contained. The capsules looked alike and were passed out to the men in envelopes. The bottles containing the supply of capsules were also labelled A, B and C and the secret of their identity was kept until the experiment had ended. A contained synthetic crystals of octacosanol in cottonseed oil, a derivative of wheat germ oil; B contained placeboes of cottonseed oil, used because it contained very nearly the same amount of vitamin E that was in the WGO; and C contained whole, fresh VioBin wheat germ oil which had been kept at a freezing temperature until used. All capsules were shipped to the base in dry ice and were kept refrigerated until used to prevent any spoilage.

This experiment was the first to use the crystalline form of the wheat germ oil, eliminating the linoleic acid and the vitamin E. The new crystalline form was named octacosanol. It was made synthetically* and a patent obtained on its biological effects. The plan of the Key West experiment was to compare the synthetic form of the supplement with the whole fresh wheat germ oil, and both against placeboes of cottonseed oil. A very hard working group of men was needed, all living together and doing the same work.

STATISTICAL TREATMENT OF DATA

The differences between T_1 (initial scores) and T_2 (final scores) were computed for every test item, and the differences were test-

---

* Made by the VioBin Corporation, Monticello, Illinois. Based partially on the basis of these experiments a patent was granted (U. S. Patent No. 3031376) and the formula for octacosanol was revealed as C_{28}, H_{56}, OH.

ed for reliability of the differences by Fisher's t technique for small samples. These differences were presumably due to the program considered as an overall situation, the one-tail t being used as changes were normally expected in only one direction.

The mean differences on each item considered between groups was also computed, and the statistical significance of the differences were determined by Fisher's small sample t, using the two-tailed distribution. These differences most critically test the value of the dietary supplements on Groups A and C as compared with B. All calculations shown are for differences between groups based upon 10, 10, 10 cases in the Groups A, B and C.

Standard errors of measurement (S.E.) were computed for each group and also for the difference obtained for each individual case (S.D. = S.E. $\sqrt{2}$).[30] Table XCIV shows the comparative differences in improvements made between the three matched groups by restricting the reliability estimates to the group at hand and using the ratio of the D./S.E. In the mile run, push-ups, squat jumps and sitting tucks all three groups made gains. On these four tests the ratio of the difference to the error of measurement was greater for the WGO and octacosanol supplemented groups.

Consideration of the number of individual cases which changed significantly using the ratio of D to S.D. gives a slight advantage to the groups which took octacosanol or WGO in the push-ups, back strength, squat jumps, sitting tucks and strength/weight.

Using the suggestion of Wilkinson[56] that in a series of reliability estimates, a certain number would become significant by chance, the probability was that .081, or 4 of the 41 test items, might be significant by chance. For this reason the D./S.E. values are presented in Table XCVI.

SUMMARY OF FINDINGS

Within Groups

In the area of physique, statistically significant improvements >.05 level were made in all three subgroups in reduction of abdominal girths (t's = 2.05 to 3.79); reduction of abdominal fat (t's = 3.72 to 6.23); and reduction of total fat index (t's = 2.83 to 8.67).

TABLE XCIV

CHANGES WITHIN GROUPS

	D (Changes Within Groups)						Significance Groups		
	Octacosanol (A)		Placebo (B)		WGO (C)		A	B	C
Test Items	Raw Score	SS[a]	Raw Score	SS[a]	Raw Score	SS[a]	(N=12)	(N=10)	(N=12)
Physique Tests									
Calf Girth (in.)	− .13	− 2.5	.03	0.5	0	0	1.32	0.42	0
Biceps Girth (in.)	.06	1.0	.07	1.0	.08	1.0	1.20	0.49	0.62
Gluteal Girth (in.)	.07	1.0	.01	0	.27	− 3.0	0.30	0.06	1.26
Thigh Girth (in.)	− .47	− 3.8	− .27	− 2.0	.15	− 2.0	3.88[b]	0.70	0.56
Inflated Chest Girth (in.)	.04	0.3	− .07	0.7	.33	2.2	0.23	0.33	1.06
Abdominal Girth (in.)	.82	3.8	.60	2.6	.42	1.9	3.79[b]	2.34[b]	2.05[b]
Chest Expansion (in.)	.38	11.9	.07	3.1	.26	8.8	2.07[b]	0.35	1.49
Expanded Chest–Abdominal Girth (in.)	.71	5.0	.54	3.8	.64	4.8	2.33[b]	1.70	1.60
Muscle Girth Index (lb.)	− .60	− 0.5	.08	0.1	− 1.30	− 1.1	0.46	0.03	0.91
Weight (lb.)	− 4.20	− 2.7	− 5.70	− 4.0	− 3.60	− 2.5	0.52	8.83[b]	1.33
Residual of Predicted Weight (lb.)	− .91	− 2.5	.51	− 1.2	1.30	3.1	1.12	0.41	0.96
Abdominal Fat (mm)	− 3.09	6.0	− 4.50	10.2	− 3.67	8.6	4.62[b]	6.23[b]	3.72[b]
Total Fat (mm)	−15.90	7.5	−28.70	10.4	−23.50	9.0	1.56	8.22[b]	3.91[b]
Fat Index (Weighted) (lb.)	−21.70	4.9	−37.70	11.4	−23.90	9.0	5.71[b]	8.67[b]	2.83[b]
Skeletal Index (lb.)	− .30	− 0.5	.60	− 0.9	− .40	− 0.5	0.24	0.18	0.21
Cardiovascular-Respiratory Tests									
T-Wave of the ECG (mm)	0.65	3.8	− 0.14	− 0.5	− 0.42	− 2.8	1.25	0.15	0.82
R-Wave of the ECG (mm)	2.60	12.0	2.65	12.2	1.37	11.5	2.34[b]	1.29	0.78
Vital Capacity (cu. in.)	4.20	1.7	3.80	1.5	6.50	2.5	0.50	0.37	0.89

Test Items	Octacosanol (A) Raw Score	SS[a]	Placebo (B) Raw Score	SS[a]	WGO (C) Raw Score	SS[a]	Significance Groups A (N=12)	B (N=10)	C (N=12)
Vital Capacity Residual (cu. in.)	13.40	5.2	18.20	7.0	15.70	6.2	0.33	3.06[b]	1.83[b]
Breath Holding (secs.)	4.66	10.0	3.65	5.0	4.00	8.0	2.55[b]	1.40	2.50[b]
Expiratory Force (mm Hg)	9.60	4.0	24.80	8.5	0.30	0	1.40	1.55	0.06
5-Min. Step Test (Brouha) (beats)	-17.20	18.0	-22.60	23.4	-17.20	18.2	3.21[b]	5.37[b]	5.22[b]
5' Terminal Pulse (Bts./Min.)	-15.60	17.0	-10.00	10.7	2.30	-1.5	3.10[b]	2.36[b]	0.39
5' Post-Ex. Diast. Blood Press. (mm Hg)	-16.10	14.0	-20.40	20.4	-5.70	5.0	3.56[b]	4.05[b]	1.20
5' Post-Ex. Syst. Blood Press. (mm Hg)	-4.80	-4.8	-5.80	-5.1	0.30	0.1	0.63	0.94	0.05
Post-Ex. Heartograph (Syst. Amp.) (mm)	2.50	9.7	5.98	23.2	4.88	18.9	4.84[b]	5.40[b]	6.32[b]
Sitting Heartograph (Syst. Amp.) (mm)	0.80	4.5	1.66	8.8	-0.41	-2.5	0.83	1.52	0.90
Schneider Index (Points)	1.58	4.9	3.60	15.0	0.58	2.3	1.79	2.32[b]	0.64
Motor Fitness Tests									
Mile Run (min.)	-1.38	17.3	-0.83	10.8	-1.14	14.8	4.06[b]	2.96[b]	4.77[b]
466-yd. Swim (min.)	-2.67	16.0	-3.00	17.7	-1.58	9.2	4.19[b]	2.91[b]	4.84[b]
Push-Ups (times)	6.54	14.0	3.85	9.5	5.13	10.0	7.39[b]	5.15[b]	2.83[b]
Chins (times)	0.33	1.1	0.48	2.5	0.13	1.0	0.55	1.23	0.23
Squat Jumps (times)	10.58	14.5	8.00	11.0	19.30	25.2	5.10[b]	2.09[b]	5.41[b]
Vertical Jump (in.)	0.84	4.9	-0.30	-0.6	-0.41	-0.8	3.06[b]	1.73	1.26
Sitting Tucks (times)	40.60	43.0	36.20	38.0	38.60	41.0	3.03[b]	1.65	3.05[b]
Right Grip Strength (lb.)	3.60	2.6	1.40	1.4	-2.00	-1.9	1.04	0.35	0.94
Left Grip Strength (lb.)	3.60	3.4	1.00	1.0	-5.30	-5.6	0.92	0.31	1.67
Back Strength (lb.)	45.40	10.2	7.70	1.4	10.10	2.6	2.44[b]	0.55	0.41
Leg Strength (lb.)	22.00	2.1	30.00	3.5	22.00	2.2	1.07	1.17	0.98
Total Strength (lb.)	74.40	7.0	39.70	5.0	17.10	2.0	2.19[b]	1.24	0.37
Strength/Body Weight	0.69	12.0	0.51	8.5	0.29	5.0	3.70[b]	1.83	0.97

[a] $6\sigma/100$ type standard scores.
[b] Requirement for significance—5 per cent level of confidence—1-tail distribution: N = 12, t = 1.80; N = 10, t = 1.84.

TABLE XCV

CHANGES BETWEEN GROUPS (MATCHED GROUPS, N = 10)

Test Item	Raw Score Difference Between Means			Significance of Difference Between Groups[a]		
	A (Octacosanol)	B (Placebo)	C (WGO)	A-B	A-C	B-C
Physique Tests						
Calf Girth (in.)	− .12	.03	0	1.18	1.33	0.29
Biceps Girth (in.)	.05	.07	.03	0.13	0.11	0.24
Gluteal Girth (in.)	.12	− .01	− .21	0.37	0.87	0.59
Thigh Girth (in.)	− .49	− .27	− .06	0.36	1.42	0.29
Inflated Chest Girth (in.)	.01	− .07	.24	0.41	0.58	0.85
Abdominal Girth (in.)	− .91	− .60	− .36	0.92	1.32	0.81
Chest Expansion (in.)	.46	− .07	.41	1.93	0.13	1.42
Expanded Chest—Abdominal Girth (in.)	.80	.54	.47	0.53	0.46	0.12
Muscle Girth Index (lb.)	− .28	− .08	− 1.08	0.09	0.40	0.46
Weight (lb.)	− 4.57	− 5.69	− 3.43	0.98	1.24	1.56
Residual of Predicted Weight (lb.)	− .73	− .51	1.51	0.09	1.14	1.17
Abdominal Fat (mm)	− 3.20	− 4.50	− 3.20	0.73	0	0.76
Total Fat (mm)	−16.90	−28.70	−24.35	1.55	0.76	0.39
Fat Index (lb.)	−22.80	−37.70	−22.62	1.47	0.01	1.00
Skeletal Index (lb.)	− 1.47	− 0.58	− 0.71	0.35	0.22	0.03
Cardiovascular-Respiratory Tests						
T-Wave of the ECG (mm)	0.23	− 0.14	− 0.20	0.40	0.37	0.06
R-Wave of the ECG (mm)	1.74	2.65	1.23	0.61	0.34	0.81
Vital Capacity (cu. in.)	0.90	3.80	7.60	0.22	0.39	0.27
Vital Capacity Residual (cu. in.)	11.10	18.20	16.40	0.51	0.28	0.14
Breath Holding (secs.)	5.75	3.65	3.75	0.65	0.76	0.03
Expiratory Force (mm Hg)	12.70	24.80	10.20	0.67	0.27	0.91
5-Min. Step Test (Brouha) (beats)	−12.50	−22.60	−17.70	1.96	0.56	0.71
5′ Terminal Pulse (beats/min.)	−13.60	−10.00	0.20	0.59	1.63	1.60
5′ Post-Exercise Diast. Blood Pressure (mm Hg)	−18.33	−20.40	− 7.11	1.09	1.52	1.95
5′ Post-Exercise Syst. Blood Pressure (mm Hg)	− 1.40	− 5.80	− 0.60	0.36	0.06	0.62
Post-Ex. Heartograph (Syst. Amplitude) (mm)	2.23	5.98	5.26	2.21	2.19	0.56
Sitting Heartograph (Systolic Amplitude) (mm)	0.64	1.66	− 0.49	0.82	0.71	1.97
Schneider Index (points)	2.00	3.60	− 0.10	0.80	1.18	2.03
Motor Fitness Tests						
Mile Run (min.)	− 1.59	− 0.83	− 1.10	1.67	2.31	0.73
466 yd. Swim (min.)	− 2.85	− 3.00	− 1.70	0.81	1.42	1.11
Push-Ups (times)	6.60	3.85	5.35	1.99	0.93	2.39

Test Item	Raw Score Difference Between Means			Significance of Difference Between Groups[a]		
	A (Crystals)	B (Placebo)	C (WGO)	A-B	A-C	B-C
Chins (times)	0.30	0.48	0.35	0.16	0.06	0.20
Squat Jumps (times)	11.70	8.00	17.90	0.91	1.54	1.80
Vertical Jump (in.)	0.75	− 0.30	− 0.35	1.57	1.58	0.08
Sitting Tucks (times)	43.50	36.20	44.40	0.32	0.06	0.41
Right Grip Strength (lb.) .	4.50	1.40	− 3.20	0.55	1.79	1.36
Left Grip Strength (lb.)..	2.40	1.00	− 7.80	0.20	1.71	2.00
Back Strength (lb.)	61.60	7.70	− 9.20	1.84	2.52	0.82
Leg Strength (lb.)	17.50	30.00	20.10	0.32	0.07	0.23
Total Strength (lb.)	86.00	39.70	− 1.60	0.93	1.44	0.70
Strength/Body Weight	0.79	0.51	0.14	0.97	1.74	0.98

[a] Requirement for significance—5 per cent level of confidence—2-tail distribution: $N = 10$, $t = 2.262$; 10 per cent level of confidence, $N = 10$, 1.833; 15 per cent level of confidence, $N = 10$, 1.608.

TABLE XCVI

COMPARATIVE DIFFERENCES OF MATCHED GROUPS ON
DIETARY SUPPLEMENTS

	Group A (Octacosanol)		Group B (Placeboes)		Group C (Wheat Germ Oil)	
[a]5 per cent t > 2,262 1 per cent t = 3.250	5%	1%	5%	1%	5%	1%
Mile Run	5[a] improved	4[a]	6[a] improved	4[a]	5[a] improved	3[a]
sd = 0.381	0 lost	0	1 lost	0	0 lost	0
r_{11} = 0.89	D/sE = 5.89		D/sE = 3.07		D/sE = 4.07	
Push-ups	2 improved	1	1 improved	0	2 improved	1
sd = 3.525	0 lost	0	0 lost	0	0 lost	0
r_{11} = 0.89	D/sE = 2.64		D/sE = 1.54		D/sE = 2.14	
Back Strength	1 improved	0	0 improved	0	0 improved	0
sd = 61.340	0 lost	0	0 lost	0	1 lost	0
r_{11} = 0.76	D/sE = 1.42		D/sE = 0.18		D/sE = −0.21	
Squat Jumps	2 improved	0	1 improved	0	4 improved	2
sd = 8.502	0 lost	0	0 lost	0	0 lost	0
r_{11} = 0.78	D/sE = 1.94		D/sE = 1.33		D/sE = 2.96	
Sitting Tucks	8 improved	7	7 improved	7	6 improved	6
sd = 6.771	0 lost	0	1 lost	1	0 lost	0
r_{11} = 0.92	D/sE = 9.06		D/sE = 7.54		D/sE = 9.25	
Chinning	1 improved	0	1 improved	0	0 improved	0
sd = 1.762	1 lost	0	0 lost	0	0 lost	0
r_{11} = 0.89	D/sE = 0.24		D/sE = 0.38		D/sE = 0.28	
Strength/Weight	1 improved	0	0 improved	0	1 improved	0
sd = 0.620	0 lost	0	0 lost	0	1 lost	0
r_{11} = 0.69	D/sE = 1.80		D/sE = 1.16		D/sE = 0.32	

[a] Number of individuals in each group, which improved, or lost, *significantly*.

$$t = \frac{T_2 - T_1}{SD} \text{ and } sd = sE\sqrt{2}$$

In the area of cardiovascular-respiratory tests, statistically significant differences $>.05$ level were shown in these groups in the five-minute Brouha Step Test (t's = 3.21 to 5.37); in the increase of the post-exercise amplitude of the heartograph after a one-minute run in place at 180 steps per minute (t's = 4.84 to 6.32); and in the reduction of post-exercise diastolic blood pressure (t's = 3.56, 4.05, respectively) for the A and B groups only (on dietary supplements of octacosanol crystals and cottonseed oil).

In the area of motor fitness tests all groups made statistically significant standard score improvements $>.05$ level, averaging 14.3 in the mile run (t's = 2.96 to 4.77); 14.3 in the 466-yd. swim (t's = 2.91 to 4.84); 11.16 in push-ups (t's = 2.83 to 7.39); 16.9 in squat jumps (t's = 1.10, 2.09 and 5.41, respectively); and 40.7 in sitting tucks (t's = 3.03, 1.65 and 3.05, respectively) in groups A, B, and C.

Between Groups

Comparatively, between groups the improvements in standard scores in the composite scores on the five dynamic muscular ability events (mile run, push-ups, squat jumps, sitting tucks, and chins) averaged respectively: 17.98 (group A), 14.36 (group B), and 18.40 (group C). The trend of advantage was with the dietary supplemented groups but the differences between groups were not significant. In the mile run group A (octacosanol crystals) reduced the time by 1.59 minutes, group C (WGO) reduced it by 1.10 minute, and group B (cottonseed oil placeboes) reduced it by 0.83 minute. These differences between the A-B and C-B groups do not quite meet the .05 level of significance. However, group A reduced the mile run time significantly more than group C (t = 2.31 $>.05$), indicating that the octacosanol crystals produce a greater effect than whole, fresh wheat germ oil. Also, in back lifting strength group A was significantly greater in improvement than group C (t = 2.31 $>.05$), indicating that the octacosanol crystals produce a greater effect than whole, fresh wheat germ oil. Also, in back lifting strength group A was significantly greater in improvement than group C (t = 2.52 $>.05$). In back strength group A was better than group B (control) at the .07 level (t = 1.84). In push-ups the improvements also favored group A over group B (t = 1.99 at .08 level); and favored the WGO group over the placeboes (t = 2.39 >.05).

DISCUSSION

The overall advantage is shown to be with group A (on octacosanol), in the all-out type of muscular endurance events which lasted over one minute, and there is also some advantage in total strength (sum of 4 tests), and in back strength as tested on the dynamometer. While the differences in these events are large enough to be very desirable and of practical value, the significance levels obtained do not reach the standard of laboratory controlled experiments.

In an event like the mile run, for instance, the difference in favor of group A over group C is significant at t = 2.52, which indicates that the group on octacosanol crystals differed significantly from the WGO group at the .036 level. The difference between A and B groups is significant at t = 1.67 (.138 level). An analysis of the actual differences shows that group A on octacosanol crystals improved 1.59 minute, the control group B on cottonseed oil improved 0.83 minute, and the WGO Group C improved 1.10 minute. The difference between the crystals group and the placebo group was 0.76 minute. This is calculated as being worth about 573 feet in the 5,280 foot run, or 10.85 per cent (based upon an average 7 minute mile, equivalent to 754 feet, per minute). Likewise, the advantage of the WGO group C over the placebo group B is 0.27 minute, equivalent to 204 feet.

What can be said is that the advantage of the dietary supplements is large enough for the groups at hand to be of some practical importance. Considering all the motor tests, the level of .05 significance is obtained 9 times for the octacosanol group, 5 times for the WGO group, and 4 times for the placebo group. The tabulation for this is as follows:

Mile run—All groups changed significantly, 5 per cent level, A, B and C.

466-yard swim—All groups changed significantly, 5 per cent level, A, B and C.

Push-ups—All groups changed significantly, 5 per cent level, A, B and C.

Squat jumps—All groups changed significantly, 5 per cent level, A, B and C.

Vertical jump—Only group A (octacosanol) had a significant change.

Sitting tucks—Group A and group C changed significantly.

Back strength—Only group A changed significantly.

Total strength—Only group A changed significantly.

Strength/weight—Only group A changed significantly.

This listing includes all the motor type events which change significantly at the .05 level, Fisher one-tailed t standard. It is apparent that the group on octacosanol crystals has an advantage.

Considering only the five events used in originally matching the groups (mile run time, push-ups, squat jumps, sitting tucks and chins) the average standard score in overall improvement for group A was 17.98; for group C, 18.40; and for group B, 14.36.

In view of other experiences with these supplements it is felt that five weeks is a very minimum for bringing out the influence of these supplements, whereas, in Tuma's[53] much longer experiment, the results seem to be more definitely in favor of the dietary supplements.

It is also reasonable to accept the level of .15 for experiments with human subjects involving maximal exertion tests, where the human motivation factor is so variable. It is clear that training changes dominate the results, whereas the dietary supplement is a lesser secondary factor.

REFERENCES

1. Berrafato, Peter R.: The effect of various physical education service classes on all-around muscular endurance of university students. Unpublished master's thesis, University of Illinois, 1953.
2. Bookwalter, K. W.: Critical analysis of achievements in the physical fitness program for men at Indiana University. *Res. Quart.*, 14:184-93, 1943.
3. Bourne, G. H.: Vitamins and muscular exercise, *Brit. J. Nutrition*, 2:261-63, 1948. Also in Bicknell, F. and Prescott, F. *Vitamins in Medicine*. London, Heinemann, 1948.
4. Brown, V. L.: Educational achievements in motor fitness. Unpublished master's thesis, University of Illinois, 1944.

5. Cureton, T. K., Jr.: Improvement in motor fitness associated with physical fitness clinic work. *Res. Quart.*, 14:154-57, 1943.

6. Cureton, T. K., *et al.: Endurance of Young Men.* Washington, D. C.: National Society for Research in Child Development, 1945.

7. Cureton, T. K., *et al.:* Effects of wheat germ oil and vitamin E on normal human subjects in physical training programs. *Amer. J. Physiol.*, 179:628, 1954.

8. Cureton, T. K., *et al.:* Influence of wheat germ oil as a dietary supplement in a program of conditioning exercises with middle-aged subjects. *Res. Quart.*, 26:391-407, 1955.

9. Cureton, T. K., *et al.:* Diet related to athletics and physical fitness. *J. Phys. Educ.*, 57:27-30, 1959; 59-62, 1960.

10. Cureton, T. K., *et al.:* Science aids Australian swimmers. *Ath. J.*, 37: 40-44, 1957.

11. Cureton, T. K., *et al.:* Wheat germ oil, the wonder fuel. *Schol. Coach*, 24:36-37, 67-68, 1955.

12. Cureton, T. K., *et al.:* Observations at Melbourne (swimming and diving), *Swim. Age*, 31:87, 1957. Also, *Ath. J.*, 37:40-44, 1957, and *Schol. Coach*, 24:36-37, 1955.

13. Cureton, T. K., *et al.:* What about wheat germ? *Schol. Coach*, 29:24-26, 1959.

14. Cureton, T. K., *et al.:* New training methods and dietary supplements are responsible for many of the new records. *Ath. J.*, 42:1-4, 1962.

15. Cureton, T. K., *et al.:* Effects of longitudinal physical training on the amplitude of the highest pre-cordial T-wave of the ECG. *Med. Sportiva*, 12:259-81, 1958.

16. Cureton, T. K., *et al.:* Effects of physical training and a wheat germ oil dietary supplement upon the T-wave of the ECG and the bicycle ergometer endurance test. *Med Sportiva*, 13:490-505, 1959.

17. Cureton, T. K., *et al.:* Supplementing the diet with wheat germ derivatives. *Wychowanie Fiz. i Sport*, 4:276-85, 1960.

18. Cureton, T. K., *et al.:* The electrocardiogram as a test of fitness. *Physical Fitness of Champion Athletes.* Urbana, University of Illinois Press, 1951.

19. Cureton, T. K., *et al.:* Rating cardiovascular condition by the heartometer pulse wave tests. *Physical Fitness Appraisal and Guidance.* St. Louis, C. V. Mosby, 1947.

20. Cureton, T. K., *et al.:* The brachial pulse wave as a measure of cardiovascular condition. *Amer. J. Physiol.*, 159:566, 1949.

21. Cureton, T. K., *et al.:* Physical fitness improvements made by four matched groups of boys in the University of Illinois sports-fitness school on different dietary supplements. Paper presented in the Research Section, Mid-West Convention, American Association of Health, Physical Education, and Recreation, April, 1959.

22. Cureton, T. K., *et al.*: Sympathetic versus vagus influence upon the contractile vigor of the heart. *Res. Quart.*, 32:553-57, 1961.
23. Cureton, T. K., *et al.*: Anatomical, physiological and psychological changes induced by exercise programs (exercises, sports, games) in adults. *Exercise and Fitness*. Chicago, The Athletic Institute, 1960.
24. Cureton, T. K., *et al.*: What the heartometer measures that is of special interest and importance to physical educators and physical fitness directors. *Phys. Educ. Today*, 7:10-14, 1960.
25. Cureton, T. K., *et al.*: Post-exercise blood pressures in maximum exertion tests and relationships to performance time, oxygen intake, oxygen debt and peripheral resistance. *The Journal-Lancet* (Minneapolis), 27:81-82, 1957.
26. Douglas, L. N.: Some results of an ASTP program in physical education. *J. Health Phys. Educ.*, 15:254-90, 1944.
27. Erschoff, B. H. and Levin, E.: Beneficial effect of an unidentified factor in wheat germ oil on the swimming performance of guinea pigs. *Fed. Proc.*, 14:431-32, 1955.
28. Fordham, S. S.: Effect of selected physical education activities on muscular endurance test scores. Unpublished master's thesis, University of Illinois, 1949.
29. Goldman, M. S. and Ramey, E. R.: Non-endocrine aspects of stress. *Perspectives Biol. Med.*, 1:33-47, 1957.
30. Gulliksen, H.: *Theory of Mental Tests*. New York, John Wiley and Sons, 1950.
31. Henschel, A.: Diet and muscular fatigue. *Res. Quart.*, 13:280-85, 1942.
32. Heusner, W. W., Jr.: Progressive changes in the physical fitness of an adult male during a season of training for competitive swimming. Doctor's thesis, University of Illinois, 1955.
33. Hughes, F. O.: Test results of the University of Michigan physical conditioning program. *Res. Quart.*, 13:498-511, 1942.
34. Johnson, Ralph H.: Military athletics at the University of Illinois. *Res. Quart.*, 14:378-89, 1943.
35. Joranko, F. L.: Relationship of improvement in muscular endurance to body types. Master's thesis, University of Illinois, 1953.
36. Keys, Ancel: Physical performance in relation to diet. *Fed. Proc.*, 2:164-87, 1943.
37. Kistler, J.: Study of results of eight weeks of participation in a university physical fitness program for men. *Res. Quart.*, 15:23-28, 1944.
38. Kong, Moonie H.: Physical fitness improvement of varsity swimmers from a season of swimming. Unpublished master's thesis, University of Illinois, 1954.
39. Kristofek, C. J.: Effect of endurance training on an adult subject. Unpublished master's thesis, University of Illinois, 1951.
40. Kroeker, E. J. and Wood, E. H.: Comparison of simultaneously recorded

central and peripheral arterial pressure pulses during rest and exertion and tilted position in man. *Circ. Res.*, 3:623, 1955.

41. Michael, E. D., Jr. and Gallon, A. J.: Pulse wave and blood pressure changes occurring during a physical training program. *Res. Quart.*, 31:43-59, 1960.

42. Michael, E. D., Jr. and Cureton, T. K.: Effects of physical training on cardiac output at ground level and at 15,000 feet simulated altitude. *Res. Quart.*, 24:446-52, 1953.

43. Moore, George C.: An analytical study of physical fitness test variables. Doctoral dissertation, University of Illinois, 1954.

44. Nakamura, Paul K.: Contributions of swimming to the physical fitness of an adult male. Master's thesis, University of Illinois, 1950.

45. Nelson, H. E.: Evaluation of the relative contribution of service courses to physical fitness. Master's thesis, University of Oregon, 1949.

46. Reindell, Herbert: Der Kreislauf dee Trainierten. *Diagnostik der Kreislauffrüh-Shäden*. Stuttgart, F. Enke, 1949.

47. Roby, F. B.: Effect of exercise on regional subcutaneous fat accumulations. Doctoral dissertation, University of Illinois, 1959.

48. Samples, C. A.: The workmeter as a diagnostic test of physical fitness states. Master's thesis, University of Oregon, 1959.

49. Sigerseth, Peter O.: Some effects of training upon young and middle-aged men. *Res. Quart.*, 22:77-83, 1959.

50. Simonsen, E., Henschel, A. and Keys, A.: The electrocardiogram of man in semistarvation and subsequent starvation. *Amer. Heart J.*, 35:584-602, 1948.

51. Surles, L. A.: Contributions of a fundamental physcial education course toward physical fitness. Master's thesis, University of Oregon, 1952.

52. Thompson, C. W., Buskirk, E. R. and Goldman, R. F.: Changes in body fat, estimated from skinfold measurements of college basketball and hockey players during a season. *Res. Quart.*, 27:418, 1956.

53. Tuma, James S.: Influence of exercise and diet supplement (wheat germ oil and octacosanol) on fitness changes during training. Doctoral dissertation, University of Illinois, 1959.

54. Warner, H. R., *et al.*: Quantitation of beat to beat changes in stroke volume from aortic pulse contour in man. *J. Appl. Physiol.*, 5:495-507, 1953.

55. Wilbur, E. A.: Comparative study of physical fitness indices as measured by two programs of physical education: the sports method and the apparatus method. *Res. Quart.*, 14:326-32, 1943.

56. Wilkinson, Bryan: Statistical consideration in psychological research. *Psychol. Bull.*, 48:156-58, 1951.

57. Yakovlev, N. N.: *Nutrition and Restoration of Work Capacity of Sportsmen*, Leningrad, State Publishing House, 1959.

58. Yakovlev, N. N.: The importance of vitamins for sportsmen. *Theory and Practice in Physical Education*. Moscow, State Publishing House, 1958.

A Ballistocardiographic Investigation of Cardiac Responses of Boys to Physical Training and Wheat Germ Oil

CEDRIC WARREN DEMPSEY[*]

PURPOSE

THE purpose of this study was to determine the changes in cardiac function induced by a systematic physical training program with the addition of a dietary supplement.

Ten subjects from each of the experimental groups were selected in an effort to gain a broader interpretation of the progressive training program and cardiac responses. Records were kept on a weekly basis and the results were presented in case study form.

RESEARCH METHODS

The basic data were acquired from an Arbeit d-v-a ballistocardiograph. Records were interpreted as a complex of waves caused by known physiologic events. Related cardiac and anthropometrical measurements were included to aid the understanding of the ballistocardiographic waves in terms of the total circulation. Special attention was focused on the reliability of the ballistocardiographic waves and their interrelationship with other cardiac variables.

Two experimental groups and one control group were formed to test the basic purpose of this study. The latter group had twenty subjects, whereas, the former each had twenty-eight boys. Analysis of covariance was used to analyze the data since the groups were unable to be statistically matched prior to the experiment. The Duncan Multiple Range Test was selected to determine the differences between treatment means. Data were col-

[*] Department of Physical Education, University of Illinois, 1963. (Sponsor: T. K. Cureton.)

lected during the first and last weeks of the eight-week training experiment. The experimental subjects were members of the University of Illinois Sports Fitness School, and the testing was in conjunction with the Physical Fitness Laboratory at the University of Illinois. The control group consisted of selected volunters from Champaign and Urbana, Illinois. These subjects were tested during the second week of the experiments and retested eight weeks later.

SUBSTANCES FED

Ten 6-minim capsules of fresh, whole WGO to the experimental group and same of devitaminized lard placeboes to the control group.

The Sports Fitness School was in operation four days per week from 1:30 PM to 4:30 PM, Monday through Thursday. The endurance program consisted primarily of interval training sessions. The amount, the intensity and the severity of the exercise program progressed weekly. The wheat germ oil feeding occurred one-half hour prior to the endurance program. A blind-feeding routine was followed with both experimental groups receiving ten capsules; one group consumed sixty minims of wheat germ oil, and the other group received a devitaminized lard placebo. The dietary supplement was distributed four days per week.

CONCLUSIONS

Both experimental groups showed substantial improvement in ballistocardiographic force measurements. Except for the velocity I wave amplitude, all of the ballistocardiographic amplitude measurements increased significantly at the .05 level of significance as tested by the Duncan Multiple Range Test. All Test VIII amplitude measurements revealed increments which were in contrast to previous findings by Knowlton and McCubbin. In working with adults both of their studies described decrements in amplitude measurements after training. Sherman found insignificant changes in ballistocardiographic force measurements of boys after a minimal training program.

The increase in the K-wave amplitude also was in contrast with previous experimental training studies. Evaluated with respect to the cardiovascular system as a closed hemodynamic circuit, the increased K-wave suggested an increase in blood flow in the descending aorta. Clinical references have corroborated this interpretation.

Other variables pertinent to cardiac systole produced similar increases as a result of the training program. Stroke output and sympathetic tone, as expressed by the systolic amplitude, were shown to improve. The lying heartograph systolic amplitude increases proved statistically significant at the .01 level of reliability. Although an apparent trend favoring the training program was indicated by the sitting and standing systolic amplitude measurements, irrefutable evidence was not found. Group A (taking WGO) showed an increase of 2.29 mm and Group B (taking placeboes) a 2.12 mm increase in the heartograph sitting systolic amplitude; whereas, Group C showed relatively small change, a .09 mm increase. Significant reduction in the change in systolic amplitude from sitting to standing gave significant evidence at the 5 per cent level that splanchnic ptosis was improved.

The significant reduction in heart rate at the .01 level of significance supported the results indicating that the training program produced a training effect. The heartograph lying pulse rate reduced 10.17 beats per minute in Group A (taking WGO) and 5.82 in Group B (taking placeboes). An increase of 1.94 beats per minute was found in the control group.

Although the all-out treadmill run time did not prove significantly different, a favorable change toward the training program was noted. Group A improved one minute in running time, and Group B showed an increase of fifty-five seconds to an improvement of twenty-five seconds for Group C. This trend, in addition to the significant change in pulse pressure after the treadmill run, indicated a favorable trend in improving the dynamic strength of the heart, although not statistically significant.

DISCUSSION

Changes between group A and group B were not irrefutably significant at the .05 level of significance in all of the variables but a supporting trend favoring the use of wheat germ oil was shown.

The heartograph lying pulse rate produced the most significant change. The training program group supplemented with wheat germ oil showed a decrease of 10.17 beats per minute over their pretraining test mean, whereas, the training group had only a 5.82 beats per minute decrease from Test I. This difference between groups was found to be significant at the .01 level of significance by the Duncan Multiple Range Test. This finding suggested that wheat germ oil and the training program had a beneficial effect in stimulating a greater venous return, a greater stroke volume and a slower pulse rate.

Evidence supporting wheat germ oil as an aid to withstand all-out physical performance was found in several variables. Group A (on WGO) proved to have a significant advantage at the 1 per cent level over group B in pulse pressure post-all-out treadmill run test. The treadmill run time showed a five-second advantage toward group A which although not at the .05 level of significance further supported the trend that wheat germ oil was a beneficial supplement in improving the dynamic strength of the heart.

Findings were also noted in the ballistocardiographic measurements. The velocity ballistocardiographic variables showed certain beneficial effects of wheat germ oil as a nutrient supplement during training. The H-wave amplitude, the I-wave amplitude and the M.R. ratio (I plus J amplitude/I plus J duration), all proved statistically significant at the .01 level of significance favoring WGO over the placeboes. The favorable findings were contrasted to the insignificant changes found in the acceleration ballistocardiographic record.

The velocity M.R. ratio (I plus J amplitude/I plus J time), significant at the .01 level of significance, and the same acceleration measurements, although not significant, suggested that the wheat germ oil supplement produced favorable results upon the functional capacity of the heart. This measurement as suggested in the related literature is an indirect measure of the work and strength of the heart (i.e. $F = Ma$).

The positive correlation between the I plus J-wave amplitude and the K-wave amplitude was supported by the serial measurement recordings. The acceleration I plus J-wave amplitude correlated 0.674 with the K-wave of the same wave and the velocity I plus J-wave amplitude related 0.660 with the velocity K-wave amplitude. This evidence suggested that an increase in stroke volume as indicated by the increase in the $\frac{I+J}{t}$ amplitude produced an increase in cardiac ejection force in boys.

RECOMMENDATIONS FOR FUTURE STUDY

The investigator recommends that the effects of wheat germ oil be further explored. To isolate the effects of wheat germ oil the experimental design should provide for a control of the total diet of the subjects. If changes occur as suggested by the study at hand, scientific inquiry should be made also to determine the dosage of wheat germ oil necessary to produce alterations in cardiac functions.

The investigator recommends that a ballistocardiographic training study be initiated with simultaneous records of the velocity and acceleration determinations and the electrocardiogram and heartogram determinations. With this procedure more precise information regarding the relationship of these records to one another may be obtained.

The investigator recommends that different types of training be evaluated in terms of their energy requirement so that their relative effect on cardiovascular variables can be more fully understood. In order to evaluate the efficiency of the various training techniques, a satisfactory method of energy assessment is needed.

The investigator recommends that a study be initiated showing the statistical relationship of the K-wave of the ballistocardiogram and indirect measures related to peripheral resistance and venous return of the blood. Discrepancies in recent investigations involving the effects of exercise upon the K-wave could be more adequately interpreted.

The investigator recommends that further studies observing the ballistocardiographic responses of children to various training techniques be explored. Also needed are studies relating stroke volume to measures of the ballistocardiogram of children. The findings in the present study represent evidence that the Arbeit d-v-a ballistocardiograph can be a valuable tool in measuring cardiac response in children.

Experiment 23

An Investigation of the Effect of Physical Training and Wheat Germ Oil on All-Out Treadmill Run Times for Young Boys

WHEI-CHU CHEN[*]

PURPOSE

THE purpose of this investigation was to compare performance as measured by all-out treadmill run time, of a group of young boys using a wheat germ oil dietary supplement with a group using placeboes, after a strenuous physical training program lasting eight weeks.

The experimental sample included seventy-four boys between seven and thirteen years of age who attended the Summer Sports Fitness sessions at the University of Illinois from 1957 through 1962. Only the wheat germ oil group and placebo group are treated in the analysis. In 1959 wheat germ oil was not utilized and in 1961 the treadmill run was not administered. Therefore, the years 1959 and 1961 were not included in this study.

RESEARCH METHODS

$D = T_2-T_1$ (in seconds), the difference between post-test and pretest of each individual is used in the analysis. The experiments conducted at different times (1957, 1958, 1960 and 1962) were regarded as one dimension of analysis in the two-way analysis of variance. Whether the data from one year differs from that of another year is not of primary interest in this study. It is used as a factor simply to cut down the error term and thus, is helpful in detecting the effect of the treatment.

When the frequencies in the subclasses are unequal, the computation of the sum of squares becomes very complex. A simple ap-

[*] Urbana, M.S. thesis, Physical Education, University of Illinois, 1964. (Sponsor: T. K. Cureton.)

proximate method suggested by Walker and Lev was followed by the author.

CONCLUSIONS

The treatment mean square corresponds to a comparison between the means for the wheat germ oil group and the placebo group. Computed over the four years, this is significant, which leads us to conclude that the wheat germ oil treatment results in a superior average compared with the placebo group.

The nonsignificant interaction (treatment year) mean square indicates that treatment differences have not been found to vary from year to year. In other words, the trend is consistently in favor of wheat germ oil groups.

RECOMMENDATIONS

It is recommended that the effects of wheat germ oil to improve physical performance be further explored. Much additional information is needed regarding the amount of wheat germ oil which should be fed as a dietary supplement.

It is recommended that the young boys should be well rested before the performance of all-out endurance events. Good motivation should be provided and several trials used with the best being considered as the endurance score.

THE STATISTICAL MODEL USED FOR COMBINING RESULTS

Table XCVII shows the arrangement of subjects and treatments for four experiments conducted at different times, 1957, 1958, 1960 and 1962. Each experiment involves two levels of

TABLE XCVII

COMBINING THE RESULTS OF FOUR EXPERIMENTS
PERFORMED AT DIFFERENT TIMES

	Placebo Group	Wheat Germ Oil Group
1957	6	5
1958	7	6
1960	6	8
1962	19	17

Note: Each cell is a sample of n_i subjects.

independent variable (wheat germ oil and placebo) and two groups of unequal number of subjects.*

ANALYSIS OF DATA

Table XCVIII shows the analysis variance in a two-way layout with unequal numbers of cases in the subclasses.

---

* Ray, W. S.: *An Introduction to Experimental Design.* New York, Macmillan, 1960, pp. 228-229.

TABLE XCVIII

SYMBOLIC DESCRIPTION OF ANALYSIS OF VARIANCE IN A TWO-WAY LAYOUT WITH UNEQUAL NUMBERS OF CASES IN THE SUBCLASSES

Source of Variation	Degrees of Freedom	Computational Formula for Sum of Squares
Total	$N-1$	$\sum_i \sum_j \sum_\alpha X_{ij\alpha}^2 - \dfrac{T^2}{N}$
Rows	$r-1$	$\sum_i \dfrac{T_{i.}^2}{n_i c} - \dfrac{T^2}{N}$
Columns	$c-1$	$\sum_j \dfrac{T_{.j}^2}{n_j r} - \dfrac{T^2}{N}$
Interaction	$(r-1)(c-1)$	$\sum_i \sum_j \dfrac{T_{ij}^2}{n_i} - \sum_i \dfrac{T_{i.}^2}{n_i c} - \sum_j \dfrac{T_{.j}^2}{n_j r} + \dfrac{T^2}{N}$
Within Classes ..	$N-rc$	$\sum_i \sum_j \sum_\alpha X_{ij\alpha}^2 - \sum_i \sum_j \dfrac{T_{ij}^2}{n_i}$

N: The total number of cases.

T_{ij}: The sum of the scores in the subsample which is located in the ith row and the jth column.

$T_{i.}$: The sum of all the scores in the ith row.

$T_{.j}$: The sum of all the scores in the jth column.

T: The sum of all the scores.

TABLE XCIX

TWO-WAY ANALYSIS OF VARIANCE OF DATA IN TABLE XCVIII

Source of Variation	Sum of Squares	Degrees of Freedom	Mean Squares	F	F
Treatments	1176.23	1	1176.23	4.02*	3.99
Years	10527.70	3	3509.23	11.98*	2.75
Interaction	1157.48	3	525.83	1.80	2.75
Error		66	292.91		
Total	156480.38	73			

* F significant at 5 per cent level.

TABLE C

NUMBER OF BOYS IN WHEAT GERM OIL GROUP AND PLACEBO
GROUP IN EACH OF FOUR YEARS IN AN EIGHT WEEK SUMMER
SESSION AND MEAN SCORE OF THE DIFFERENCE BETWEEN
T_2 AND T_1 (D) ON TREADMILL RUN TIME (IN SECONDS)
FOR EACH SUBGROUP

Year	Item	Placebo Group	Wheat Germ Oil Group	Sum
1957	N	6	5	11
	ΣD	63	131	194
	D	10.5	26.2	
1958	N	7	6	13
	ΣD	237	349	586
	D	33.86	58.17	
1960	N	6	8	14
	ΣD	79	103	182
	D	13.17	12.88	
1962	N	19	17	36
	ΣD	213	265	478
	D	11.21	15.59	

Whether the data from one year differs from that of another
year is not of primary interest in this study, except that it may
enter a bias. In other words, the dimension of year is used as a
factor simply to cut down the error terms and thus become helpful in detecting the effect of the treatment.

Experiment 24

The Effects of an Octacosanol Dietary Supplement Upon the Total Body Vertical Jump Reaction Time

THOMAS K. CURETON AND R. W. WIGGETT[*]

PURPOSE

THE purpose of this experiment was to determine and examine the effects of an octacosanol dietary supplement upon the total body vertical jump reaction time.

Tests were administered to two male subjects, both trained athletes.

RESEARCH METHODS

A new dietary supplement called *octacosanol*, a derivative of wheat germ oil was administered to two male subjects, both trained athletes, for six months after a month of preliminary testing for stabilization, elimination of educational effect and standardization until a plateau had been reached in both subjects. The whole experiment extended over six months during which 231 tests were made of the experimental subject's total body response time, and 471 tests made of the control subject, contrasting normal with the "warmed-up" state. No other such longitudinal experiment on this same type motor test, with or without dietary supplementation, has been known. Tests were given on seventy-seven different days.

The many repetitions during the preliminary phase of the experiment were used to determine the standard errors of the overall test procedure, these are as follows:

	Visual Reaction	*Auditory*	*Combined*
For R.W. (the control subject) ...... 20 trials	0.004 seconds	0.003	0.004
For M.B. (the experimental subject) .. 20 trials	0.003 seconds	0.003	0.003

$$\text{S.E.}_{\text{Meas.}} = \sqrt{\frac{s}{N-1}}$$

---

[*] Physical Fitness Research Laboratory, University of Illinois, Urbana, 1965. (Special Investigative Project.)

TABLE CI

COMPARISON OF THE CONTROL AND THE EXPERIMENTAL
TAKING OCTACOSANOL

	Control Subject R.W.			Experimental Subject M.B.		
	Visual	*Audi-tory*	*Com-bined*	*Visual*	*Audi-tory*	*Com-bined*
At Beginning	0.254	0.235	0.255	0.227	0.247	0.263
(Av. of first five tests)	(72)	(76)	(71)	(77)	(74)	(64)
At start of feeding	0.215	0.208	0.210	0.243	0.233	0.244
	(79)	(78)	(80)	(76)	(76)	(69)
At end of feeding	0.196	0.199	0.197	0.198	0.190	0.199
	(83)	(80)	(83)	(83)	(82)	(83)

Summary of Improvements from Point of Leveling Off (Adjusted Level)

R.W. (the control)   Sig. Ratio
　Visual .... from 0.2148 to 0.1960 = 0.0188/.004 = 4.70
M.B. (the experimental)   0.2426 to 0.1976 = 0.0450/.0035 = 12.86
R.W. (the control)
　Auditory .... from 0.2086 to 0.1986 = 0.0100/.004 = 0.312
M.B. (the experimental)   0.2330 to 0.1902 = 0.0428/.003 = 16.46
R.W. (the control) .... from 0.2102 to 0.1966 = 0.0136/.004 = 3.09
M.B. (the experimental)   0.2438 to 0.1990 = 0.0448/.003 = 17.92

CONCLUSION

The advantage is very decidedly in favor of the octacosanol supplemented subject. The best advantage is in the total body combined signal reaction where the gain was 14 SS for the supplemented experimental subject compared to a gain of 3 SS for the nonsupplemented control subject. This is statistically significant difference by the $D/_{\text{S.E.}_{\text{diff.}}}$ technique.

Experiment 25

Effects of Training and Dietary Supplements on Selected Cardiac Intervals of Young Boys

Linda B. Cundiff[*]

PURPOSE

THIS study was designed to determine the effects of the eight week University of Illinois Sports Fitness School training program plus dietary supplements on selected cardiac intervals in fifty-three young boys.

The fifty-three boys were placed in groups on the basis of an initial 600-yard run.

RESEARCH METHODS

Simultaneous recordings of the brachial pulse wave, acceleration ballistocardiogram and the electrocardiogram were utilized for the five basic measures taken. These five variables were as follows: a) Q to the brachial pulse upstroke, b) pulse transmission time, c) systolic amplitude, d) Q to the peak of the G-wave in the ballistocardiogram and e) the R to R interval on the electrocardiogram. Records were obtained at rest, 1½, 5 and 10 minutes recovery after a two-minute step test on a sixteen-inch bench at the rate of 30 steps per minute. Each subject was tested before and after the conclusion of the University of Illinois Sports Fitness School.

A statistical analysis consisting of the values of *t* computed from the differences of the three group means were carried out. Reliability coefficients were obtained from a test-retest of twenty young boys in the fourth and fifth week of the University of Illinois Sports Fitness School, while they were in the exercise program, therefore, they are not as dependable as ideal reliability

---

[*] Master's thesis, Physical Education, University of Illinois, Urbana, Illinois, 1966. (Sponsor: Dr. T. K. Cureton.)

testing procedures (i.e. test-retest situations where no experimental variable is allowed between tests), as the program possibly changed some of the boys.

One group received devitaminized lard placeboes, the second group received wheat germ, and the third group received wheat germ oil as a dietary supplement.

TABLE CII

GROUP MEANS FOR THE CARDIAC CYCLE INTERVALS,
SYSTOLIC AMPLITUDE AND 600 YARD RUN

Group Q to BPW		*Rest*		*1'30" Post-exercise*	*5' Post-exercise*	*10' Post-exercise*
Placebo	T_1	.212		.176	.196	.206
	T_2	.186†	.024	.165	.185	.190*
Wheat Germ	T_1	.205		.173	.188	.206
	T_2	.191*	.014	.168	.181	.189†
Wheat Germ Oil	T_1	.208		.176	.199	.210
	T_2	.188†	.020	.170	.185†	.189†
Pulse T. T.						
Placebo	T_1	.049		.030	.035	.037
	T_2	.023*	.026	.017	.029	.035
Wheat Germ	T_1	.048		.033	.036	.046
	T_2	.030*	.018	.025	.026	.000*
Wheat Germ Oil	T_1	.054		.036	.046	.050
	T_2	.030†	.024	.028	.031*	.033†
Systolic Amplitude						
Placebo	T_1	3.25		2.66	2.90	3.03
	T_2	2.82	−0.43	2.67	2.73	2.83
Wheat Germ	T_1	3.20		2.91	2.93	3.07
	T_2	2.75	−0.45	2.63	2.41*(18SS)	2.69
Wheat Germ Oil	T_1	2.93		2.81	2.64	2.75
	T_2	3.08	+0.15	2.71	2.89*(gain)	2.86
R to R (ECG)						
Placebo	T_1	.81		.83	.76	.73
	T_2	.91	+.10	.91	.86*	.88*
Wheat Germ	T_1	.87		.86	.78	.77
	T_2	.89	+.02	.91	.84	.82
Wheat Germ Oil	T_1	.84		.86	.78	.76
	T_2	.88	+.04	.87	.82	.82

600-Yard Run		*Mean*	*D (sec.)*	*SS Change*	
Placebo	T_1	151 Sec.		61	
	T_2	131 Sec.	20	75	+14
Wheat Germ	T_1	149 Sec.		62	
	T_2	132 Sec.	17	70	+08
Wheat Germ Oil	T_1	154 Sec.		58	
	T_2	130 Sec.	24	76	+18

* *t* value significant 5 per cent level of confidence.
† *t* value significant 1 per cent level of confidence.

RESULTS

Table CII is a summary of the means for the variables which showed significance. The asterisks are placed next to the variables which showed significant *t* values.

Q to the brachial pulse upstroke interval shortened in all groups from T_1 to T_2. There was a significant shortening in all groups at rest. The group receiving the wheat germ supplement shortened significantly at five minutes recovery and again all groups shortened significantly at ten minutes post-exercise.

All significant changes consisted of a shortening in the pulse transmission time interval. The placebo group shortened significantly at rest; the group receiving the wheat germ supplement shortened significantly at both rest and ten minutes post-exercise; the group receiving the supplement of wheat germ oil shortened significantly at rest, five and ten minutes post-exercise.

The systolic amplitude showed a significant increase in the group receiving the wheat germ oil supplement at five minutes post-exercise. A significant decrease in systolic amplitude was obtained in the group receiving the wheat germ supplement at five minutes post-exercise.

The Q to peak of G (acceleration BCG) did not show significant changes in the three groups at any time this interval was recorded.

The R to R (ECG) showed a significant change in the placebo group (lengthening) which is indicative of a slower pulse rate.

CONCLUSIONS

The following conclusions are based on the results obtained.

1. There is a shortening of the interval of Q to brachial pulse upstroke due to sympathoadrenergic influence, but in the WGO experimental group, there was relatively less shortening than in the placebo or wheat germ group.
2. There was a shortening of the pulse transmission time (using G to brachial upstroke) due to more tone in the brachial artery, but relatively less shortening than in the wheat germ or WGO experimental groups.
3. There was a gain in systolic amplitude at five minutes post-

exercise in the group on wheat germ oil supplement attributable to exercise plus the wheat germ oil supplement, whereas, there was a loss in amplitude in the wheat germ and placebo groups.

4. There was a lengthening of the R to R (ECG) interval as result of the training only.

Experiment 26

Longitudinal Effects of Training and Wheat Germ Oil on Total Body Reaction Time

GARY A. JOHNSON

PURPOSE

THE purpose of this experiment* was to conduct a longitudinal experiment with repetitious testing of total body reaction time (Garrett-Cureton Test), the average of visual, auditory and combined signals, with testing 2-5 times each week for sixteen weeks, and to compare the two matched groups, one taking WGO capsules (VioBin) and the other taking similar capsules of devitaminized lard (with vitamin E added to equal that in WGO), thus to see if there would be a difference developed between the two groups as time proceeded.

The subjects were volunteer middle-aged men, 25-50 years of age, who were regular participants in the Adult Fitness Program of the University of Illinois, directed by Professor T. K. Cureton. Nine men took part in the experiment.

RESEARCH METHODS

The nine men were tested two to three times per week for six weeks to adjust them to the test, obtain reliability data on the test, and to determine a "plateau of learning." The data were averaged and plotted each week, and after the plateau was clear for two weeks, the WGO was fed daily to the experimental group of four subjects and the placeboes to the five control subjects. All subjects took the one hour per day of physical training 3-5 times per week, this consisting of calisthenics, interval walk-jog routines and muscular endurance exercises, a mixture but continuous for an hour 3-5 days per week, and after the first six weeks

---

* Urbana, M.S. thesis, Physical Education, University of Illinois, 1966, p. 48. (Sponsor: T. K. Cureton.)

461

were tested, twice each week at noon in the Physical Fitness Research Laboratory (75-80 F, 50 to 80% relative humidity). The data were averaged for each subject, and ranked, then alternately placed in the experimental and control groups, which groups were then proved to be equated by testing the significance between the means, resulting in an insignificant statistical difference.

VioBin WGO was used with the experimental group, ten capsules of the 6-minim size, seventy capsules per week, taking them daily; and likewise with the control group taking placeboes. Details of these substances are given elsewhere in the report. The data are given in Table CIII. Each case is plotted in the study.

RESULTS

By group statistics, and using the small sample t there were insignificant differences between the two groups being compared:

1. The WGO group mean improved from the beginning average of 0.314 second to a plateau level of 0.290 second, a gain of 0.024 second.

2. The placebo group improved from a beginning average of 0.311 second to a plateau level of 0.283 second, a gain of 0.028 second.

3. All but one of the four individuals in the WGO group improved significantly (by the Gulliksen formula for retesting an individual, H. Gulliksen, *Theory of Mental Tests*, New York, Wiley, 1950, p. 40) at the 0.05 level.

4. Two of the five individuals in the control group failed to improve significantly by the same method as above.

5. In the plotted average results, no advantage appears for the WGO group compared to the control group from the first to the twelfth week and then there did develop an advantage for the WGO group. Only one of the WGO subjects failed to improve after the plateau and this one very nearly improved at the 0.05 level.

6. The sample is too small to state that the differences are unequivocally in favor of the WGO-fed subjects but the trend is slightly that way.

7. Matched subjects are compared in Table CIII based upon the initial baseline values at the start of the feeding, with

TABLE CIII

DIFFERENCES BETWEEN AND WITHIN GROUP MEANS
IN TOTAL BODY AVERAGE REACTION TIME

Testing Period	WGO Group N = 4	Placebo Group N = 5	Between Groups	Within Groups WGO	Placebo
Baseline	°.314	.311	.003		
T1	.315	.307	.008	+.001	−.004
T2	.303	.303	—	−.011	−.008
T3	.306	.299	.007	−.008	−.012
T4	.301	.297	.004	−.013	−.014
T5	.295	.298	.003	−.019	−.013
T6	.295	.292	.003	−.019	−.019
T7	.291	.291	—	−.023	−.020
T8	.293	.292	.001	−.021	−.019
T9	.290	.287	.003	−.024	−.024
T10	.292	.293	.001	−.022	−.018
T11	.295	.284	.012	−.019	−.027
T12	.283 (N = 3)	.283	—	−.031	−.028
T13	.279	.291 (N = 4)	.012	−.035	−.020
T14	.278	.288	.010	−.036	−.023
T15	.279	.290	.011	−.035	−.021

Two testing periods per week from T1 to T10.
One testing period per week from T11 to T15.
° Measured in fractions of a second.

the result that the WGO made greater gain twice, and once
a tie, and the placebo group won once.

8. No final conclusions can be reached, except that the physical training improved the total body reaction time as an
average.

It is recommended that the experiment be repeated with rigid
dietary controls and a greater number of randomly drawn subjects (which are impossible conditions amongst the subjects available from the University of Illinois).

The loss of a subject during the sixth week of supplementation limited the interpretation of results to individual changes
during the remaining weeks of the experiment. Individual comparisons between groups were made by matching two subjects
(one subject from each group) on the basis of beginning reaction time (baseline value). Table CIV presents the individual
changes of the matched subjects.

TABLE CIV

LARGEST INDIVIDUAL GAINS IN TOTAL
BODY AVERAGE REACTION TIME

Subject	Largest Gain	Subject	Largest Gain
I (WGO)	0.023	III (WGO)	0.039*
V (Placebo)	0.006	VIII (Placebo)	0.057*
VI (Placebo)	0.014		
II (WGO)	0.043*	IV (WGO)	.041*
VII (Placebo)	0.038*	IX (Placebo)	.041*

* .01 level of confidence.

A nonparametric rank test was used to determine significant differences in the between-group means and significant changes in the within-group means. Individual changes were evaluated by the "reliability of a single case," based on the standard error of measurement; the formula was as follows:

$$t = \frac{D}{s\sqrt{2N}}$$

where:

D = difference between T_1 and T_2 means
s = standard error of measurement
N = 1

Experiment Relating WGO and Wheat Germ Cereal to Flicker Fusion Frequency

Thomas K. Cureton and B. Don Franks[*]

PURPOSE

THE purpose of this experiment[*] was to match the sixty-three young boys in the Sports Fitness School in the summer of 1967 in three groups to compare the effects of wheat germ (Kretchmer, toasted fresh), wheat germ oil (VioBin) and place-boes of devitaminized lard (with E) on the flicker fusion frequency test (Krasno-Ivy Apparatus).

Sports Fitness School for boys, 7-13 years of age, three groups of twenty each.

RESEARCH METHODS

The three groups were satisfactorily matched in the principal variable, i.e. the flicker fusion frequency, twenty subjects in each group initially. Analysis of covariance was used to determine the matching and the significance of the differences in the improvements. There were insignificant differences between the groups in age, height and weight.

RESULTS

The criterion test, flicker fusion frequency, changed the most in the placebo group (113.45 f/second), next in the wheat germ cereal group (33.35 f/second) and lastly, in the wheat germ oil group (1.50 f/second) ($F = 3.23$). The between groups F was 3.23, significant at the .05 level.

In the 600-yard run group the largest improvement was in the placebo group (13.58 second) compared to the wheat germ oil group (11.11 second) and then lastly, the wheat germ cereal group (9.89 second). All differences were statistically insignifi-

---

[*] Staff experiment, summer term, 1967.

cant between groups (F = 0.21). The placeboes were devitaminized lard, 15 × 3 minim capsules per day.

Advantage appeared five times each for the wheat germ cereal
and wheat germ oil groups, four times for the cereal and once
for the wheat germ oil. No differences were statistically significant at the 5 per cent or 1 per cent level, except in one item, the
flicker fusion frequency test in which the placebo group changed
more than the cereal or the wheat germ oil group at rest (F =
3.23, significance at .05). The interpretation of this might be that
the wheat germ cereal and wheat germ oil groups were relatively
more relaxed than the placebo group, but all three groups increased in flicker fusion frequency, which would indicate that
the effect of the training had improved the retinal circulation in
all groups (it improves with increased sympathoadrenal stimulation). The groups which took the dietary supplements were
more adapted at rest, following eight weeks of strenuous phys-

TABLE CV

CHANGES OF INDIVIDUALS IN WHEAT GERM OIL GROUP
IN TOTAL BODY AVERAGE REACTION TIME

Testing Period	Subject I	Subject II	Subject III	Subject IV
Baseline	.269	.318	.333	.338
T1	.281	.336	.324	.320
T2	.268	.314	.313	.316
T3	.266	.329	.322	.309*
T4	.267	.298	.322	.315
T5	.264	.295	.327	.297†
T6	.270	.291*	.313	.307*
T7	.261	.278†	.317	.308*
T8	.263	.294	.315	.300†
T9	.259	.290*	.310	.300†
T10	.251	.310	.307	.298†
T11	.256	.307	.311	.305*
T12	.263	.292	.294†	
T13	.255	.275†	.307	
T14	.246	.280†	.307	
T15	.258	.280†	.298†	

Two testing periods per week from baseline to T10.
One testing period per week from T11 to T15.
Numbers represent thousandths of a second.
* .05 level of confidence.
' 01 level of confidence.

TABLE CVI

CHANGES OF INDIVIDUALS IN PLACEBO GROUP
IN TOTAL BODY AVERAGE REACTION TIME

Testing Period	Subject V	Subject VI	Subject VII	Subject VIII	Subject IX
Baseline	.268	.278	.331	.335	.344
T1	.269	.296	.318	.320	.331
T2	.283	.280	.318	.309	.327
T3	.271	.265	.314	.313	.330
T4	.273	.270	.319	.301*	.324
T5	.268	.279	.316	.303*	.326
T6	.274	.273	.316	.287†	.311*
T7	.265	.277	.308	.278†	.325
T8	.278	.275	.315	.286†	.308†
T9	.273	.270	.298*	.284†	.312*
T10	.265	.278	.307	.290†	.323
T11	.272	.264	.299*	.281†	.304†
T12	.262	.266	.297*	.285†	.303†
T13		.271	.297*	.293†	.303†
T14		.271	.294†	.286†	.300†
T15		.277	.293†	.279†	.310*

Two testing periods per week from baseline to T10.
One testing period per week from T11 to T15.
Numbers represent thousandths of a second.
* .05 level of confidence.
† .01 level of confidence.

ical training in a hot summer, finishing with lower pulse rates and flicker fusion frequency than the placebo control group.

DISCUSSION

The fact that the training experiment, which included about three hours of activity work per day, including one period of conditioning gymnastics and one period of running endurance, improved the 600-yard run time *in all groups* is of some significance. The differences are large in terms of converting the times to distance in feet. The advantage with the placebo group was statistically insignificant.

If the program left the boys with higher relative sympatho-adrenergic condition, at least this persisting through the period of the final tests, T_2, we might expect to find somewhat faster pulse rates and higher c.f.f. and brachial pulse waves. This has typically been the case and such stimulation has been shown to

TABLE CVII

1967 SPORTS FITNESS SCHOOL EXPERIMENT

Variable	Placebo Group (C) T_1	T_2	Change	Cereal (Wheat Germ) (B) T_1	T_2	Change	Wheat Germ Oil (A) T_1	T_2	Change	F^*
Age (years)	9.95 N = 20			10.0 N = 20			10.8 N = 20			
Height (inches)	56.63 N = 19	56.94	0.31	57.21 N = 19	57.78	0.57	57.52 N = 19	58.10	0.58	
Weight (lb)	82.63 N = 19	82.84	0.21	89.21 N = 19	90.47	1.26	90.05 N = 19	89.89	− 0.16	
18 Item Motor Test (SS)	52.36 N = 19	58.94	6.58	55.0 N = 19	58.15	3.15	48.15 N = 19	54.10	5.95	.23
Softball Throw (ft)	87.05 N = 19	85.05	− 2.0	93.47 N = 19	95.73	2.26	91.94 N = 17	91.94	0	1.22
Sit-Ups (20')	109.26 N = 19	217.31	108.05	93.93 N = 16	218.5	124.57	102.05 N = 17	171.94	69.89	1.45
Pull-Ups	1.66 N = 18	2.00	0.34	2.52 N = 17	2.94	0.42	2.38 N = 17	2.83	0.45	.03
Broad Jump (inches)	55.68 N = 19	56.84	1.16	56.84 N = 19	58.57	1.73	56.78 N = 19	58.84	2.06	.23
50-Yard Dash (sec)	9.17 N = 19	8.94	− 0.23	9.16 N = 19	9.0	− .16	8.81 N = 19	8.68	− .13	.30
600-Yard Run (sec)	148.73 N = 19	135.15	−13.58	144.73 N = 19	134.84	− 9.89	150.05 N = 18	138.94	−11.11	.21
Flicker Frequency (f/min)	2573.77 N = 20	2687.22	113.45	2632.15 N = 20	2665.50	33.35	2633.95 N = 20	2635.45	1.50	3.23*

* Reliability levels (F for analysis of covariance): = 1.43, p <.25; 2.42, p <.10; F = 3.18, p <.05.
In this experiment, the cereal (wheat germ) and WGO had the advantage in five tests and the placebo group in two.

last for a week or more in some boys. However, after two or three weeks, almost every boy was shown to have relaxed to slower pulse rates. It is admitted that the intensity of the program in the last week or two built up some cumulative fatigue. The supplemented groups with wheat germ and WGO were more relaxed (held hemostasis better at rest) than the placebo group.

Pull-ups have also been shown to give similar insignificant results in all other similar short-term training groups, as in our experiment on the Underwater Scuba (Swimming) Group at the United States Naval Base, Key West, on young men.

DIRECTIONS FOR USE OF FLICKER PHOTOMETER

1. The subject should not smoke (2 hours), drink alcohol (4 hours), or take vasodilator drugs (24 hours) prior to test.
2. Subject rests in dark room at least ten minutes.
3. If glasses are normally worn, then they should be used during test.
4. Record machine used (A or B), name, date, age, weight, height, activity for the previous twenty-four hours.
5. Turn on machine.
6. Subject seated one yard from machine with eyes approximately horizontal to the small window in the front of the machine.
7. Make sure that there are no distractions in the room—it is important for the subject to concentrate solely on the window.
8. Hand the stop button to the subject and instruct him to push it as soon as he sees the first flicker.
9. Set the dial at the back at 1600 and turn it on (a trial run to let the subject see the flicker and press the button to stop it).
10. Give three trials (setting the dial at 3100, 2900 and 3000, respectively, unless his threshold is above one of these).
11. Record each trial, total and average scores.
12. If the trials are extremely variable (more than 150-200 difference on any two trials), then have the subject rest for a few minutes and repeat.

Experiment 28

Effects of Training with and without Wheat Germ Oil on Basal Metabolism and Selected Cardiovascular Measures of Middle-Aged Men

Jacques J. Samson[*]

PURPOSE

THE purpose of this study was to measure and examine the effects of training with and without wheat germ oil on basal metabolism and certain cardiovascular measures of a group of middle-aged men.

Twenty-four men, 25 to 63 years of age, were used, six of whom were nonexercising controls. They were volunteers and no claim is made that they were a random sample.

RESEARCH METHODS

The objective is to see if the WGO affected the group at hand. For ten weeks the men were training progressively (following Cureton's rhythmic continuous exercises). It would normally be expected that the basal metabolism would increase due to the stress of the progressive low to middle gear program, as has been shown to occur in several other programs, without full adaptation ever being reached when it would have been expected that the BMR would decrease after first rising. The program was led by a good leader. At the end of ten weeks, the men were tested on the mile run, and divided into three groups of six each.

Eighteen of the twenty-six men followed the training program and six did not. The eighteen men taking the exercises were divided into three groups of six men each after the first ten weeks. The training itself, for this period of time made changes in all three groups, compared with the controls: a) lowered the BMR

* Urbana, M.S. thesis, Physical Education, University of Illinois, 1968, p. 123. (Sponsor: T. K. Cureton, assisted by B. Don Franks.)

with relation to the controls, b) did not change the R-wave with respect to the controls, Lead V_4, c) had no effect on the K-wave of the BCG with respect to the controls, d) lowered the angle of obliquity with respect to the controls, e) appreciably increased the rest/work ratio of the heartograph with respect to the controls.

EFFECT OF WGO

The more important part of the experiment was the effect of WGO in the second ten weeks from T_2 to T_3. The subjects took ten capsules of whole, fresh WGO, seven days per week. None were taking anything else.

Group A—6 men, training on WGO capsules (10×6 minims daily)

Group B—6 men, training on placeboes (10×6 minims daily)

Group C—6 men, training without the addition of capsules.

The tests given at T_1 were repeated within a week without training in between to permit the usual r_{11} (retest) reliability check, and from these data the S.E.$_{\text{meas.}}$ = $\sigma_1 \sqrt{1-r_{11}}$ was computed. The reliability check used was the ratio of D (difference between T_2 and T_3)/S.E.$_{\text{meas.}}$ If this ratio was as large as 2.0 or 3.0, the difference was considered reliable enough to guarantee a real difference over and above the errors of measurement, corresponding to the 5 per cent or 1 per cent level, respectively.

RESULTS

The group A taking WGO improved more than the other groups. The R-wave (V_4 lead) improved 2.4 mm in amplitude, and the group C taking no capsules at all improved 1.0 mm, and the group B taking placeboes improved 0.7 mm. The application of analysis of variance type of sampling reliability failed to show a difference between the WGO group and the placebo group better than the 0.10 level but comparison of the difference (1.7 mm) with the S.E.$_{\text{meas.}}$ ± 0.47 gave a T ratio of 3.62, indicating that the WGO was effective with the group at hand. No generalizations to a universal sample can be made.

The group A taking WGO improved the BMR (in %) 2.50 compared to 4.67 for the group B taking placeboes, and 16.50

taking no capsules at all. Both the WGO and the placeboes act to depress the BMR relatively, which may be interpreted as holding closer to homeostasis than the group taking nothing. Since the program increased in intensity progressively, this may be taken to indicate that the WGO group resisted the stress better and showed less sympathoadrenergic effect from the training, whereas, the group taking nothing was upset the most. This also indicates that the placeboes were not "true" neutral placeboes but had some effect. The T ratio between the WGO group and the placebo group was $T = 1.612$; and the T ratio between the WGO group and the group taking nothing was $T = 10.43$. The WGO had an effect.

Groups A and B both decreased the angle of obliquity and also the diastolic blood pressure (supine) more than the group taking nothing. These differences were slight and may be considered insignificant.

The I (acceleration) wave of the arbeit ballistocardiogram increased in amplitude 3.2 mm in the WGO group A, but improved only 0.2 mm in the group taking placeboes, and improved 0.6 mm in the group taking nothing. The advantage of the WGO group over the placebo group is significant in terms of the group at hand ($T = 3.0/0.114 = 26.35$) (Cf. Exp. 22).

The use of the S.E.$_{meas.}$ is applied strictly to this experiment. It reflects the combination of all variable errors attributable to the subject, the operator and the test situation. No attempt has been made to generalize the small amount of data to 95 out of 100 experiments, as the data were not randomly drawn for any group of six subjects, nor were the data normally distributed. The application of variance and the "t" test are of nebulous worth in this type of experiment.

The Effects of Training with and without Wheat Germ Oil on the Precordial T-Wave and Other Selected Fitness Measures of Middle-Aged Men

Jerry L. Mayhew

PURPOSE

THIS study[*] investigated the effects of progressive rhythmical endurance exercises with and without wheat germ oil as a dietary supplement on the precordial T-waves and other selected fitness measures on middle-aged men.

Twenty-five sedentary male volunteers, 24 to 62 years of age, were used as subjects. Nineteen of these participated in a 20-week long rhythmical endurance program, following Cureton's program (cf. *Physical Fitness and Dynamic Health*, New York, Dial Press, 1965). Six subjects served as a nontraining control group as a check upon environmental changes.

RESEARCH METHODS

In the first ten weeks the nineteen subjects were tested (T_1) and progressively conditioned for ten weeks, and at the end of this time were randomly assigned to three groups: a) WGO experimental group, N = 6, b) placebo training group, N = 6, c) training group without supplements or placeboes. All were tested at this point (T_2). All three groups continued to train on the Cureton program for ten more weeks, and then tested again (T_3). Subjects forewent all other types of physical work on the days of testing, and went without food for three hours before taking the tests. The overall program extended from November until March.

The tests given included the ECG (lead V_4) on a physiograph at the Physical Fitness Research Laboratory, 7:00 to 9:00 PM,

---

[*] Urbana, M.S. in Physical Education, University of Illinois, 1968, p. 128. (Sponsor: T. K. Cureton.)

taken in a sitting position on the ergometer bicycle, following a 15-minute rest in position. Then the subject rode for 2 minutes (25 kg-m/second at 60 r.p.m.) and recordings taken during the last 10 seconds. The graph included ECG, notations about the subject and a time calibration record. The motor tests were then given for total fat, total proportional strength (sum of four dyna-mometer tests), three flexibility tests, agility run, breath holding after 1-minute step test, chins, dips and vertical jump. All tests were repeated at T_1, T_2 and T_3, at 0, 10 and 20 weeks, respectively.

The dietary supplements were fed at the end of each day's work, 10 × 6 minim capsules of VioBin WGO and ten similar capsules of devitaminized lard.

RESULTS

At the end of the ten weeks of physical training the nineteen subjects made the following changes in the amplitude of the T-wave, significance >0.05 level:

Sitting resting T-wave amplitude ...... 1.95 mm increase
Immediately after the 2-minute ride ..... 0.58 mm increase
During the second minute of recovery ... 1.85 mm increase
During the third minute of recovery .... 1.43 mm increase

At the end of the ten weeks of physical training the WGO experimental group (N = 7) made the following changes (without supplementation):

During the second minute of the 2-minute ride 0.58 mm gain
During the second minute of recovery .... 1.85 mm gain
During the third minute of recovery ...... 1.43 mm gain

And at twenty weeks of physical training the changes were as follows: (over T_1)

Sitting rest, amplitude of the ECG T-wave .. 2.14 mm gain
During second minute of the 2-minute ride .. 0.99 mm gain
During the second minute of recovery ...... 1.82 mm gain
During the sixth minute of recovery .... 1.15 mm gain
During the tenth minute of recovery .... 2.57 mm gain

The comparison between the experimental WGO group and the control group at T_3, using T_1 measures as covariates, gave the following results on the T-wave: WGO group improved 0.99, control group −0.41.

During the fifth minute of recovery, the WGO experimental group was better than the placebo group by .... 0.94 mm

During the second minute of exercise, the experimental group was better than the placebo group by 1.40 mm

At twenty weeks of physical training the training group had improved significantly greater in changes than the control group (which did not exercise): strength/weight >0.01 level; Illinois agility run >0.001 level; trunk flexion >0.05; expiratory force >0.05 level; and vertical jump >0.05 level (N = 19).

Another comparison was made between the training group (N = 7) and the controls (N = 6) at T_3 using the T_1 measures as the covariates. The training group was significantly better in total strength (0.05 level); strength/weight 0.01 level; Illinois agility run 0.05 level; and breath holding after exercise, 0.05 level.

It was shown that the placebo group (N = 6) had a greater influence on strength, the placebo group having greater gain in strength than the WGO group by 85.50 lb (significance >0.05).

DISCUSSION

Regarding the effects of progressive physical training on the T-wave, this study agrees with Cureton's study (*Medicina Sportiva*, 13:490-505, Oct., 1959). It is also known that "pressure situations" such as competitions in the same week as taking ECG

TABLE CVIII

RELIABILITY COEFFICIENTS*

Variable T wave	*Reliability Coefficients*
Sitting rest	0.802
Last ten seconds of first minute of ride†	0.748
Last ten seconds of second minute of ride†	0.717
Last ten seconds of first minute of recovery	0.995
Last ten seconds of second minute of recovery	0.991
Last ten seconds of fourth minute of recovery	0.974
Last ten seconds of fifth minute of recovery	0.729
Last ten seconds of sixth minute of recovery	0.867
Last ten seconds of seventh minute of recovery	−0.423
Last ten seconds of eighth minute of recovery	0.876
Last ten seconds of ninth minute of recovery	0.967
Last ten seconds of tenth minute of recovery	0.896

* N = 6, with one week between tests.
† Two-minute bicycle ergometer ride (25 kg-m/sec at 60 rpm).

TABLE CIX

MEANS, STANDARD DEVIATIONS, AND MEAN CHANGES OF GROUPS USED FOR DETERMINING THE EFFECTS OF TWENTY WEEKS OF TRAINING

Group	Variable T wave	Units	T-1 Mean	T-1 S.D.	T-2 Mean	T-2 S.D.	T-3 Mean	T-3 S.D.	Changes in Mean from T-1 to: T-2	T-3
Training control	Sitting rest	mm	4.00	.43	6.28	1.11	6.14	1.86	2.28	2.14
			3.83	1.83	3.83	1.16	3.50	1.22	0.00	-0.33
Training control	1 minute exercise	mm	2.70	2.16	4.14	2.91	5.57	2.99	1.44	2.87
			4.66	2.50	4.16	2.63	5.00	3.34	-0.50	.34
Training control	2 minutes exercise	mm	3.72	2.56	4.30	0.93	4.71	1.60	0.58	0.99
			2.86	1.02	2.50	0.48	2.45	0.38	-0.36	-0.41
Training control	1 minute recovery	mm	6.15	3.47	4.81	1.42	5.71	1.49	-1.24	-0.44
			3.70	1.46	3.30	1.32	2.78	0.97	-0.40	-0.92
Training control	2 minutes recovery	mm	6.00	.60	7.85	1.67	7.42	1.39	1.85	1.82
			4.66	1.21	5.83	0.98	5.16	0.75	1.17	.50
Training control	3 minutes recovery	mm	3.72	3.26	5.15	3.54	5.57	2.99	1.43	1.85
			3.33	1.36	2.00	0.30	4.33	.37	-1.33	1.00
Training control	4 minutes recovery	mm	5.22	3.72	6.74	2.95	7.47	1.50	1.52	2.25
			5.36	1.45	6.13	0.69	5.86	1.26	0.77	0.50
Training control	5 minutes recovery	mm	8.15	2.56	6.85	1.81	6.62	0.91	-1.30	-1.53
			4.28	0.98	5.28	0.96	5.10	1.41	1.00	0.82

TABLE CX

MEANS, STANDARD DEVIATIONS, AND MEAN CHANGES
OF CONTROL AND TWENTY-WEEK TRAINING GROUPS*

	T-1 Mean	S.D.	*T-3* Mean	S.D.	Change in Mean From T-1 to T-3
Rest (Sitting)					
Cycle time (sec)					
Training	0.851	0.196	0.949	0.115	0.098
Control	0.805	0.118	0.763	0.108	−0.042
Diastole (sec)					
Training	0.492	0.167	0.563	0.098	0.071
Control	0.443	0.099	0.408	0.084	−0.035
Isovolumetric Contraction Period (sec)					
Training	0.057	0.007	0.059	0.006	0.002
Control	0.058	0.005	0.056	0.004	−0.002
Ejection Period (sec)					
Training	0.252	0.026	0.276	0.020	0.024
Control	0.248	0.022	0.244	0.024	−0.004
Per Cent Diastole in Cycle Time					
Training	56.4	7.1	60.2	4.7	3.8
Control	54.5	4.4	53.0	3.7	−1.5
Per Cent Electrochemical Lag in Cycle Time					
Training	6.3	1.7	5.5	0.7	−0.8
Control	7.1	1.4	7.3	1.3	0.2
Per Cent Isovolumetric Contraction Period in Cycle Time					
Training	6.9	1.3	6.2	0.6	−0.7
Control	7.4	1.2	7.5	0.8	0.1
Per Cent Ejection Period in Cycle Time					
Training	30.4	4.6	29.3	2.6	−1.1
Control	31.0	2.2	32.2	2.0	1.2
Diastolic Blood Pressure (mm Hg)					
Training	80.4	6.8	76.0	7.5	−4.4
Control	83.6	7.6	86.4	6.4	2.8
Systolic Blood Pressure (mm Hg)					
Training	129.5	17.4	125.0	15.6	−4.5
Control	134.4	7.1	140.2	4.7	5.8
Systolic Amplitude of Brachial Pulse Wave (cm)					
Training	1.02	0.35	1.16	0.39	0.14
Control	0.90	0.13	0.80	0.16	−0.10
Total Peripheral Resistance (mm Hg/mm SA/beat)					
Training	11.01	3.04	9.42	2.84	−1.59
Control	12.45	2.44	14.72	2.99	2.27
Per Cent Electromechanical Lag in Cycle Time					
Training	7.7	1.1	6.4	0.8	−1.3
Control	8.6	1.4	8.3	1.5	−0.3
Diastolic Blood Pressure (mm Hg)					
Training	80.6	13.3	76.9	12.8	−3.7
Control	84.9	9.1	86.4	9.5	1.5

	T-1		T-3		Change in Mean From
	Mean	S.D.	Mean	S.D.	T-1 to T-3
Systolic Blood Pressure (mm Hg)					
Training	139.0	18.0	137.4	16.4	−1.6
Control	151.5	6.6	154.5	4.8	3.0

* Only conditions of sitting rest, during the last ten seconds of the ride, and 30 seconds post-exercise at T-1 and T-3 data on variables which were significantly different (0.10 level) at T-3 were reported. All significant differences favored the twenty-week training group (N = 8) over the control group (N = 10).

tests will usually depress the amplitude of the T-wave. This was also shown in Cureton's study at the Underwater Swimmer's School, U. S. Navy (*The Research Quarterly*, 34:440-453, Dec., 1953). In general, the type of physical training used in this study will improve the amplitude of the T-wave but this may be over-shadowed by unusual stress having been taken within a few days of the ECG test.

In the tenth to twentieth week of training the group which was supplemented with WGO was a bit lower at T_3 than at T_2 but the depression was not as great as that in the control group taking placeboes. This depression in both of the training groups, T_2 to T_3 is unquestionably associated with the increasing diffi-culty of the program, this getting gradually more and more in-tensive and also longer. The WGO, then, acts to help the men resist the stress, and this is what several other experiments show.

MATERIALS FED

Although the WGC was uncamouflaged, the feeding of the VioBin WGO and P was double-blind. The three treatments were fed four days/week in the following dosages:

WGO .... 15 6-minim capsules
Placeboes (P) .. 15 6-minim capsules of devitaminized lard
(with vitamin E equal to WGO)
WGC .... 1½ ounces, dry cereal form

The subjects were tested each week of the eight-week period.

TABLE CXI

SIGNIFICANT DIFFERENCES AMONG TRAINING GROUPS WITH WHEAT
GERM OIL, PLACEBOES AND NO SUPPLEMENTATION

Variable	Significance Level		Significant Differences in Adjusted Group Means*		
	T-2	T-3	TW	TP	TO†
Electromechanical Lag					
Rest (sitting)	—	0.05	0.055	0.054	0.053
Last 10 seconds of ride	—	0.05	0.043	0.041	0.041
30 secs post-exercise	—	0.10	0.048	0.046	0.046
5 mins post-exercise	—	0.05	0.056	0.053	0.053
Isovolumetric Contraction Period					
Rest (supine)	—	0.10	0.055	0.054	0.053
30 secs post-exercise	—	0.01	0.042	0.039	0.040

* T-3 means adjusted for the linear effect of the covariates (T-2 measures). Significant differences were determined by Duncan's multiple range. All means underlined by the same line are *not* significantly different (0.10 level). Means not underlined by the same line are significantly different.

† TW = training with wheat germ oil group (N = 7); TP = training with placebos group (N = 7); TO = training only group (N = 8).

STATISTICAL TREATMENT

Owing to the inequality of the group n's at the eighth week (one subject in the WG group dropped out), it was considered inappropriate to use the analysis of variance for a randomized block design as originally planned, since it would decrease each n_k by one. Instead, the planned comparisons, WGO versus placeboes and WG versus placeboes were made on the eight week differences by using the *t*-test for correlated samples. Although multiple *t*-tests increase the probability of a type I error in proportion to the number made, making two planned *t*-tests produces the least possible increase in the probability of a type I error and would not appear to vitiate the results. An *a* level of .15 was decided upon.

RESULTS

The mean, SD and SE_m at the pretest and at the eighth week is given for each group in Table CXII. The three group means were nearly identical at the pretest.

TABLE CXII

DESCRIPTIVE STATISTICS FOR TREATMENT GROUPS—PRETEST AND
EIGHTH WEEK TOTAL BODY REACTION TIME (MILLISECONDS)

	WGO Group		Placebo Group		WG Group	
	Pretest	*Eighth Week*	*Pretest*	*Eighth Week*	*Pretest*	*Eighth Week*
X̄	313.0	238.2	313.7	253.6	313.5	253.4
SD	41.64	30.11	44.25	41.82	17.47	14.46
SEₘ	12.7	9.52	13.26	13.22	5.38	4.70

	T-1		T-3		Change in Mean From T-1 to T-3
	Mean	S.D.	Mean	S.D.	
During Last Ten Seconds of Ride (Sitting)					
Cycle Time (second)					
Training	0.449	0.050	0.516	0.049	0.067
Control	0.461	0.055	0.452	0.058	-0.009
Diastole (second)					
Training	0.168	0.034	0.218	0.034	0.050
Control	0.182	0.040	0.184	0.039	0.002
Isovolumetric Contraction Period (second)					
Training	0.026	0.005	0.029	0.003	0.003
Control	0.027	0.005	0.025	0.005	-0.002
Ejection Period (second)					
Training	0.217	0.017	0.229	0.017	0.012
Control	0.213	0.021	0.205	0.024	-0.008
Per Cent Diastole in Cycle Time					
Training	37.3	3.8	42.0	3.1	4.7
Control	39.1	4.7	40.4	4.3	1.3
Per Cent Electromechanical Lag in Cycle Time					
Training	8.6	1.1	7.7	0.7	-0.9
Control	8.8	1.6	8.7	1.3	-0.1
Per Cent Ejection Period in Cycle Time					
Training	48.5	3.0	44.5	2.6	-4.0
Control	46.4	3.3	45.5	3.0	-0.9
Thirty Seconds Post-Exercise (Sitting)					
Cycle Time (second)					
Training	0.563	0.087	0.700	0.113	0.137
Control	0.546	0.076	0.553	0.091	0.007
Diastole (second)					
Training	0.283	0.060	0.382	0.041	0.099
Control	0.268	0.049	0.281	0.068	0.013
Electromechanical Lag (second)					
Training	0.043	0.006	0.045	0.005	0.002
Control	0.046	0.004	0.045	0.004	-0.001
Isovolumetric Contraction Period (second)					
Training	0.033	0.005	0.037	0.004	0.004
Control	0.033	0.007	0.031	0.007	-0.002
Ejection Period (second)					
Training	0.204	0.023	0.236	0.026	0.032
Control	0.199	0.022	0.196	0.023	-0.003

Effects of Training with and without Wheat Germ Oil on Cardiac Intervals and Other Fitness Measures of Middle-Aged Men

JACK F. WILEY*

PURPOSE

THE purpose of this study was to determine the effects of endurance training with and without wheat germ oil on the ICP and EML pre-ejection intervals of the heart cycle of the left ventricle.

RESEARCH METHODS

Thirty-two sedentary male volunteers, twenty-four to sixty-two years of age, were tested at 0 weeks (T_1), 10 weeks (T_2) and 20 weeks (T_3) of the experimental training period on the ICP (isovolumic contraction period) and EML (electromechanical lag period) of the ECG. The data were obtained from simultaneous records of the carotid pulse wave, phonocardiogram and electrocardiogram at rest (sitting), and during the last ten seconds of a five-minute submaximal ergometer bicycle ride (5000 ft. lb/minute at 40 r.p.m.); and also at thirty seconds and five minutes post-exercise, sitting. The apparatus is described in the following two papers: B. D. Franks and T. K. Cureton, Jr., Effects of Training on Time Components of the Left Ventricle, *J. Sports Med.*, 9:80-88, June, 1969; and Orthogonal Factors and Norms for Time Components of the Left Ventricle, *Medicine and Science in Sports*, 1:171-176, Sept., 1969, and in the thesis of Wiley.

Twenty-two of the subjects participated in a mixed calisthenics and running program for twenty weeks, and ten served as non-training controls. At T_2 the training groups were divided into three groups on the basis of their mile run time: a) A continued

* Urbana, Ph.D. thesis, Physical Education, University of Illinois, 1964, p. 200. (Sponsor: T. K. Cureton.)

TABLE CXIII

MEANS, STANDARD DEVIATIONS AND MEAN CHANGES OF GROUPS USED FOR DETERMINING
THE EFFECTS OF WGO AND TRAINING

Group	Variable	Units	T-1 Mean	T-1 S.D.	T-3 Mean	T-3 S.D.	Changes in Mean from T-1 to T-3
WGO	Total fat	mm	139.33	33.84	109.33	20.96	— 30.00
Placebos			105.16	27.85	102.83	23.99	— 2.33
Training			112.28	23.24	103.57	15.87	— 8.71
WGO	Total strength	lbs	948.00	149.62	878.33	182.31	— 69.67
Placebos			1035.33	173.01	1120.83	99.36	85.50
Training			932.57	189.98	969.28	113.17	36.71
WGO	St/wt		5.19	0.25	5.20	0.73	0.01
Placebos			6.07	1.59	6.79	1.09	0.72
Training			5.17	1.06	5.46	0.53	0.29
WGO	Trunk flexion	ins	13.51	3.71	9.30	1.76	— 4.21
Placebos			10.25	2.47	10.15	3.59	0.10
Training			11.85	3.63	11.18	3.59	— 0.67
WGO	Trunk extension	ins	11.41	2.67	12.55	1.57	1.14
Placebos			12.81	6.54	14.73	6.04	1.92
Training			13.62	2.42	14.41	2.39	0.79
WGO	Shoulder extension	ins	10.90	5.80	13.76	6.23	2.86
Placebos			12.80	5.97	13.71	5.44	0.91
Training			11.25	3.49	13.11	4.45	1.86
WGO	Illinois agility run	secs	20.20	1.98	19.06	1.78	— 1.14
Placebos			19.25	0.82	17.86	0.98	— 1.39
Training			20.01	1.63	18.90	1.37	— 1.11

Measure	Units					
Vital capacity residual WGO	c ins	−38.79	44.21	−10.93	38.18	27.86
Placebos		15.77	37.06	18.98	41.35	3.21
Training		−50.10	29.24	−47.36	32.32	2.74
Expiratory force WGO	mm Hg	120.50	24.52	135.33	22.79	14.83
Placebos		160.16	16.52	172.33	16.31	12.17
Training		144.28	14.39	149.57	20.09	4.29
Breath-holding after exercise WGO	secs	15.53	1.48	15.88	3.08	0.35
Placebos		19.58	11.47	27.28	12.16	7.70
Training		14.37	4.20	18.01	2.47	3.64
Chins WGO		3.16	1.72	4.16	2.48	1.00
Placebos		4.50	1.04	5.50	1.87	1.00
Training		4.00	2.16	4.28	1.97	0.28
Dips WGO		4.00	2.28	5.66	4.13	1.66
Placebos		5.16	4.07	6.83	5.41	1.67
Training		7.14	4.25	6.57	2.69	0.57
Vertical jump WGO	ins	17.83	2.56	18.16	3.12	—
Placebos		18.83	4.02	19.33	3.66	0.33
Training		18.57	2.87	18.85	2.85	0.50

training group (N = 7) with WGO added as a dietary supplement; b) A continued training group on a dietary supplement of devitaminized lard placeboes (N = 7); and c) A continued training group without supplementation (N = 8). The group taking WGO took ten capsules of the 6-minim size (VioBin) whole, fresh oil; and the placeboes were similar capsules, undistinguishable from each other, fed in double-blind fashion, given in the T_2 to T_3 period of ten weeks.

RESULTS

Analysis of covariance was used for determining significance among groups. Analysis of variance was used to compare the groups initially. The first comparison was made between the ten-week training group (N = 22) and the nontraining controls (N = 10) at T_2 using the T_1 measures as the covariates to determine the effects of the first ten weeks of training. In the measures being considered as critical, at T_2 the training group had made significantly greater changes than the control (nontraining) group in the following measures: *at rest*—increased ICP time, and cycle time, increased systolic amplitude of the brachial pulse wave and lower diastolic blood pressure. *During exercise*—increased cycle time, diastole, ICP period and ejection period; *during recovery*—increased cycle time, diastole, EML lag, ICP, ejection period and systolic amplitude of the brachial pulse wave.

At T_3 the above listed training changes were still present, and the control nontraining group did not make greater changes than the experimental group on any of the variables at T_1 or T_2.

At T_2 there were no significant differences between the two training groups or on supplements. The training affected them equally.

At T_3 the WGO experimental group had made significantly greater increases at the 0.10 level in: a) the EML at rest (sitting) in the last ten seconds of the ergometer bicycle ride and at thirty seconds of recovery and five minutes of recovery; b) in ICP contraction period at rest (supine) and at thirty seconds of recovery. These changes were in the same direction as, but greater than, the effects of training alone.

TABLE CXIV

SIGNIFICANT DIFFERENCES AMONG TRAINING GROUPS
WITH WGO, PLACEBOS AND NO SUPPLEMENTATION

Variable	Significance Level T-1	T-3*	Significant Differences in Adjusted Group Means†		
Total strength	—	0.05	891.13 (TW)‡	990.31 (TO)	1087.01 (TP)
St/wt	—	0.05	5.35 (TW)	5.62 (TO)	<u>6.49</u> (TP)
Vital capacity residual residual	—	0.05	−24.36 (TO)	−17.08 (TP)	<u>2.02</u> (TW)

* The testing periods were at ten (T-2) and 20 (T-3) weeks of the training period.

† Determined by *Duncan's multiple range.* All means underlined by the same line are *not* significantly different (0.10 level). Means not underlined by the same line are significantly different.

‡ TW = training with wheat germ oil (N = 6); TP = training with placebos (N = 6); TO = training only (N = 7).

CONCLUSIONS

Both the ten and twenty weeks of physical training caused an increase in cardiovascular fitness at rest, during and after exercise.

Supplementation of the physical training with WGO in the usual manner from the tenth to the twentieth week of the training program caused a significantly greater lengthening than training with placeboes or training only in resting exercise and recovery EML; and in resting and recovery ICP time.

Experiment 31

The Effects of Wheat Germ Oil and Wheat Germ on Total Body Reaction Time on Young Boys in Matched Groups

Chris A. Milesis, Thomas K. Cureton and Peter Richter[*]

PURPOSE

THE purpose of the experiment[*] was to determine the effects of wheat germ oil (WGO) and wheat germ (WGC) on the total body reaction time (TBRT) in 10-13-year-old boys undergoing sports-fitness training at the University of Illinois.

The subjects were young boys, 10-13 years, in the University of Illinois Sports Fitness School.

RESEARCH METHODS

One week prior to the eight-week experimental period, the total sample ($N = 30$) was pretested on TBRT, using the methods and equipment described by Tillman. TBRT as used here will refer to the mean of five trials each of visual reaction time, auditory reaction time and combined visual-auditory reaction time. The pretest was the basis for arranging the thirty subjects into ten blocks of three, with each of the three subjects in a given block assigned to one of three dietary treatments: WGO, WG or placebo (P). This was carried out as follows (each number in the three treatment columns represents a ranked subject):

		TREATMENTS		
		WGO	WG	P
Block	1	1	2	3
Block	2	6	5	4
Block	3	7	8	9
.		.	.	.
.		.	.	.
.		.	.	.
Block	10	30	29	28

[*] Physical Fitness Research Laboratory, University of Illinois, Champaign, Illinois, Summer, 1968.

486

Materials Fed

Although the WG was uncamouflaged, the feeding of the VioBin WGO and P was *double-blind*. The three treatments were fed four days/week in the following dosages:

WGO .... 15 6-minim capsules

Placeboes ...... 15 6-minim capsules of devitaminized lard (with vitamin E equal to WGO)

WG .... 1½ ounces, dry cereal form

The subjects were tested each week of the eight-week period.

Statistical Treatment

Owing to the inequality of the group n's at the eighth week, (one subject in the WG group dropped out), it was considered inappropriate to use the analysis of variance for a randomized blocks design as originally planned, since it would decrease each n_k by one. Instead, the planned comparisons WGO vs. placeboes and WG vs. placeboes were made on the eighth week differences by using the *t*-test for correlated samples. Although multiple *t*-tests increase the probability of a type I error in proportion to the number made, making two planned *t*-tests produces the least possible increase in the probability of a type I error and would not appear to vitiate the results. An *a* level of .15 was decided upon.

RESULTS

The mean, SD, and SE_m at the pre-test and at the eighth week is given for each group in Table CXII. The three group means were nearly identical at the pre-test, whereas at the eighth week the means were 238.2, 253.4 and 253.6 msec. for the WGO, WG and P groups, respectively. The weekly performances for the groups are shown in Figure 47.

It is interesting to note the marked slowing of TBRT that occurred at the sixth week in all three groups, the reason for which is indeterminate. *It is also interesting to note that the WGO and P groups did not differ appreciably until the last four weeks of the experiment;* in fact the difference between the two groups became larger during weeks six through eight. This may give a clue as to the time required for WGO to become effective.

The *t* value for WGO versus placeboes was 1.262 (p < .15) with nine degrees of freedom, while the *t* value for WG versus P was 0.019 (p > .15) with eight degrees of freedom.

CONCLUSIONS

Within the limits of this study the following conclusions seem warranted:

1. The feeding of fifteen of the 6-minim capsules of WGO four days per week to physically active 10-13-year-old boys causes a reduction in total body reaction time significantly greater (.15 level) than that of the group of placebo controls.
2. There was no evidence that similar feeding of 1½ ounces of WG had any effect on total body reaction time when compared (.15 level) with placebo controls.

Appendix A

RELIABILITY OF TESTS AND CALCULATIONS FOR STATISTICAL SIGNIFICANCE

Reliability and Validity of Tests

THE tests used are described in various sources, along with reliability and validity coefficients. The reliability has to do with the reproducibility of the tests by the same operator under the same conditions. References are given in detail in each chapter dealing with a particular test, or group of tests, as to the material; usually the needed data are given in the abstracts of each study, shown in Part Two. The principal tests[8, 9, 12-14] used are grouped as follows:

Endurance. Time in the 600-yard run (boys), mile run (men), all-out treadmill run, 8.6 per cent slope, 7 mi/hr (motor driven), muscular endurance tests (push-ups, chinning the bar, squat jumps, sitting tucks, sit-ups, etc.).

Peak oxygen intake capacity and net debt. Tested on an ergocycle or on a treadmill, done to the limit of one's ability, usually taken by Douglas bag method with separate bag for the intake sample and one or several bags for the oxygen debt samples. Breath holding after exertion is sometimes taken as proportional to the net oxygen debt, as it has a correlation with it of about 0.75.

Total body reaction time (the Garrett-Cureton test). Done by reaction time jumps from a specially designed platform, hung like a flat box with very sensitive micro-switches between the lid and the bottom part of the box. Reactions are timed (actually movement times) in response to visual, auditory and combined signals.

Strength tests. Usually measured on suitable calibrated dynamometers for maximal strength on each test: hand grips (right and left), back lift and leg press.

Precordial T-wave. Taken from the electrocardiogram in a given standardized position. The highest T-wave of the precordial lead is taken, using the standardized CR$_{II, IV, V}$ positions.

Ballistocardiogram, brachial pulse wave (Sphygogram). As taken on the arbeit direct body (shin-bar) type BCG, and on the Cameron heartometer, or by electronic pick-up apparatus. These deflections have to do with the "vigor" of the heart as transmitted through movements of the body (BCG) or by pulsations through the large arteries (pulse).

Pulse rate (sitting, standing, during work or during recuperation). Taken usually by electrical recording, or by counting the wrist pulse rate, or by stethoscope counting (auscultation). The Schneider index is based upon five subtests of pulse rate and one of systolic blood pressure. The pulse ratio is the ratio of the two-minute recuperative pulse taken as soon as possible after a standardized work load. The pre-ejection intervals are fractional parts of the heart cycle (beat) divided at the first heart sound into electromechanical (EML) and isovolumic (ICP) intervals. The latent period is from the Q to the beginning of the up-stroke of the pulse, usually taken at the carotid artery position (angle of the jaw) by a Brecht-Bauke pick-up electrode.

Basal (and sitting) metabolism. Taken usually by Douglas bag method so that the RQ may be determined, which helps to tell if the subject is normally rested and undisturbed mentally. Appropriate corrections are made by the Smithsonian tables (temperature, pressure, dry, and surface area). The temperature of the room is also observed.

Flicker fusion frequency. Taken on the Krasno-Ivy machine as the amount of flicker which can be seen, alternating up and down the scale, an average of ten readings.

Composite criterion. A criterion composed of several tests averaged or totaled after the raw scores are changed into standard scores by appropriate tables. Standard scores may be averaged but this is impossible when several tests are at hand, measured in different units. A common unit must be used before averaging, or adding to a total.

ERRORS OF MEASUREMENT IN OXYGEN INTAKE DATA

A principal error of the constant type is in the type of valve and hose used for collecting the gas. Theron *et al.* has described a valve with half of the resistance of the Hans-Rudolph or Otis-McKerrow valve (cf. Theron, J. C., Zwi, S. and McGregor, M.: A low resistance respiratory valve, *Lancet*, 1:415, 1958). The individual differences and S.E.$_{meas.}$ are given in Moncrief's article, *J. Sports Med.*, 153-157; and a timing error is described by Phillips, Ross from San Diego, Timing error in determining maximal O_2 intake, *The Research Quarterly*, 38:315-316, May, 1967.

Moncrief (*J. Sports Med.*, 8:153-157, 1968) summarized Taylor's results in 1944 (C. Taylor, Some properties of maximal and submaximal exercise with reference to physiological variation and the measurement of exercise tolerance, *Amer. J. Physiol.*, 142: 200-212, 1944) and also those of Henry, *et al.* and Jere Mitchell. He quotes the Taylor results giving 0.70 for the reliability of the L/min of O_2 intake, a test-retest of 0.264 liters/minute and S.E.$_m$ = 0.013 L/minute based upon thirty-one males, 19-26 years of age. Henry's results give r from retest data 0.51 for slow movements and 0.35 for fast movements for peak O_2 intake, open circuit method. The reliability of the all-out run was 0.95. He concluded that there was a large intra-individual oxygen consumption error and that this was the principal source of the unreliability.

RELIABILITY OF THE EXPERIMENTS ON HUMANS

The most important type of reliability is the consistency (reproducibility) of the experiments from year to year. This may be determined by the number of times reliability by the accepted research standards was obtained. If, for instance, seven experiments of a given type were run, in different years and with different subjects, how similar would the results be, year to year? (refer to Fig. 9, Part Two) showing seven years of work with small boys).

The most important immediate step taken to determine reliability was to arrange for retests of the subjects, regardless of who they were, so that at least two determinations were available on the same subjects, taking the same tests under the same operators (testers). These data make it possible to determine the actual differences, case by case, from the retest data. Such variations are called "chance variations." They are usually squared and summed, then averaged, and the square root extracted. The result is s (or σ, sigma). This s may then be related to the number of cases used, and divided by the probability correction $(\sqrt{N-1})$ if the number of observations is 20 or over, and by $\sqrt{N-2}$ if 10-19 in number, or by $\sqrt{N-3}$ if under 10.[5] This result is called the S.E.$_{meas.}$ (standard error of measurement). It may be computed theoretically from the formula, S.E.$_{Est.} = \sigma \sqrt{I-r_{11}}$, where, r_{11} is the coefficient of reliability,[4] and σ is the S.D. (standard deviation) of the whole experimental sample of cases. This result (or S.E.$_{Est.}$) tells us how much variation was present in the basic testing. Many types of variation exist,[2] day to day fluctuations, variable time to meals, variable feeling of the subjects, attendance, etc.

The usual preferred measure of reliability is the t, described in the Fisher statistics of small samples. It is computed from a formula applicable to retests from paired scores, which we generally have used in this work:[6] $t = \dfrac{T_2-T_1}{s\sqrt{2N}}$, where N = the number of paired retests available in the data, and s = $\sqrt{\dfrac{d^2}{2N}}$

However, there are certain problems about this statistic, the most important limitation being that of the requirement of a randomly drawn or distributed sample. Very frequently with volunteer subjects, the sample is *not* random, but is "packed" (all subjects too nearly alike), or skewed (subjects too poor or too good, causing an imbalance in the normal distribution, which more technically is called skewness), a flat distribution being platykurtic; and if too peaked, is called leptokurtic, or L-shaped, or square shaped. Data may take many shapes, so it is basic to plot the data (number of cases versus the variable) to determine what shape the distribution is at hand. A normal curve may be quickly graphed over the obtained data to see if it is a reasonable fit, or more exactly, if the number of cases are relatively large, a Chi square determination may be calculated to give a quantitative value to the fit or mis-fit. With very small samples this is seldom done, so *t* test results are not always exactly meaningful, although commonly computed. It is more important in the work done in this volume to note the number of times a meaningful result was obtained in different experiments. This is shown in Table VI, which shows the thirty-one experiments tabulated to three degrees of reliability results: a) *significant, t <* .10 level of probability, which means that in one hundred experiments, ninety of them would yield results as good as obtained in the one experiment at hand. More strict levels are written as reliable at the .05 level (95 times out of 100 reproducible) or .01 (99 times out of 100 times reproducible). The reasonable standard for our experiments is .10 level, classified as field experiments. Geigy[7] in referring to such field experiments, with human subjects in pharmocological research, states that the .20 level (80 per cent reproducible) is the lowest permissible level, and that usually taken. A higher standard may be taken but unless the human subjects are on rigorous diet control, and kept always under laboratory observation, unreliability may usually be the result because of the many conditions which interfere with any given human experiment. Human subjects are very variable. Each Chapter shows the results from the several experiments of one type classified as a) *significant <* .10, b) *favorable trend in the right direction for improvement* and c) *no experimental result of value (NER), negative or not worth considering at all.* These results are given in Tables VI, XIV, XXII, XXVIII, XXIX and XXXIII.

THE SIGNIFICANCE OF THE DIFFERENCE BETWEEN TWO MEANS, MATCHED GROUPS

It is customary to find the ratio of the obtained difference (D) to the standard error of the difference (S.E.$_{\text{diff.}}$). This ratio, D/S.E.$_{\text{diff.}}$, is designated T. The degrees of freedom are the N-1 cases for each group being compared and summed. The table is used then to determine the T for that many degrees of freedom (Guilford, p. 136-37).[18]

The differences are usually taken as the difference between the means, i.e. T_2-T_1 = difference between the means. This is the numerator of the T formula.

The S.E._diff. is usually obtained by computing the S.E._Mean from the formula, $S.E._M = \dfrac{s}{\sqrt{N-1}}$ or if the cases are from 10 to 19, the radical is $(N-2)$ or with cases numbering 1 to 9, it is used as $(N-3)$. If the error is obtained for each mean, then the mean difference error is $\sqrt{S.E._{M_1}^2 - S.E._{M_2}^2}$, which assumes the data to be uncorrelated. A somewhat softer standard may be used if there are enough cases to justify a stable intercorrelation between the T_1 and T_2 series. In this case the formula is as follows:

$$S.E._{M_{diff.}} = \sqrt{S.E._{M_1} - S.E._{M_2} - 2\, r_{12}\, \sigma_{M_1}\, \sigma_{M_2}}$$

When the subjects all change proportionately, and the two sets of data, T_1 and T_2 are perfectly correlated $(r_{12} = 1.0)$ then we may omit the last term in the formula above.[5]

An alternate method is to take the actual differences between the T_1 and T_2 series, for each retest as paired, then determine the σ of these differences, and compute σ_{d_M} as has been done in our experiments at times:

$$\sigma_{d_M} = \sqrt{\dfrac{(T_2 - T_1)^2}{2(N-2)}}$$

The significance ratio, t is then D/σ_{d_M}.

FURTHER COMMENT ON RELIABILITY

As a whole the reliability of the tests used for endurance are remarkably good, as the retest r_{11} has been computed in various experiments to be usually better than 0.80 and in the boys' work was around 0.88 for the 600-yard run and even slightly better for the all-out treadmill run. An elaborate study of the reliability of the tests of the type used in this study has been made in another report, namely, *Improving the Physical Fitness of Youth* (Cureton and Barry) 1964. The cardiovascular tests are not as reliable as the motor tests: T-wave 0.765, and 0.745; R-wave 0.750, 0.781; the heartograph area 0.631, systolic amplitude 0.765; pulse rate 0.700; strength between 0.752 and 0.904; Schneider index 0.522; total body reaction time 0.723 to 0.745. Young boys are quite unstable.

The reliability coefficients are better for adults, and are quoted in Cureton's *Physical Fitness Workbook, Endurance of Young Men, Physical Fitness Appraisal and Guidance, Physical Fitness of Champion Athletes* and *The Physiological Effects of Exercise Programs on Adults.*

There are many ways of destroying an experiment. If the subjects are absent, sick, or refuse to cooperate, or the groups become badly unbalanced for any one of the many possible reasons, then the experiment may develop excessive variability. If tests are given when the subjects are tired, the results may be worse on T_2 than on T_1. Subjects sometimes become involved in extraneous activities other than what they are held responsible for in the experiment, and this may drain their energy, so that they do poorly on tests or do not practice properly. Probably the most important "built-in" uncorrectable error is *biological individuality,* meaning that some subjects do not use the WGO, OCTCNL, etc.

In the results it may be noted how many times results have come up to the desired level of significance, how many times the results are favorable but not enough cases were used to show statistical significance at an acceptable level of reliability. If there was no evidence at all, no trend in the right direction, then the symbol NER is used, meaning "no evidence revealed," not even a trend. If in a given column significance was obtained at a satisfactory level several times, the dietary supplement has an effect upon the test, which can be reproduced in other experiments. Then, if there are, in addition, several positive trends, the effect is potentially in the WGO, the OCTCNL or the WGC, and higher reliability may usually be obtained by running the experiment over with more cases and with greater care. If there are some exceptions, the job is then to pin down what was wrong with the experiment. If control of an experiment is lost, this should not be blamed upon the oil (or any other dietary supplement).

When the feeding of the WGO was for less than a month (Exp. 12), the results are usually not significantly large enough to bring up a large enough ratio in the $D/S.E._{meas.}$ relation, or in the $D/\sigma_{diff.}$ ratio.[23] A failure may be due to a D too small, or to the denominator (error) being too large. When the D is so small that it is meaningless, there is no reason to pursue the matter with elaborate calculations which mean nothing in the end. For instance, in one experiment the change in chinning was a fraction of one chin. There is no meaning to reliability calculations of such a meaningless difference.

In Ganslen's work (Exp. 6, 1951) the difference from T_2 to T_3 was relatively large in terms of net oxygen debt but the variability error for oxygen debt was so large, that the large difference was not reliable. The reliability of the "peak" O_2 intake test has been shown to vary from 0.56 to 0.86 for the r_{11}, and this is quite variable. It would take a large number of cases to prove anything, and also much better control over the subjects.

Only one thesis study was excluded from the summary, namely, that of E. I. Marx, for no reason related to Mr. Marx at all. This study was done in 1952 when a swimming coach was retiring. Perhaps he anticipated retirement and let up in his efforts, so the team lost all meets. Gross irregularities developed in the time spent in practice and some men did not come at all. The study was carried out and finally finished but the results were so unusual, in that many of the men were much lower in the tests at the end of the season than they were at the start of the season, that the results were not reasonable. The halves of the team, which had been matched on the times in a 100-yard "drop-off" type swim became very unbalanced as some men stopped practice. For this reason this study has been excluded.

Several references are given to standard books on statistics, which were used in this work. Unfortunately, many data taken in physical fitness work on humans are not normally distributed. Ehrlich[20] demonstrated on a sampling taken from students at the City College of New York, using nine tests most commonly used in physical fitness performances (dips, chins, standing broad jump, running broad jump, bar vault, sprint (dash), leap, bar snap and maze run) that all were curvilinear and resulted in skewed distributions. Items having to do with strength, speed or power are usually skewed. This is also true with O_2 intake test (L/minute) and many other variables. Improvements become harder as the ability increases, resulting in skewed data and negative parabolic distributions. Such data, if samples do not accommodate to the Fisher t test.[15] It is necessary to use only

D/S.E.$_{meas.}$ for evaluation of reliability or resort to nonparametric statistics, as has been done in some of our experiments.

CURVILINEARITY AND CORRELATIONS

If the *exact* relationship is sought between measures of the BCG and measures of the HGF, a correlation of a velocity BCG measure with a velocity HGF measure may not yield the true relationship. The reason is that a correlation may reveal the angular relationship between two straight lines but not between two curvilinear lines. Since all velocity and acceleration data are *not* straight lines, which may be easily determined by plotting the data, one variable against another, the correlation (Pearson coefficient) usually underestimates the true relationship. Therefore, all of the correlations given are probably underestimates. Even so, the canonical correlations are relatively high, compared to the simple intervariable correlations. The results from factor analysis are always rather vague because the intercorrelations are not true relations, all are usually underestimates. This is doubly true in all dynamic problems of relationships between velocity and acceleration data. Engineers would never think of using correlations, as the first rule in dealing with empirical data is to plot the data and then fit the data with mathematical curve fitting. Neither correlations nor factor analysis will reveal *true* relations in relating velocity, acceleration, force or power data.

The calculation of the "irrefutable levels" of sampling reliability have followed the customary Fisher type statistics[6] but a great penalty is usually paid for small samples, in that the statistical "inferred" reproducibility is extended to samples of infinite size. Even with this method the calculated "t" values are usually better than the 0.10 level. No important generalizations have been made when "T" has been less than 2.0, or close to this according to the number of cases used. In some of the smaller samples the "t" has been avoided due to lack of normality of the data.

REFERENCES

1. Holzinger, Karl J.: *Statistical Tables for Students in Education and Psychology.* Chicago, The University of Chicago Press, 1950, 11th printing.
2. de Beer, E. J. (Ed.): The place of statistical methods in biological and

chemical experimentation. *Ann. N. Y. Acad. Sci.*, 52:789-942, March 30, 1950.

3. Goodwin, H. M.: *Elements of Precision Measurements and Graphical Methods.* New York, McGraw-Hill Book Co., 1930.

4. Odell, C. W.: *Educational Statistics.* Errors of estimate and of measurement. New York, The Century Co., 1925, pp. 230-244.

5. Peters, C. C. and Van Voorhis, W. R.: Reliability of differences and of statistics. *Statistical Procedures and Their Mathematical Bases.* New York, McGraw-Hill Book Co., 1940, pp. 126-190.

6. Fisher, R. A.: *Statistical Methods for Research Workers* (5th ed.). Edinburgh and London, Oliver and Boyd, 1934.

7. Geigy Pharmaceuticals: *Scientific Tables* (6th ed.). Ardsley, N. Y., Ed. by Konrad Diem, Geigy Chemical Foundation, 1962, pp. 156-158 on Significance Tests, recommends using 0.20 level of reliability in testing human subjects.

8. Scott, M. G. and Cureton, T. K., *et al.: Research Methods Applied to Health, Physical Education and Recreation.* Washington, D. C., American Association for Health, Physical Education and Recreation, 1949, pp. 301-314, Experimental group methods of research (by Elizabeth G. Rodgers and Hyman Krackower); and pp. 459-477, Errors in measurement (by F. M. Henry, T. K. Cureton, J. E. Hewitt and R. F. Jarrett).

9. Cureton, T. K.: *Physical Fitness Appraisal and Guidance.* St. Louis, C. V. Mosby Co., 1947.

10. Gulliksen, H.: *Theory of Mental Tests.* New York, Wiley, 1962, p. 486.

11. Larson, L. A., Rodgers, E. G., Clarke, H. H. and Cureton, T. K.: *Measurement and Evaluation Materials in Health, Physical Education and Recreation.* Washington, D. C., 1201 16th St., 1950, p. 138. 138.

12. Larson, L. A. and Yokum, R. D.: *Measurement and Evaluation in Physical, Health and Recreation Education.* St. Louis, C. V. Mosby Co., 1951, p. 507.

13. McCloy, C. H.: *Tests and Measurements in Health and Physical Education.* New York, F. S. Crofts Co., 1942, p. 412.

15. Walker, H. M. and Lev, J.: *Statistical Inference.* New York, Holt, Rinehart and Einston, 1953, p. 510.

16. Peters, C. C. and Van Voorhis, W. R.: *Statistical Procedures and Their Mathematical Bases.* New York, McGraw-Hill Book Co., 1940, p. 516.

17. Brozek, J. and Alexander, H.: Components of variation and the consistency of repeated measurements. *Res. Quart.*, 18:153-166, May, 1947.

18. Rosemeir, R. A.: The use of an exaggerated alpha in a test for the initial equality of groups. *Res. Quart.*, 39:831-832, Oct., 1968.

19. Guildford, J. P.: *Fundamental Statistics in Psychology and Education.* New York, McGraw-Hill Co., Inc., 1942.
20. Ehrlich, Gerald: An analysis of the mathematical curves underlying some physical education test items. *Res. Quart.,* 17:270-275, Dec. 1946.

Appendix B

A STATEMENT ON SIGNIFICANCE PROBABILITY

Philip J. Rasch[*]

WHEN I taught research courses, I used to ask the class:
"If (one of the class) came in and said he had seen an accident on the freeway, would you believe him?"

The answer, of course, was always "Yes." Then I would ask:

"If the same person came in and said he saw a flying saucer land on the freeway, would you believe him?"

Here, of course, the answer was "No." Then I would ask:

"Why not? The evidence is exactly the same in both cases!"

The answer, once more, is that the more unlikely the statement the greater the proof required.

Statistically, if the experimenter is interested in showing that no difference exists, he uses a small value for the significance probability; if he is interested in showing that a difference exists, he uses a larger value. But even here there are grounds for disagreement. Bill Pierson and I submitted a paper to *Ergonomics* reporting no significant difference at the .01 level. It came back with a notation that it would be accepted if we recalculated our data to report the significance at the .05 level. Fortunately, this made no difference; it was not significant at that level either. If it had been, we would have been in the position of being required to report something as significant when it was our belief that it was not.

The editor has a point in that in the medical and biological fields the significance level is conventionally .05. But even this is not a self-evident truth. *Documenta Geigy* scientific tables show

---

[*] Head of Physiology Division, Naval Medical Field Research Laboratory, Camp Le Juene, North Carolina, personal correspondence.

examples of sequential analysis which gives only a .10 level and specifically approves this level by stating:

> However, even though a difference has significance probability in large samples of only 0.1 it is permissible in some circumstances (for example with drugs which are life-saving) to reject the null hypothesis. The physician would willingly take the risk that in one case out of ten he has failed to administer a better drug. The tendency in medical and biological investigation is to use *too small* a significance probability (p. 156).

Unfortunately the history of investigations of dietary supplements is a bad one. The minute anything even appears useful someone starts to manufacture and promote it, usually without valid justification. The evidence rather strongly suggests that nutrient deficiencies decrease performance; that harder work requires more nutrients but that the quantities necessitated are still well within the levels resulting from an adequate diet; that supplementing nutrients over and above the levels resulting from an adequate diet does not improve performance. In the last *Journal of Sports Medicine and Physical Fitness,* Kraut observes that, "Unless the diet is abnormally unbalanced, it also contains enough vitamins and mineral salts." (I am not here concerned with the argument that the trainer has no way of telling whether the man is getting an adequate diet and should administer nutrients as a precautionary measure, as this represents an entirely different approach.)

The picture this gives is something like that of drugs—supplements can be prescribed intelligently only after competent bioassay. For that reason most of us have worried primarily about committing a Type I error in our investigations of these substances. From your standpoint, however, I think you could argue with reasonable justification for acceptance of the .10 level. Speaking personally, I would be decidedly hesitant to reject out-of-hand any of your studies that attained this level. Because of the "biological individuality" to which you refer, I would concede you twice the usual figure.

Sensational, nutritional discoveries seem to blossom and then fade away. Ershoff (*Proceedings of the Society of Experimental Biology and Medicine,* 77:488, July, 1951) made startling claims for the benefits of whole liver powder. This attracted considerable attention for a while, but now seems forgotten. If I were to collect all of these claims I could probably compound a substance which would be "guaranteed" to improve performance 400 per cent or 500 per cent. But there is an inherent fallacy. I have before me at the moment a study of vitamin E by Janet Travell and others (*Circulation*, 1:288, February, 1950). They found improvement in 37 per cent of their subjects and 27 per cent of their controls, and comment that Evans and Hoyle found improvement in 40 per cent of their controls. This brings us up short.

If some of your scientists will accept the .20 level, this is an example of the point raised in my first paragraph. Actually there is no logically defensible reason for accepting any given level. If .20 is accepted, why reject .21 per cent. All I can say is that in the classroom you pass a student with 70 per cent and fail one with 69 per cent and the difference between the two scores is certainly not significantly great.

I do not know whether this is exactly the type of answer you want or not. At best it is only a statement of opinion as to what I would or would not be willing to accept.

Appendix C

BIOCHEMICAL INDIVIDUALITY

Roger J. Williams

BIOCHEMICAL individuality is the possession of biochemical distinctiveness by individual members of a species, whether plant, animal or human. The primary interest in such distinctiveness has centered in the human family, and in the distinctiveness within animal species as it might throw light on human biochemistry.

While it has been known for centuries that bloodhounds, for example, can tell individuals apart even by the attenuated odors from their bodies left on a trail, the first scientific work which hinted at the existence of substantial biochemical distinctiveness in human specimens was the discovery of blood groups by Landsteiner about 1900.

A few years later Garrod noted what he called "inborn errors of metabolism"—rare instances where individuals gave evidence of being abnormal biochemically in that they were albinos (lack of ability to produce pigment in skin, hair and eyes), or excreted some unusual substance in the urine or feces. To Garrod these observations suggested the possibility that the biochemistry of all individuals might be distinctive.

About fifty years later serious attention to the phenomenon of biochemical individuality resulted in the publication of several articles and a book on this subject. These reported evidence indicating that every human being, including all those designated as "normal," possesses a distinctive metabolic pattern which encompasses everything chemical that takes place in his or her

Note: From *Encyclopedia of Biological Sciences*, Edited by Dr. Peter Gray, Head, Department of Biology, University of Pittsburgh, Reinhold Publishing Corp., New York, 1961.

body. That these patterns, like the abnormalities discussed by Garrod, have genetic roots is indicated by the pioneer explorations of Beadle and Tatum in the field of biochemical genetics in which they established the fact that the potentiality for producing enzymes resides in the genes.

Biochemical individuality, which is genetically determined, is accompanied by and in a sense based upon anatomical individuality, which must also have a genetic origin. Substantial differences, often of large magnitude, exist between the digestive tracts, the muscular systems, the circulatory systems, the skeletal systems, the nervous systems, and the endocrine systems of so-called normal people. Similar distinctiveness is observed at the microscopic level, for example in the size, shape and distribution of neurons in the brain and in the morphological "blood pictures," i.e. the numbers of the different types of cells in the blood.

Individuality in the biochemical realm is exhibited with respect to a) the composition of blood, tissues, urine, digestive juices, cerebrospinal fluid, etc.; b) the enzyme levels in tissues and in body fluids, particularly the blood; c) the pharmacological responses to numerous specific drugs; d) the quantitative needs for specific nutrients—minerals, amino acids, vitamins—and in miscellaneous other ways including reactions of taste and smell and the effects of heat, cold, electricity, etc. Each individual must possess a highly distinctive pattern, since the differences between individuals with respect to the measurable items in a potentially long list are by no means trifling. Often a specific value derived from one "normal" individual of a group will be several times as large as that derived from another.

The implications of this individuality are extremely broad. For medicine they suggest that susceptibility to all disease—infective, metabolic, degenerative, mental or unclassifiable (including cancer) probably has its roots in biochemical individuality and that the differences in responses to drugs including alcohol, caffeine, nicotine, carcinogens and morphine derivatives, which are well authenticated, have a sound and discoverable basis. It is a well-known fact that conditions which will produce disease in certain individuals will not do so in others. The basis for this observation has hitherto not been recognized; it doubtless has its roots in bio-chemical individuality—a development which has received little attention. People definitely possess what may be called "biochem-ical personalities" and it seems extremely likely that these are meaningful in connection with the numerous and increasing per-sonality disorders and difficulties which afflict men and women in modern life.

Biochemical individuality offers a sound scientific basis for recognizing the existence in every individual of a unique make-up in the broadest sense. For centuries "individuality" has been writ-ten about and its place in the scheme of things has been dis-cussed, but the knowledge of what individuality consists of and how it manifests itself has indeed been scanty. Only in recent years have we had a basis for understanding it in a definitive way.

The understanding of individuality is basic to the understand-ing of human behavior. It is not enough to know the ways in which all human beings respond alike to certain stimuli; it is fully as important to know also why different people confronted with about the same stimulus react very differently. Since bio-chemistry underlies many of our moods and our reactions to dif-ferent types of stimulus, and since it is in the area of biochemistry that individuality is most definitively recognized, biochemistry merits inclusion as one of the most important of the so-called "behavioral sciences."

Because biochemical individuality points the way toward in-dividuality in the broadest sense of the word, it has profound implications not only in medicine, psychiatry and psychology but also in human relations, education, politics and even philos-ophy.

REFERENCE

1. Williams, Roger J.: *Biochemical Individuality*. New York, Wiley, 1956.

Appendix D

STATISTICS, MEASUREMENT AND
EDUCATIONAL RESEARCH

Henry F. Kaiser

I SHOULD like to make a short survey of some random ruminations and polemical personal pontifications regarding educational measurement and statistics, and point out possible implications of my remarks with respect to the scientific study of education.

Preliminary Thoughts

Because of a failure to distinguish measurement problems from statistical problems, traditional training has often confused and thus confounded these two distinct aspects of quantitative methodology; witness the unfortunate synonymous use of "reliability" and "significance." Current thought attempts to react against the earlier confusion to separate, probably to too large an extent, measurement from statistics. For in one sense such a distinction is a little artificial: almost invariably in educational research the problem of devising measurement instruments on one hand and the statistical problems of sampling and design cannot each be considered in isolation.

I think it could be said that the problem of measurement is closer to the concerns of the educational researcher than is statistics. Statistics, as an independent discipline, is only a formal set of procedures for analyzing data, while the scientist must take upon himself the principal responsibility of devising his own measurement tools—for only he knows, however vaguely, the concepts with which he is concerned.

In educational research, perhaps the largest methodological difficulties stem from a failure to plan ahead with sufficient care. Once we perceive a problem, we are tempted to blast forward in

506

an ill-conceived fashion to attempt to solve it. Oftentimes, technical problems of measurement and statistics are only vaguely conceived of *a priori,* being dismissed with the thought, "We can cross that bridge when we come to it." It is found only later that data so enthusiastically gathered cannot be analyzed in a systematic fashion. Some people who have been denied this allegation, suggesting that if enough data is gathered with enough enthusiasm, solutions to problems will surely come forth like a bolt from the blue. Perhaps so; but quite likely these solutions will be to the wrong problems. Rather than "cross the bridge when you come to it," a better maxim would be, "Look before you leap." Careful thought on what to measure and how to measure it, considered simultaneously with appropriate methods of statistical analysis, is the sound way to do business. Yet also I would never suggest that such planning should inhibit subsequent effort; one should not be stunned into silence because of difficulties in planning. A struggling start is certainly better than no start at all.

Let us think about statistics in a little more detail. As I suggested before, statistics is an independent discipline, having nothing necessarily to do with any science. From this viewpoint, statistical methods are capable only of providing us with decisions about the probability distributions of random variables. It is the responsibility of the scientist, as a scientist and not as a statistician, to consider the relationship of statistical decisions to scientific decisions in education. In playing the role of statistical consultant, there is nothing more distressing to me than having a purported scientist ask me to state his problems; who am I to speak with authority about the problems of the administration of secondary school guidance for curriculum workers in a laboratory school setting?

Scales of Measurement

The relationship of kind or level of scale of measurement of the educator's data to statistical procedures appropriate for working with these data persists as a topic of great controversy. In one school statistics is considered as above: formal discipline which bears no necessary relationship to the real world. This school of thought—to which I must admit for the most part I adhere—asserts that consideration of scales of measurement are irrelevant to statistical procedures. Actually, this is more than an assertion: it is a fact. Statistically, we can do anything we please perfectly "legally"—so long as the formal statistical assumptions are more or less met. But, whether the statistical results have any scientific meaning is an entirely different question, and should be thought of as such. For example, we have often heard the statement that a variable must be measured on an interval scale in order to compute a mean; really, this is hogwash. However, for our scientific *interpretation* of a mean, such considerations *may* be of importance. Pertinent here is the distinction between a scientific and a statistical hypothesis. While statistical hypothesis is nothing more than a statement about the probability distribuion of a random variable, a scientific hypothesis is a statement about something in the real world. For example, the question, "Are boys smarter than girls?" is not a statistical hypothesis. However, corresponding to this, as scientific hypothesis, there may be a reasonable isomorphism to a statistical hypothesis; in this case, it could be the assertion that the population mean IQ of boys is greater than that of girls, given that IQ both for boys and girls is normally distributed and that each of these distributions has the same variance. This statistical statement obviously leads to a traditional *t*-test. What it appears that we do in practise, then, as scientists using statistics, is first to state a scientific hypothesis, then translate this to a seemingly reasonable statistical hypothesis, formally test this statistical hypothesis, make a statistical decision, and finally make a corresponding, equally reasonable or useful scientific decision. In making these reasonable translations, it would appear that in some not-well-defined way measurement considerations are of importance.

The other school of thought on the question on the relationship of scales of measurement to statistical procedures is due to S. S. Stevens, who is responsible for the insightful taxonomy of scales of measurement into nominal, ordinal, interval and ratio scales. Although after the fact, this taxonomy seems particularly obvious, it was not fully articulated until the late '40s. It may surely be considered one of the major landmarks in the theory of measurement. However, it would seem that Stevens has gone a wee bit too far. This is represented by his pontifications on what you *can't* do. For example, you can't do a *t*-test unless the variables are measured on an interval scale. As suggested above, of course you can; what I think Stevens means to say is if you want to make scientific sense out of the results of your *t*-test it is really sufficient that the variables be measured on an interval scale—and it may be necessary.

Perhaps my disenchantment with these prescriptions stems from the experience of dealing with educationists who have taken Stevens too literally, i.e. I have often been confronted with insecure and terrorized consultees with hollow and haunted eyes, so frightened that they will do something "wrong" that they are inclined catatonically to do nothing. After all, many of us are scientists first and statisticians second. To allow statistics to repress our ideas is an anathema of the worst kind. The tail should never wag the dog.

To the extent that research conclusions hold up, one has pragmatic evidence of the efficacy of his scaling assumptions. For example, the massive weight of evidence would indicate that most intelligence tests are essentially measured on an interval scale. As an educational psychologist I would say with a high degree of confidence, that a difference in IQ of 75 and 85 may be considered the "same" as the difference between 100 and 110. To have established this statement *a priori* is like proving the existence of God. On the other hand, if one were newly to devise a rating scale, say, and handle the data as if it were on an interval scale, the generalities of the scientific translations could well be suspect —although the statistics were perfectly dandy.

Thus it would seem that the critical issue in scaling is the scientific generality of the resulting conclusions. The more general the scaling, the more general the scientific (as opposed to statistical) results will be. A careful consideration of levels of measurement would then seem essential to scientific conclusions, although such cogitations are irrelevant to statistical procedures.

Significance Testing

Let me turn now to some comments on the applications of statistics. In reading the research literature in education, I am impressed—I might say appalled—by the relative frequency with which tests of significance are performed as a matter of thought-less ritual. Although I have strained for years to understand the meaningfulness of the seemingly ever-popular significance test, I remain convinced that there is little relationship in this ritual-istic procedure to the scientific thinking of educational investi-gators. First, typically one tests a null hypothesis against all pos-sible alternatives. Appealing to subjective probability, such hy-potheses are simply absurd. What scientist, on this green earth, would ever state that girls and boys are exactly equally bright? Or that the Dandy-Dan method of teaching arithmetic is ex-actly as effective as the Johnson-Kleinsohn procedure? Testing such closely specified null hypotheses against omnibus alterna-tives simply doesn't make sense, for such null hypotheses will be rejected, or not, simply as a function of the sample size and the power of the test used. Even were boys much, much brighter than girls, a sample of size two would rarely show significance; or, if boys and girls were essentially equally bright—but not quite—a sample of size 4,000,000 would almost certainly pick up the negligible difference. Significance testing is a myopic way of doing business.

It seems to me that the only time when testing procedures in statistics are valid is for the purpose of final adjudication between two or more equally specific theories, where each can be trans-lated into statistical hypotheses of the same dimensionality in the parameter space. Thus, rather than having "everything-else" al-ternatives, the scientist should state a particular difference which he, as a scientist, considers to be educationally significant. Once this is done, he should assert precisely what sort of risks he is willing to take for all possible errors. Then, the standard appli-cation of statistics (à la Neyman-Pearson) will do the deed. But in areas such as education and psychology—the behavioral sci-ences generally—studies which are concerned with such final ad-judication would seem rare indeed.

It is just that in the vast majority of educational research, theory has not reached a level of sophistication which allows sci-entists to make precise quantitative predictions for alternative hypotheses. For these studies, a more appropriate statistical pro-cedure would be to estimate the differences of interest or the degree of relationship rather than dichotomously succeeding, or failing to succeed, to see "truth." Thus, the first concern would be a point estimate of the parameter for the problem in question. (I must admit that this major interest would seem implicit in the somewhat irrational defenses of so-called "descriptive" statistics.) After this primarily important point estimate is made, it would seem nice to jazz it up by putting an interval about it and indicate the degree of confidence which we have in the interval. Finally, but least important, we might sneak a peek to see if our interval covers zero. It is most unfortunate that many popular texts emphasize significance testing first—not last. . . .

Nonparametric Methods

At this point, it seems appropriate to comment on the recent rise of nonparametric methods in educational statistics. I consider the stampede to these procedures unfortunate. First, most nonparametric methods emphasize the significance testing viewpoint. Usually, in nonparametric procedures, distributions are computable only under a traditional null hypothesis—have you ever heard of the sampling distribution of the rank-order correlation coefficient for a population rank-order coefficient different from zero?—and thus, to a certain extent, my previous diatribe about the thoughtless use of significance testing applies. A second consideration is related to the question of scales of measurement. For there are many poor souls who are driven into a dark corner by the imprecations of the overly serious scales of measurement boys and are unwilling ever to accept the notion of an interval scale and thus, at best, apply the much less informative nonparametric methods to their safe and sure ordinal data. Third, we often hear the cry that it is so important to meet the formal assumptions in statistical procedures. The question, "Have the assumptions for the *t*-test been met?" is an example of the watchword of these folk. Well, of course, the statistical assumptions have not been met. Nor have the assumptions of the corresponding nonparametric approach been met. For the assumptions in a formal statistical model are abstract assumptions and never can exactly be met in the real world. There is no such thing as normal distribution in Nature. Or, for most nonparametric methods, who ever heard of a continuous distribution existing in Nature? The correct question of "just" meeting assumptions is somewhat more difficult. It is simply a matter of how closely one comes. And to assess how close one must be seems a subjective, almost arbitrary decision. Fortunately, the problem of meeting statistical assumptions—considering that they never can be met exactly—is not really so bad for many traditional procedures using metric data. Empirically it is well known that standard, very useful things are robust, i.e. relatively insensitive to the underlying statistical assumptions, and thus one can blatantly go forward with only slight distortion in his probabilistic conclusions.

Multivariate Analysis

In the often encountered situation in the behavioral sciences where there are a number of criterion or dependent variables, there has been built up in recent years a large number of techniques subsumed under the general title of multivariate analysis. Unquestionably the most common multivariate procedure in use today is factor analysis, a technique which, at the exploratory level, has probably done more than anything to bring some sort of preliminary order out of chaos.

I cannot resist the opportunity to get in a plug for some recent developments in traditional factor analysis. First, regarding the communality problem, Chester Harris of Wisconsin has recently published some remarkable results linking the important statistical work of Rao with the important psychometric work of Guttman. His paper has clearly demonstrated the crucial notion of *scale-free solutions*—solutions which are metric invariant, so that we are no longer tied to the traditional normalization of observations. With regard to the transformation problem, Harris and I have invented methods which can yield all possible solutions—involving correlated or uncorrelated factors—using orthogonal transformations only. This seems important, for we can now attack the general problem with tractable machinery, for the first time. Finally, a mathematical statistician, Karl-Gustav Jöreskog of Uppsala, has begun to look at the "right" problems in factor analysis (from a psychometrician's viewpoint) and those things that we have been doing with such great gusto for so many years are now being annointed with the propriety of sampling distributions, etc.

But, of course, factor analysis is not the only multivariate technique. Generalizations of the *t*-test and of the analysis of variance have been made to the multivariate case. The ultimate fruitfulness of these approaches is probably yet more or less an unknown quantity. In educational research, undoubtedly the most vigorous activity in the application of the multivariate analysis of variance has been led by Professor Darrel Bock of the University of North Carolina. It will surely be interesting to continue to watch the progress of this provocative area of statistical methodology in education.

Name Index

515

Subject Index